Medical Writing

Robert B. Taylor

Medical Writing

A Guide for Clinicians, Educators, and Researchers

Third Edition

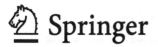 Springer

Robert B. Taylor
Oregon Health & Science University
Portland, OR, USA

ISBN 978-3-319-70125-7   ISBN 978-3-319-70126-4   (eBook)
https://doi.org/10.1007/978-3-319-70126-4

Library of Congress Control Number: 2017958546

Printed on acid-free paper

This Springer imprint is published by Springer Nature
The registered company is Springer International Publishing AG
The registered company address is: Gewerbestrasse 11, 6330 Cham, Switzerland

For Francesca, Masha, Jack, and Annie

Preface

This book is intended to make you a better medical writer. This is true whether you are a clinician in a busy practice, an educator teaching students in the health professions, or a researcher who conducts and reports randomized clinical trials. It is for the physician, physician assistant, or nurse practitioner who sees patients and who also wants to contribute to the medical literature. It is for the medical educator writing articles and book chapters to share new information and, incidentally, to attain promotion and tenure. And it is for the investigator whose career success depends, in large measure, on critical skills in developing research protocols, preparing grant applications, and writing articles describing the eventual research findings.

It has been 6 years since publication of the second edition of this book. The landscape of medical writing has changed in many ways, and I will cover much of the new territory in this third edition. But the aim of the book remains unchanged: to improve your writing skills, whether you are a clinician, educator, or medical researcher.

So what exactly has happened in the past 6 years? Although there had been some early rumblings when the second edition was written, the intervening years have seen the evolution of pay-to-publish open access journals, predatory publishers, highjacked journals, and bogus book reviews. The International Committee of Medical Journal Editors has changed its *Uniform Requirements for Manuscripts* to an updated version: *Recommendations for the Conduct,*

Reporting, Editing, and Publication of Scholarly Work in Medical Journals. In this third edition, I cover these topics, as well as add new sections on altmetrics, parachute studies, bacronymic article titles, peer review fraud, how to find permission-free illustrations for your work, and ways to avoid common mistakes in writing and submitting a research report.

Medical writing is different from composing a short story or a novel. Although all authors should strive for accuracy, clarity, and simplicity, medical writing has certain rules—some unwritten and others found in the *Instructions to Authors* that seem to differ just a little from journal to journal—that seem to encourage complexity rather than a pleasing flow of words. Yet, despite the need to be precise and often to include p-values, confidence intervals, and other foes of an elegant literary style, medical writing can still be readable and sometimes even *natural.*

If you are new to medical writing or even if you have been the author of some articles or book chapters and seek to improve your abilities, this book can help you. Who am I that I can make this assertion and write this book, both fairly presumptuous acts? Here's my reasoning. As a practicing physician and medical educator, writing has been my avocation. Over 14 years in private practice and 39 years in academic medicine, I have written using all the major models described in this book: review articles, case reports, editorials, letters to the editor, book reviews, book chapters, edited books, authored books, research protocols, applications for grant support, and reports of clinical research studies. Most items submitted for publication have been published. Not all. Perhaps my most noteworthy qualification is not that I have managed to produce a lengthy curriculum vitae. In my opinion, what is more important for you, the reader, is that I have made all the errors. That's right, the mistakes. Over the years, I have jumbled spelling, mixed metaphors, tangled syntax, wandered away from my own outline, written on unimportant topics, submitted grant requests that seemed to befuddle reviewers, and offered articles to the wrong journals. But along the way, I have published 33 medical books and added several hundred papers and book chapters to the literature. This book is written to share what I have learned—what works and what doesn't in medical writing.

This book aims to help clinicians, educators, and researchers translate their practice observations, pedagogical innovations, wise thoughts, and investigational data into written form and eventually into print. In striving to achieve this purpose and as (I hope) a good educator, I have written the book with four learning objectives in mind. Upon completion of this book, the reader should:

- Understand more about the art of medical writing, including motivation, conceptualization, composition, and frustrations
- Know how to use different models of medical writing, such as the review article, report of clinical research, and more
- Recognize how to get a manuscript published
- Realize that writing can be fun

The book's content is a blend of personal experience and research on the Web and in printed sources. Throughout all chapters, I have attempted to follow the time-honored principle of supporting theory with examples, some from actual published materials and some simply created to help illustrate the ideas presented. Most of the examples presented are "good examples"; a few are illustrations of what not to do.

In Chap. 1, I challenge authors to consider three questions before beginning work on an article or book: *So what? Who cares? Where will it be published?* As the author, I believe that I should answer the three questions in regard to this book. The "So what?" question asks what is new and different, and I think that the answer lies in the fact that I address medical writing knowledge and skills from the viewpoint of the clinician and medical educator, not that of the journal editor or professor of English literature. The "Who cares?" issue concerns the potential reader; for this book, that is the reader who aspires to write for publication in the medical literature. This is, in fact, a surprisingly large number of persons—all competing for limited space in print. In regard to the "Where will it be published?" question, I am pleased that this book is published by Springer Publishers, the world's leading publisher of scientific books and journals, with whom I have had an author–publisher relationship since 1976.

As a clinician and/or perhaps a medical educator or clinical investigator, you have a tremendous source for writing ideas—the patients, students, or research subjects you see each day. Think about the possible significance of a cluster of uncommon problems you have observed recently, the unlikely manifestation of a common disease, your curricular innovation that others could implement, or the extraordinary courage displayed by one of your patients or study participants. Perhaps you have found a new way to use an old remedy, have your own thoughts about a recently published study, or even have a pile of data from a clinical investigation you recently completed. This book is about helping you recognize the reportable idea, organize your information, and *write it up*.

Happy writing!

Virginia Beach, VA   Robert B. Taylor

About This Book

True ease in writing comes from art, not chance,
As those move easiest who have learn'd to dance.
English Poet Alexander Pope (1688–1744)

Together we are embarking on a journey through the ins and outs of writing in general and of medical writing in particular, with all its idiosyncrasies. This short introduction tells a little about the book's organization and its own peculiarities, including word use, reference styles, and the examples and allusions you will encounter. In the end, our common goal is to find some true ease in writing, through consideration of both current theory and samples from the literature and by looking at what constitutes excellent and not-so-good writing.

The book progresses from the theoretical to the practical. It begins with basic writing topics and skills. Next comes a consideration of the various models for medical writing, from the review article to the report of a research study. There are chapters on writing a research protocol, how to get grant funding for your research (or other project), and how to write a report of a research study. The final chapter discusses how to get your work into print, longer in this third edition because of the recent emergence of new models of publication and perils for the author. The appendix has some handy tools that may help you along the way, including a glossary of medical writing terms, proofreaders' marks, commonly used abbreviations that you may use in your own writing, and definitions of methodological and statistical terms used in research reports.

In the early chapters on basic writing skills, I use the word *article*, even though later in the book the principles of authorship described will also apply to editorials, letters to the editor, research protocols, grant proposals, and research reports.

Within chapters, you will also note some shorthand reference citations, presented in parentheses. These identify articles and books used as examples to illustrate enviable (and sometimes deplorable) titles, organizational structure, and prose. Although I believe few readers would actually want to consult these writings, I have provided abbreviated citations, just in case. With the information provided, you could find most of the articles on the Web. This third edition presents some newer examples of good and bad medical writing and also retains a few classic gems.

At the end of each chapter are references to sources pertinent to ideas described in the text. These are presented in the style of the "Recommendations for the Conduct, Reporting, Editing and Publication of Scholarly Work in Medical Journals," a very useful guide that will be discussed in later chapters. Using this reference style for the book models the way you will generally prepare citations for your medical articles.

I have done my best to make this book a pleasure to read. This includes using short, strong words and, at times, colorful images. I have included allusions to medical history, classical writing, mystery novels, opera, sports figures, comics, and a few very odd creatures. We will visit Hippocrates and Frau Roentgen, Shakespeare and Hemingway, Princess Turandot and Pogo, and zombies and clones. As you read along, you will also learn some medical information, such as whether or not the use of probiotics can reduce crying episodes in infant colic and the relationship between the exposure to aircraft noise and cardiovascular mortality. All the examples in the book help illustrate points about medical writing that I consider important.

I hope that what follows will help you master the art of writing, to "move easiest" by learning—not really new dance steps—but some guidance on how to walk the path from idea to print. I wish that I could promise that having read this book, your next writing effort will be so inspired and luminous that everything else in print will seem drab by comparison. In fact, this is unlikely to occur. But I do earnestly believe that, as stated in the Preface, using the principles and tips presented here will make you a better medical writer.

Contents

Chapter 1
Getting Started in Medical Writing

[W]ords are things, and a small drop of ink,
Falling like dew, upon a thought, produces
That which makes thousands, perhaps millions, think

British poet Lord Byron (1788–1824), Don Juan

Does being a clinician or holding a faculty appointment make you or me a capable medical writer? No, it doesn't, any more than being a physician or even an inspiring educator qualifies me to be a good stock picker, business manager, or even vacation planner. It only means that I have medical knowledge and skills and am trained to care for patients or perhaps have some gift for teaching or research. On the other hand, just because you are a clinician who sees patients daily or a researcher concerned with protocols and statistical significance does not mean that you cannot become a capable, even great, writer. And, yes, even the classroom or bedside teacher can learn to write well. Being that great writer requires knowledge, practice, experience, the capacity to endure rejection, and a strong will to succeed.

© Springer International Publishing AG 2018
R.B. Taylor, *Medical Writing*,
https://doi.org/10.1007/978-3-319-70126-4_1

The knowledge part includes both medical and "writing" knowledge. Let us assume that, by virtue of your clinical practice, you have the medical knowledge. Then what you must master are the body of information and the technical skills that can help you become a great writer. You must know how to assemble and use basic writing resources. You also need to understand key issues in medical writing such as how to get started and how to get finished, the various models of medical writing, how to prepare a manuscript, and how to get your work published. Acquiring this knowledge is no small task, but it can be done.

Writing for the medical literature has its own special considerations. Composing vibrant prose is not usually the key issue and at times may appear to be disadvantageous. By that I mean that editors of scientific journals tend to favor densely written articles that put specificity ahead of clarity. Rew has written, "A fog has settled on scientific English. Well-written English effortlessly communicates the writer's intent to the reader. Unfortunately, far too often, science is written in a form that renders the content hard to understand, and which makes unreasonable demands on the reader" [1]. It seems that many medical articles, notably reports of clinical research studies, are written chiefly to be published and cited, and readability is a minor consideration. I hope that you and I can aspire to a level of literacy acceptable to your editors and that readers will appreciate the enhanced readability of our work.

The ability to endure rejection is a must. I began medical writing in the early 1970s while in a small-town private practice. I had some early success in conducting clinical studies and seeing the results in print in respected journals. I also wrote some articles for controlled circulation, advertiser-supported journals, such as *Medical Economics*. Not everything I wrote was published. I also began writing health books for nonmedical people, what the editors call the "lay audience." Here I collected so many rejection letters that I could have wallpapered a room with them. Only when I began writing and editing medical books did my acceptance rate become favorable. However, after 40 years of medical writing experience, I still receive rejections for clinical papers, editorials, and book proposals. And, yes, it still hurts.

If you aspire to be a medical writer, you will need determination. Being a writer takes a lot of effort, and you really need to want to see your work in print. But if you develop the itch to write, it can only be relieved by the scratch of the pen—or today by the click of the computer keyboard. If you begin to see yourself as a writer working on a project, as I am working on this book today, then you will think about the project whenever you have a spare moment, and as ideas occur, you will capture them on a scrap of paper, index card, or smartphone. There is tale, perhaps apocryphal, that Scottish poet Sir Walter Scott (1771–1832), while once struggling with a sentence, went hunting. The ideal wording popped into head. Scott quickly shot a crow, plucked a feather, and used the bird's blood to record the prose before it faded. Some of my best thoughts have been scribbled on paper napkins. You will log the concept or phrase when and where you can, just so it doesn't get away, because that is what writers do.

Why We Write

For years I have periodically conducted writing workshops for clinicians and medical educators. Presenting writing workshops, of course, guarantees an audience that is self-selected to be more interested in writing than those in competing workshops on how to perform a no-scalpel vasectomy or ways to code office visits to receive maximum reimbursement. Generally, most of the participants are previously published medical authors, at least to some degree. Each of these workshops begins with the same question: Why do we write? The answers, while diverse, tend to be the same in each workshop and are listed in Table 1.1. I am going to discuss a few of these.

First, let's consider and dismiss the final entry on the list— earn income. Medical writing is not lucrative. Advertiser-supported publications (more about them later) often pay a

TABLE 1.1 Reasons why we write

Gain intellectual stimulation
Share ideas
Report research
Express an opinion
Generate discussion
Advance one's discipline
Assert "ownership" of a topic
Attain promotion/tenure
Report a case
Enhance one's personal reputation
Achieve some small measure of immortality by publishing our ideas
Earn income

few hundred dollars for an article. Book royalties are generally meager compared to what a health professional earns in his or her "day job." Book chapters, editorials, and research reports pay little or nothing and are written for reasons other than financial gain. If your goal is wealth, you should add more clinical hours to your schedule or buy stocks that go up—something other than medical writing.

What about the other reasons we write? For those in academic medicine, promotion and tenure are very important, and publications are the key to success. As medical schools become increasingly dependent on clinicians seeing patients for economic survival, it would seem that this clinical effort would be rewarded with the carrots of career achievement— promotion to the next rank and, where applicable, tenured faculty positions. This, however, is not the case. In 1988, a study at Johns Hopkins Medical School reported, "Those who were promoted had had about twice as many articles published in peer-reviewed journals as those who were not promoted" [2]. I have not seen a recent similar study, but I don't believe that anything has changed, and an academic faculty member who bets his or her career on advancement without publications is taking a dangerous path.

I tell young faculty members that, as a broad generalization, it takes at least two publications a year to be considered as "satisfactory" in scholarly activity when it comes time for promotion. Some can be clinical reviews or case reports, but others must be research reports published in refereed journals. Also, you must be the first author on your share of the papers, not always second or third author. Faculty members who chiefly see patients often do not get this message. Beasley and Wright surveyed faculty in 80 medical schools in 35 states. They differentiated between clinician investigators (the research faculty) and clinician educators (the patient care faculty) and concluded, "Clinician educators are less familiar with promotion guidelines, meet less often with superiors for performance review, and have less protected time than clinician investigator colleagues" [3].

Another benefit of medical writing is the in-depth knowledge it brings. Think of it as a self-education program. If you or I plan to conduct research (which requires various phases of writing such as the research protocol, grant application, and ultimately the research report) or develop a clinical review or book chapter on a topic such as hyperthyroidism or ovarian cancer, then we will necessarily learn a lot about the topic during the process. In academic medicine, the way to really get to know a field is to contribute to it, and those who contribute by means of publication need current, evidence-based knowledge if their writing is to be credible.

In my opinion the most enduring reason to be a medical writer is the intellectual stimulation. Medical writers have a lot of fun learning about their topics, rummaging in their imaginations for the best way to present material and finding just the right words to say what is important. And what you write can stimulate discussion. For example, I published an article on leadership with the premise that leadership skills can be learned. A reader disagreed, stating that my article had "missed the mark" and that the top leaders have inherited abilities and character traits. I had an enjoyable time composing my reply.

There is also the pleasant side effect of getting known. As an editor of a number of medical reference books, I have had the heartwarming experience of visiting clinics in Asia,

Europe, and South America and having young doctors exclaim, "Doctor Taylor, I have read your book." On a practical level, if you are a referral physician who specializes in, for example, refractive surgery of the eye or the management of Parkinson's disease, publishing articles on these topics helps assure referrals.

In the end, however, when the going gets tough and your paper has been rejected again, what will sustain you is not the discussion with readers, the occasional recognition, or the clinical referrals. It is the simple joy of writing.

Why We Don't Write

If writing is such a joy, why don't we write? And for those in academic medicine and whose career advancement depends on publications, isn't it curious that so many resist writing?

In my workshops on medical writing, the second discussion question is "Why don't we write?" Table 1.2 lists some of the answers received over the years.

What about the resource issues cited in the list? Time to write is always mentioned early in the discussion. No one in private practice has revenue-generating time that is allocated to writing. Those in academic practice soon find that they don't either. For academicians, time to do research and to

TABLE 1.2 Reasons given for not writing

Not enough time
Nothing to write about
No one to work with in writing
Shortage of secretarial support
Lack of knowledge as to how to research information
No mentor for writing activities
No motivation
No self-confidence
Don't know how to start
"I hate writing!"

write must be "bought" by obtaining funding (which is why grant proposal writing is important). For the rest of us, writing time is going to be carved out of personal time. When I was in private solo practice, my writing time was in the early morning, before breakfast and when my family was asleep. For others, the time will be weekend mornings or late at night. In workshops, sometimes I have encountered vocal— sometimes even angry—disagreement with my "writing on your own time" beliefs, but most experienced medical writers and editors will tell you this is the way it is.

Whatever time you designate as writing time must be vigorously protected. In practice, patients will get sick and call; this is the virtue of writing in the early morning or late-night hours when the telephone is quiet. In academic medicine, you may need to close the door while writing or go to the library to prevent colleagues from coming to discuss problem residents, curriculum changes, or patient referrals—anything but writing.

How about the lack of ideas, lack of secretarial support, absence of like-minded colleagues, and so forth? Any clinician seeing 15–25 patients a day encounters a wide variety of clinical phenomena that could present the idea for an article: common causes of pelvic pain, ways to manage the patient with a low back strain, an unusual manifestation of lupus erythematosus, herbal therapy in the treatment of depression, and much more. The variety you see depends on your specialty. Your writing ideas will come from your clinical experience. This is as it should be, because it brings immediacy to your writing and provides the credibility you need to write on the topic. Later in the book, we will discuss how to develop clinical observations into writing topics, outlines, and articles.

In my opinion, laments about lack of secretarial help, collegial support, and research access are not as valid as they once were. Why? Because of the computer and the Internet. Not too many years ago, I was highly dependent on secretarial support; I dictated my articles and made corrections by hand to be changed on computer by my typist. Today I use the Microsoft Word program on my computer, doing the typing myself; the computer's efficiency has led me to change my writing methods. With e-mail, coauthors are also readily available. In fact, I can pass documents back and forth with colleagues across the country by e-mail just as readily as with those down the hall.

The World Wide Web has revolutionized research, making information needed for writing readily available to anyone with a computer and Internet access. Because knowing how to use the available resources is so important to medical writers, we will shortly spend time learning about what is online and how to use it. Basically, you can learn just about anything you need to know while sitting at your desk, if only you learn how to do it.

The lack of self-confidence is quickly overcome after a few publications, which may also help to spark motivation.

Regarding the last entry on Table 1.2, I can't do much for those who really hate to write.

Random Thoughts About Medical Writing

Writing as History

In 1912 the citizens of the village of Caledonia, New York, placed a large boulder as a monument commemorating the historic treaty between Chief Ganaiodia, representing the Native Americans in the area, and the local villagers and farmers. As a civic leader, my grandmother had an idea. She dispatched my mother, then aged 9, to the grocery store to buy a tin of cookies. Yes, those were the days that cookies came in tin boxes, and one could safely send a 9-year-old child alone to the grocery store. When my mother returned, grandmother removed the cookies, which I am sure were put to good use. What she wanted was the metal box, into which she placed several items, including a copy of the village's weekly newspaper. The box was then buried beneath the boulder as a time capsule. I believe that it is still there beneath the boulder.

Your writing is a time capsule. It shows what you and your colleagues think today about important issues such as diagnosis, treatment, prevention, prognosis, clinical correlations, health policy, practice management, and much more. As readers, we use medical writing to look back in history.

Think about the historic figures in medicine. Who comes to mind? Hippocrates, Galen, Maimonides, Paracelsus, Vesalius, Harvey, Osler, and more (I am sure that, in choosing just a few to discuss briefly, I have omitted many favorites, but I am going to try to make a point). Three centuries before the Common Era (CE), the words of Hippocrates were recorded in *On Hemorrhoids*, *On Fractures*, *On Ulcers*, *On the Surgery*, *On the Sacred Disease*, and the *Book of Aphorisms*. Galen, writing in Rome during the second-century CE, compiled the medical knowledge of the day into an encyclopedic work that endured as an authoritative reference for centuries. Maimonides wrote on diet, reptile poisoning, and asthma during the twelfth-century CE. Later, during the Renaissance, Paracelsus described Meniere's disease and the treatment of syphilis with mercurials; he gave us the guiding principle of toxicology: "The dose makes the poison." We know this because Paracelsus *wrote* it. Vesalius produced drawings of the body that greatly advanced the study of anatomy. Harvey, in the 1600s, wrote describing the circulation of blood in the body, and later Sir William Osler's book *The Principles and Practice of Medicine* defined the practice of medicine in the late nineteenth century [4].

Do you notice the common theme above? Is my point becoming clear? While all were undoubtedly outstanding physicians of their day, they are remembered because they *wrote*. They recorded their observations and their thoughts. In doing so, they literally helped shape the history of healing. And by writing, they created the building blocks upon which today's house of medicine stands.

You and I can do a little of this, too. At this time, none of us is likely to become the "father of medicine" or the "father of anatomy." Hippocrates and Vesalius hold those titles. But we can add small twenty-first-century contributions to the house of medicine while metaphorically tucking some of our work away in today's time capsule for someone in the future to ponder.

Writing and Reading

Reading goes with writing like ice cream goes with apple pie—one just makes the other better. All writers must read if they are to be any good at medical writing, and you should read diverse items and for various reasons: for information, for ideas, for structure, for style, and for a sense of history.

All clinicians need to read the medical literature regularly to stay up-to-date in their specialties; this is part of being a good healer (later, in Chap. 3, I will describe how clinicians read the literature). Educators and researchers must read constantly to know the latest advances in their areas of interest. Your journal reading will help build bridges to your own experience.

Writers also read to seek information. For example, when writing the section above, I needed to reread parts of Sebastian's excellent reference book *A Dictionary of the History of Medicine* [4] to learn about Hippocrates, Galen, and Harvey. No, I did not have all the information in my head. Right now I have promised to write a book on the great innovations in medicine, and as I revise this third edition of *Medical Writing*, I am searching for information on the next topic I will cover.

In addition, writers read to seek general knowledge and, perhaps, to troll for ideas. Some clinical interest topics I have encountered recently include the merits of vitamin D, atypical fractures with bisphosphonate therapy, the role of alternative medicine, and new drugs for diabetes.

There is also reading for structure. By this I mean considering articles analytically. When you read an article that you like—because of the writing, not the topic or statistics—go back and reread the article looking at how the author put it together. How was the title composed? How was the abstract constructed? How did the writer organize the information so that it was clearly presented? What tables and illustrations were used, were they effective, and why were they effective? How many references were included, and what publications were cited? Reread this part of the book before going on to Chap. 2, and think about the questions I just asked as they apply to the Chap. 1 you are now reading. What are the good points and what could I have done better? In short, look at the craftsmanship of the article or book chapter, as well as the message.

Read also for style. Study examples of well-written medical literature. This may be a little hard to find, as refereed journals have increasingly become the repository for published, citable, but barely readable reports of research data. The writing in the *British Medical Journal* is better than most, and some of the best writing in US medical journals is found in editorials and opinion pieces, as described in Chap. 7.

Reading for style includes reading nonmedical books, vitally important to those who aspire to be serious writers. Here you can gain a sense of language, grammar, syntax, and the rhythm of words in good literature. I believe that a medical writer should always be reading a nonmedical book. Read some of the classics, such as the grand metaphoric prose of Herman Melville's *Moby Dick*; the powerful, yet spare journalistic style of Ernest Hemingway's *The Old Man and the Sea*; the subtle and complex style of Jane Austen's *Pride and Prejudice*; or the symbolism of Thomas Mann's *The Magic Mountain*. You might also include a Tom Clancy thriller or Patricia Cornwell medical mystery or a James Michener epic.

You and I can gain a sense of perspective by reading about our heroes and our language. To read a collection of time capsule items, try to find a copy of R. H. Major's *Classic Descriptions of Disease* [5]. To learn about the words we use, I humbly recommend my own book, *The Amazing Language of Medicine* [6]. And one should include a book on the history of our profession such as Roy Porter's *The Greatest Benefit to Mankind* [7].

Writing and You

Who Writes?

Is there a profile of the medical writer? There is no single "typical" person who chooses to write. However, there are degrees of "fit" between a person's preferences and characteristics desirable for writing. It goes beyond mere technical skills. Writing may be an opportunity for you to use your talents and may give you great satisfaction, while others describe writing as "frustrating" and "stressful." Most importantly, you need to be aware of your own preferences, strengths, and priorities. Psychological inventories, such as the Myers–Briggs Type Indicator (MBTI), have described personality types that tend to be most attracted to writing as being creative, adaptable, and eager to take on new challenges (INFP, ENFP, INTP, and ENTP, in MBTI terminology) [8].

Medical Writing as Storytelling

Who hears more stories than patient care clinicians? The patient relating a medical history is really telling his or her story. It is a narrative and often one that is rich in color, emotion, and drama. In fact, there is an appealing metaphor that characterizes the patient and the clinical narrative. It begins with the concept that the job of the healer is to help the patient manage his or her "story." And—here is the metaphor—the patient comes to the clinician with the plea: "My story is broken and I hope that you can help me fix it" [9]. Certainly among all these stories—broken and fixed, with the clinician as both actor and observer—there are limitless topics for medical writing. Abraham Verghese states, "It may take years of practice for a physician to appreciate and accept his or her role as storymaker and storyteller" [10]. One good example of such narrative writing is Howard Brody's *Stories of Sickness*, 2nd edition [11].

Writing as Creativity

Whether what you are writing is a compilation of data in a research report, an editorial about a topic that sparks your passions, or a new look at how to treat your favorite disease, your writing involves creativity. This means that you are producing something that comes from you, personally, and that did not exist before you made it. I find this both humbling and energizing. In writing this paragraph, I am putting 89 English words together in a way that no one ever did before. This is exciting.

This creativity is what can get the juices flowing. It helps focus your sense of purpose—that writing is important, especially what you are writing *now*. The creative process is more important than committees, television, the crabgrass in the lawn, and even football. Your rewards come when you have finished something and you can say, "This is great, and I created it," and from others reading the results of your literary effort— and sometimes responding—even when they disagree.

Of course, creativity is also a solitary process. Note that of the great medical writers in history that we discussed earlier, none had a Boswell to record his thoughts (from your college courses, perhaps you recall James Boswell, the eighteenth-century writer best known for recording the words of Samuel Johnson). Nor do we find coauthors listed. And none had a team of administrative assistants, research assistants, or fact-checkers. Each did it alone with parchment and quill and paper and pen.

Be aware that your medical writing will require hours spent staring into the computer screen and rummaging in books and web sites—lonely endeavors, to be sure. American author Truman Capote once wrote, "Writers, at least those who take genuine risks, who are willing to bite the bullet and walk the plank, have a lot in common with another breed of lonely men—the guys who make a living shooting pool and dealing cards" [12]. The solitude of writing will mean overcoming the tendency to wander down the hall to yak with colleagues, go for coffee, or chat on the telephone—anything to maintain contact with other humans. So be prepared for quiet time alone with your ideas. However, you may find that your ideas and your creativity are very good company.

Writing Topics and Your Career

If you are in private practice with no aspirations to an academic career or research grant funding, then you might skip this short section. However, if you are a faculty member seeking academic advancement (promotion and tenure) or a future in research, the following can be an important advice. Here it is: find your "career topic" early and stick with it as long as you can. The "career topic" will be what you write about, over and over. It will also be the subject of your research and perhaps why you receive patient referrals. For example, for years, I have written on migraine headaches. Clearly because of writing review articles and book chapters on this topic, I—as a family physician—became a leading headache referral physician in our academic medical center. In fact, I received more headache patient referrals than I really wanted, all because of writing on the topic.

Some topics I have seen young academicians developing recently include a national scorecard on women's health services, health literacy of patients, the impact of high professional liability rates on physician retention, changes in the quality of health services when patients are forced to change doctors, the integration of complementary/alternative practices into allopathic medicine, the cost efficiency of various health screening methods, racial or gender disparities in health care, and a wide variety of clinical diagnoses. The list of potential topics is endless. Take ear infection, for example, which most would describe as a mundane topic. Yet in 2011 a team from Finland published an article in the *New England Journal of Medicine* (NEJM) describing a placebo-controlled trial of antimicrobial treatment of otitis media (Tähtinen PA et al. N Engl J Med. 2011:364:116). In 2016, the *Journal of the American Medical Association* (JAMA) described the effect of cranberry capsules on bacteria/pyuria among older women in nursing homes (Juthani-Mehta M et al. JAMA. 2016;316:1879). I regret to report that cranberry capsules were no more effective than placebo.

What is important is to identify a topic that energizes you and that has the potential to endure. For example, one could write on a topic of, for example, treatment of Bartholin cyst or infant crib safety, but would soon run out of things to say and articles to write. It is much better to write on a topic of general interest, with evolving research and, if possible, high social relevance. Then, as you write on various facets of the topic in journals and books, you establish your national position as an authority in the field, which is a requirement for promotion to the rank of professor in academic medical centers.

What should you *not* write about? First of all, don't write on topics outside your area of clinical expertise. To use somewhat exaggerated examples, the psychiatrist probably shouldn't be writing about knee injuries, and the orthopedic surgeon should find a topic other than pancreatitis. Also, do not write on a clinical area in which you do not wish to receive referrals and perhaps become recognized locally as an expert. I once knew a general internist who wrote a few articles on alcoholism. He was interested in the topic because his father was an alcoholic. Before long his practice was dominated by alcoholic patients, both through referrals by colleagues and then by patients seeking out the local expert on the topic and by attorneys requesting expert testimony. This shift in practice emphasis was not at all what he had planned.

Assembling Your Resources

Because the topic of resources is so important, I am going to cover it early in the book. You must not try to write without assembling what you need to write. Without designating a writing area, acquiring books and computer resources, and learning to use key web sites, a premature foray into writing is likely to cause frustration.

Your Writing Space

What are your logistic requirements for writing? First of all, you will need a comfortable chair and desk surface. The chair must support your back and ideally will have a height adjustment that can change if your shoulders start to ache after a few hours of typing. The surface may be the kitchen table, as long as it is well lit and is large enough to accommodate papers, books, computer, and all the rest.

You will need a computer with high-speed Internet access. The days of submitting manuscripts on paper are gone. All my latest article submissions have been online, and paper was needed only for author attestations and signatures. My last six books were submitted online.

The point of the story is that you will need a computer for composition, revision, and submission. At home and work, I use both desktop and notebook computers. I find the desktop computer easier to use for long sessions of typing, chiefly because I have two large side-by-side screens. The notebook is more convenient when moving work from place to place and definitely if the computer must be taken into the shop for repair.

Other items to have handy are a telephone, notepad, pen or pencils, and a cup of your favorite beverage. Add your books, computer programs, and web sites, and you are good to go.

Books

If I were advising you a decade ago, this section would be much longer. On my bookshelf I have copies of *Dorland's Medical Dictionary* and *Stedman's Medical Dictionary*. For the most part, they are collecting dust. Almost everything I need I can find online (see below). Nevertheless, there are a few books that just might be helpful.

The *5-Minute Clinical Consult*, published by Williams & Wilkins (LWW), is a very useful reference for a wide variety of clinical conditions. Using an outline format, this "cookbook" tells what the busy clinician needs to know about a wide variety of diseases, with an emphasis on the outpatient setting. There is a version that can be loaded onto your smartphone or tablet.

The *Quick Look Drug Book* (LWW) is one of my favorites. Like several of the items noted above, Lippincott Williams & Wilkins publishes it. It is a paperback book, published annually, that is useful for checking drug generic names, brand names, and doses. The latter is vitally important for accuracy in medical writing (see Chap. 3). A computer program, described below, is available.

A little-known but very useful book is Neil Davis' *Medical Abbreviations: 32,000 Conveniences at the Expense of Communications and Safety*. All too often in medical writing, I encounter abbreviations for which I cannot find the explanation. Here are two randomly selected examples. What are the meanings of TDS and BEGA? Give up? TDS stands for traveler's diarrhea syndrome, and BEGA stands for best estimate of gestational age. TEMP can mean temperature, temporary, or temporal. This little book can help clear up the confusion in ways I seldom could achieve looking in the indexes of my big reference books. I buy mine online at www.medabbrev.com.

If you are taken with using classical medical quotations to augment your own prose, a good source is Maurice B. Strauss's *Familiar Medical Quotations* (Little, Brown Publishers). It is out of print but is available from online booksellers: Search Google for Maurice Strauss AND familiar medical quotations.

Computer Programs

Thesaurus

There is no need to buy a printed thesaurus. Your Microsoft Word program has an excellent one; just highlight the word and go to Tools at the top of the desktop.

Electronic Medical Dictionary

Stedman's Electronic Medical Dictionary is an excellent choice. Lippincott Williams & Wilkins reports that Version 7.0 defines more than 107,000 terms, including 5000 new terms. LWW also tells that you can read the definition of a term, hear it pronounced, see it illustrated, and watch it in motion. I don't really value the audio pronunciations (after all, I am writing—not giving a lecture), and spare me the anatomic animations. That said, this is a very useful program to have loaded on your hard drive.

Nevertheless, when my *Stedman's Medical Dictionary* is finally out of date, I probably will not buy a new edition; I think I have found something almost as good—and for free. Since the first edition of this book was published, I have begun using *The Free Dictionary* by Farlex. This online web site is a one-stop source for both medical and nonmedical word definitions, with the advantage of supplying the etymology of each word. As a field test, I looked up the word *pterygium*. I learned that the word describes "an abnormal mass of tissue arising from the conjunctiva of the inner corner of the eye that obstructs vision by growing over the cornea." I also discovered that the word is derived from an old Greek word meaning "wing."

You can access *The Free Dictionary* at: http://www.thefree-dictionary.com/. It is also available as an app for smartphones and tablets. And, in fact, Google is also a good dictionary. I compared both *The Free Dictionary* and Google by typing in the somewhat arcane word *dysdiadochokinesia*. Both gave me the correct definition plus the origin of the word. With these sites available, you may not need a formal medical dictionary at all.

Spell-Checker

I am a huge fan of *Stedman's Plus Medical/Pharmaceutical Spellchecker*, produced by LWW. This amazing program integrates with your Microsoft Word spell-checker. Then it works while you type to verify spellings of medical and pharmaceutical words plus the everyday words on the MS Word spellchecker. The latest version has the most recently released drug names, including brand names, and virtually all medical words you will ever use. It even has a feature that allows you to add words to its base. For example, *Dorland's* (the medical dictionary described above) was not in its vocabulary, so I added the word so that it will not be underlined in red next time I use it.

Drug Reference Program

As an alternative or in addition to owning the *Quick Look Drug Book*, the *Quick Look Electronic Drug Reference* (LWW, again) can be purchased and loaded on your hard drive.

Web Sites

Web sites are where today's professionals look for information. In fact, the list of books and programs above may be wholly unnecessary a decade from now. I am going to discuss my favorite sites; I think it is best to become really familiar with just a few and learn to use them well. This is much better than cruising a large number of sites but doing so inefficiently. Also, some of the best web sites charge a subscription fee, which will put economic limits on your surfing. For example, medical schools are likely to have subscriptions to *MDConsult* and *UpToDate* (described below), as long as they are accessed from a university computer. However, you must pay a fee if you wish to use them at home. No matter which web sites you choose as your personal favorites, you must learn to use them yourself. You cannot be dependent on the expertise of a medical librarian. And to be an effective web searcher, it helps to understand Boolean searching.

Boolean Searching

Boolean logic, named for British-born Irish mathematician George Boole, refers to relationships between search terms. Fundamentally, it allows you and me to search the web for the commonality, or maybe the lack thereof, of two possibly related items. It lets you limit or widen your search. It's not difficult. In a Boolean search, you will use one of three words to link two (or more) items. The words are AND, NOT, and OR. As an example, let's assume that I want to look up current information about the treatment of migraine headaches. I would first enter the terms migraine AND treatment. This will give me only articles about migraine therapy and not information about the aura of migraine or the treatment of peptic ulcer disease. If I request migraine OR treatment, I should get a much longer list, including the treatment of migraine but also possibly including the treatment of hypertension and chronic hepatitis. The mnemonic in Boolean searching is: OR is mORe.

You can link more than two terms. The more terms you combine with AND, the shorter the list of articles created. The more terms linked with OR, the more articles on the list retrieved.

Many, but not all, web sites allow Boolean searching.

Google

Don't laugh. Google, at http://www.google.com, is an outstanding search engine. If you want a quick link to a phrase, book title, author's name, or an unfamiliar web site, try Google first. I have made it my Internet home page. The more you use Google, the better you will like it. According to a report published in 2006, Google provided 56.4% of referrals from search engines to medical articles [13].

If you have ever had an article published in an indexed journal, search your name on Google to see what you find. Google allows Boolean searching; its default is AND. Sometimes in a Google search, you may want to search for a specific phrase, which is done using double quotes. Google describes it this way: What is the difference between typing pink monkey and "pink monkey?" Because of the default Boolean AND, the pink monkey search will result in finding all documents in which both the individual words pink and monkey are present. The "pink monkey" search will only locate the documents in which the phrase *pink monkey* is present.

Google Scholar

Google Scholar, first made available in 2004, is an especially useful site when searching for a clinical citation. It seems to let me focus my query better than PubMed and will some-times even let me have access to a full paper, rather than just an abstract. When data were collected showing that Google provided more than half of all referrals to scientific articles (described above), Google Scholar was very new. Today Google Scholar includes 80–90% of all articles published in English [14]. The Google searching strategies described above apply.

MEDLINE/PubMed and MeSH

MEDLINE (Medical Literature, Analysis, and Retrieval System Online) is a service of the US National Library of Medicine (NLM). It allows you to search up to 26 million references in some 5600 life science journal articles, chiefly those in the biomedical sciences. Your search can go back to the 1950s.

You can access MEDLINE on the Internet by going to the NLM home page at http://www.nlm.nih.gov. There is no fee for use of this service and no requirement to register. You might also access MEDLINE through your medical library, public library, or a commercial web site. An example of the latter is *Medscape* (www.medscape.com), a web site for physi-cians that offers e-mail accounts and specialty-specific cur-rent medical information, as well as MEDLINE/PubMed access. Registration for *Medscape* is required, but there is no charge. The easiest access is to go directly to PubMed via http://www.pubmed.com.

PubMed can be accessed through https://www.ncbi.nlm.nih.gov/pubmed. In PubMed you have choices: You can search by title word, phrase, text word, author name, journal name, or any combination of these. PubMed allows Boolean searches. Your search will yield a list of citations to relevant journal articles, including the authors, title, publication source, and generally an abstract. PubMed will search published scientific articles, but not books.

You can also search by using the NLM controlled vocabulary, MeSH, which stands for Medical Subject Headings. MeSH is used to index articles from 5400 of the world's leading biomedical journals for the MEDLINE/PubMed® database. The NLM fact sheet describes MeSH as follows: "MeSH is the National Library of Medicine's controlled vocabulary thesaurus. It consists of sets of terms naming descriptors in a hierarchical structure that permits searching at various levels of specificity."

At the most basic level of the MeSH hierarchical structure are very broad headings such as "Anatomy" or "Mental Disorders." More specific headings are found at more narrow levels of the eleven-level hierarchy, such as "Ankle" and "Conduct Disorder." There are 27,883 descriptors in 2016 MeSH. You can learn more about MeSH at https://www.nlm.nih.gov/pubs/factsheets/mesh.html.

Are you confused yet? I am. I have always considered MeSH headings to be the medical librarians' full employment act. I don't use it. The sites described above—Google, Google Scholar, and PubMed—are sufficient for my needs.

PubMed also offers "Loansome Doc," a feature that lets you place an electronic order for the full-text copy of an article found on MEDLINE/PubMed. The source is the National Network of Libraries of Medicine (NN/LM). You will need to register. You might also be able to link to the journal publisher's web site and may be able to view a full text of an article. You may need to pay a fee. To learn more about Loansome Doc, go to https://www.nlm.nih.gov/pubs/factsheets/loansome_doc.html.

BioMedLib.com

Sometimes you may think that PubMed and other sites have too much "dead wood" in their lists. To save time, I suggest that you check out BioMedLib.com, available at http://bml-search.com. This free web site offers a much more focused response to your query than PubMed. They also offer a free online publication, *Who is Publishing in My Domain,* screening 14,000 journals for current articles pertinent to your interests.

UpToDate

I like *UpToDate* but for different reasons than I like *MEDLINE/PubMed* and *MDConsult*. *UpToDate*, subscription based, is a comprehensive clinical information source. What makes it different is that it offers state-of-the-art reviews of clinical subjects. The *UpToDate* web site (http://www.uptodate.com/home/about-us) states, "More than 6300 world-renowned physician authors, editors, and peer reviewers use a rigorous editorial process to synthesize the most recent medical information into trusted, evidence-based recommendations that are proven to improve patient care and quality."

Of course this means that *UpToDate* is composed of "review articles," and is not really taking you to primary sources, although articles contain lists of reference citations. This site is very useful for the busy clinicians seeing patients and for educators teaching residents. *UpToDate* is designed to initially search a single subject, such as "headache." Then you will be offered a menu of modifiers such as migraine, cluster, tension type, and so forth. You cannot do a Boolean search on *UpToDate*. For the medical writer, it is helpful to check current thinking on a topic. For primary sources of clinical evidence, I would look elsewhere.

ICMJE Recommendations (Previously "The Uniform Requirements")

The "Uniform Requirements" has long been the bible for the serious medical researcher, writer, and editor. The guidelines, set forth by the International Committee of Medical Journal Editors (ICMJE), have been revised, and the work is now titled *Recommendations for the Conduct, Reporting, Editing, and Publication of Scholarly Work in Medical Journals* (ICMJE Recommendations).

The Uniform Requirements were first published in 1978 by a small group of editors of general medical journals (the "Vancouver Group") who met informally in Vancouver, British Columbia. This group evolved into the International Committee of Medical Journal Editors (ICMJE). The group meets yearly and updates the document as needed, most recently in 2016. You will use this information often to answer questions, especially when writing reports of clinical trials.

What are the ICMJE Recommendations? According to the document, "The ICMJE developed these recommendations to review best practice and ethical standards in the conduct and reporting of research and other material published in medical journals, and to help authors, editors, and others involved in peer review and biomedical publishing create and distribute accurate, clear, reproducible, unbiased medical journal articles" [15]. For example, the section "Preparing a Manuscript for Submission to a Medical Journal" has excellent discussions of reporting guidelines, the various components of a research report (more on this in Chap. 11), and how to cite references that you will find very valuable when working on your manuscripts (see Table 1.3). We will return to these document preparation guidelines later in the book.

TABLE 1.3 Some topics discussed in the ICMJE Recommendations

Authorship and contributorship
Editorship
Peer review
Conflicts of interest
Confidentiality
Protection of research participants
Copyright
Overlapping publications
Fees
Electronic publishing
Clinical trial registration

Where Do I Start If I Have Never Been Published?

The Medical Writer's Three Questions

In Puccini's opera *Turandot*, Princess Turandot asks Prince Calef three questions, framed as riddles. If the lovestruck prince answers the three queries correctly, he gets the princess's hand in marriage. If he fails, an early death will be the result. For medical writers, also, there are the three key questions, mentioned in the Preface to this book, that must be answered when considering a project: So what? Who cares? Where will my article be published?

For the medical writer—whether neophyte or seasoned—these questions are vital. If you answer the three questions clearly, you have the best chance of success. On the other hand, if you fail to provide a convincing answer to one or more of the questions, you won't exactly lose your head, but the success of your paper is definitely in jeopardy.

So What?

The medical landscape is littered with published papers that, like discarded fast-food wrappers along a country lane, have accomplished little more than adding a few lines to the author's curriculum vitae. If you aspire to add to the medical literature (or *litter*-ature), I urge you to be thoughtful in considering the "So what?" question.

This question aims to determine the significance of your work. After all, undertaking a writing project is going to take you away from your patients, your family, your hobbies, or whatever else you might otherwise be doing with your time. And you are asking your audience also to commit time to reading it. So be sure the effort is worthwhile.

The "So what?" questions asks: Is what I am writing about something that hasn't been said already and perhaps said better than I will say it? Am I saying anything new? Let's assume that you are a surgeon writing for a surgical journal. If you are writing an article titled "Surgical Treatment of Acute Appendicitis: A Report of 100 Cases," my first thought is that this topic may be important, but what can you say that hasn't already been said? But if your topic is "A New Surgical Technique for Appendectomy in the Patient with Acute Retrocecal Appendicitis," then you have my attention.

Here is another example. One could study and report the diagnoses of the next 1000 patients seen in your office. But so what? On the other hand, if you studied the next 1000 patients seen with a presenting complaint of pelvic pain and followed them to the definitive diagnoses, then most generalists and gynecologists would be interested.

Who Cares?

This question has to do with relevance to the potential reader and to the universe of health-care professionals and patients who might benefit. Let us think about a paper describing how I treat sore throats empirically with saline gargles and garlic, where I found that the treated group actually fared significantly better than the control group. Although the topic seems unlikely, with good statistics this paper might be relevant to generalists who see many patients with sore throats. I recently read about pickle juice being useful in preventing leg cramps and being touted by the Philadelphia Eagles as their secret weapon in their cramp-free win over the Dallas Cowboys in a game played in over-one-hundred-degrees Texas heat (Pickle juice, food fad, or foolproof fix? Available at http://healthpsych.psy.vanderbilt.edu/pickleJuice.htm/). Is pickle juice truly useful in preventing exercise-induced cramps? Now here is a study many would care about a great deal.

On the other hand, when I was in private practice four decades ago, we often recommended that patients with peptic ulcer disease drink plenty of whole milk. Yes, things have changed. Nevertheless, at that time it seemed that, more often than I expected, many patients with peptic ulcer disease reported not liking milk. Interesting observation. Is there some pattern here? I thought of doing a study and writing it up. I asked my colleagues about this idea and learned, to my dismay, that they really didn't care. I never did the study.

Where Will My Article Be Published?

Getting an article published requires two consenting adults — an author and an editor. Of course, for refereed publications there are peer reviewers who must also nod approval. Even book publishers often have proposals reviewed by experts in the field.

When you write an innovative, relevant article, you must seek the best journal for your work. Ideally you begin with a specific publication in mind, your "target journal," and then drop back to your second and third choices only if you are not successful with your first choice.

Be careful with your target journal. Some journals have such a low acceptance rate that rejection is almost guaranteed. On the other end of the spectrum, the advertiser-sponsored publications (discussed below), while lacking the cachet of the *New England Journal of Medicine*, need a steady supply of innovative articles and offer good opportunities for the neophyte author. Some articles, by the nature of their content, are best suited for refereed journals that publish research reports; others—such as "how-to" and "five-ways-to" articles—are generally inappropriate for such journals, and sending them in is a waste of time. There is also the "gray literature," describing works presented at scientific meetings or as conference posters and thus being "published" as abstracts of the scientific congresses.

Some Early Steps

Writing Models for Beginners

As a beginning author, it would be quite difficult to write a publishable report of original research on your first or second attempt. First, you need research data, which you are unlikely to have. Second, the report of original research is the most demanding of all publication models and faces the greatest competition in the publication sweepstakes. There is, however, one way that you, the relative neophyte, can actually succeed in having your name on a research report. That occurs when you are the junior member of a research team and you participate in all phases of the project, including writing the report. This approach works even better if the team includes a senior mentor, who can guide you through the process.

In the absence of a research team, a seasoned mentor, and a pile of research data, what is the aspiring author to do? Plan to start with a writing model that offers the best chance of getting in print with the least need for expertise and the least risk to your ego. No, such a publication won't get you tenure or assure a lifelong career, but it will get you going. Also, it just might help you settle on a topic area that you can pursue in future writing.

The leading models appropriate for neophyte writers are review articles, case reports, editorials, letters to the editor, and book reviews. All are covered in depth in later chapters of this book. The review article is appealing because advertiser-supported publications, sometimes called "throwaways," have a constant appetite for content. Examples of such publications are *Postgraduate Medicine*, *Consultant*, and *Hospital Practice*. All have web sites for those who want to learn more.

Case reports are tempting and are sometimes a good way to get started as a writer. Be sure of two things: One is that you have a point to make about the case—the "So what?" question again. The second is to be sure that your target journal(s) actually publishes case reports; not all journals do so. That is the "Where will my article be published?" question once more.

Editorials allow you to express opinions, and you may be an especially appropriate author for an editorial if you hold a position that gives you some expertise in the topic. For example, if you direct a pain clinic, you are qualified to write about narcotic abuse or regarding analgesic under-prescribing for patients with pain.

Letters to the editor are a quick and easy way to get in print. Generally a letter to the editor comments on a published paper. What you have to say must offer new insights, and it must connect with the readers. Often such letters disagree with conclusions of the paper, and that is okay. Letters to the editor should be short and to the point.

Book reviews are another opportunity for publication. Never send in an unsolicited book review. On the other hand, you can write to your favorite journal and volunteer to be a book reviewer. If added to the reviewer list, you will receive a book to review. Your job will be to write the review, as described in Chap. 7. You keep the book as payment.

Book chapters are almost always invited by book editors, who try to choose prospective chapter authors from those already writing on the topic needed for the book. You may be invited to write a book chapter after publishing a few articles on your new focus area, but book chapters are usually not where a new writer begins. The same holds for writing a book. A few will succeed, but for most this is not where to start.

Mistakes We Make When Getting Started

- Trying to do it alone: If at all possible, work with someone more experienced. Your colleague may be a coauthor or someone who reads your work and offers comments.

- Trying to run before you can walk: Do not attempt to write the definitive treatise on a topic or the grand epic in your specialty. Aim early to learn the writing and publication process by getting something written and in print, however humble your early pieces may seem. In my early days, I wrote for *Medical Economics* and *Physician's Management* on topics such as "Having Regular Meetings with Your Office Staff" and "How to See Patients More Efficiently in Your Office." I don't write on practice management subjects anymore, but these articles helped me learn how to write and get published.
- Starting to write without preparation: It is a big mistake to begin writing until you have selected and refined your topic, figured out how you will structure your article, done your research, and assembled your writing tools. Without being prepared, inspiration won't carry you very far beyond page 1. Starting off unprepared will almost surely lead to an uneven product, and you will spend a lot of time doing remedial work. It is much better to be ready when you start and know where you are going.

The Value of Early Success

Do not underestimate the value of timely success in medical writing. I urge you to strive for something in print early, for your own contribution to the twenty-first century time capsule. Seeing your work in print is an exciting affirmation of your self-worth. A few initial publications will carry you through the effort of more writing and the rejections that are sure to come as you aim higher and higher. Also, try very hard to avoid a succession of early failures.

The next four chapters deal with basic writing skills that can help you win the publication race. The later chapters in the book describe the specific writing models, including "how-to" advice and problems to avoid. The last chapter has tips that can help you get your work published.

References

1. Rew DA. Writing for readers. Eur J Surg Oncol. 2003;29(7):633–4.
2. Batshaw ML, Plotnick LP, Petty BG, Woolf PK, Mellits ED. Academic promotion at a medical school: experience at Johns Hopkins University School of Medicine. N Engl J Med. 1988;318(12):741–7.
3. Beasley BW, Wright SM. Looking forward to promotion: characteristics of participants in the Prospective Study of Promotion in Academia. J Gen Intern Med. 2003;18(9):705–10.
4. Sebastian A. A dictionary of the history of medicine. New York: Parthenon; 1995.
5. Major RH. Classic descriptions of disease. Springfield: Charles C Thomas; 1932.
6. Taylor RB. The amazing language of medicine. New York: Springer; 2017.
7. Porter R. A dictionary of the history of medicine. New York: Parthenon; 1999.
8. Hammer AL. Introduction to type and careers. Palo Alto: Consulting Psychologists Press; 1995.
9. Brody H. My story is broken; can you help me fix it? Lit Med. 1994;13(1):79–92.
10. Verghese A. The physician as storyteller. Ann Intern Med. 2001;35(11):1012–7.
11. Brody H. Stories of sickness. 2nd ed. New York: Oxford University Press; 2003.
12. Capote T. Preface. Music for chameleons. New York: Vintage; 1994.
13. Steinbrook R. Searching for the right search—reaching the medical literature. N Engl J Med. 2006;354(1):4–6.
14. Trend watch. Nature. 2014;509(7501):405.
15. International · Committee of Medical Journal Editors. Recommendations for the conduct, reporting, editing, and publication of scholarly work in medical journals (ICMJE Recommendations). http://www.icmje.org/about-icmje/faqs/icmje-recommendations/

Chapter 2
Basic Writing Skills

Imagine practicing medicine without being versed in the language of medicine, including all its formal terminology and informal jargon. Without access to this specialized linguistic domain, physicians couldn't understand normal physiology or pathophysiology. They would be incapable of synthesizing findings from the history and physical, labwork, and imaging studies to make a diagnosis. Words like marasmus, fistula, and tinnitus would make no sense. Communication in any kind of meaningful way with peers or patients would be unworkable.

Chip Souba, MD, The Language of Leadership [1]

Do not skip this chapter. Yes, there will be the temptation to go directly to the chapter describing the article or research report you want to write, but that would be a mistake. It would be like attempting to build a house without a blueprint and tools. In writing an article or a book chapter, the topic is what you want to "build." The structure is your blueprint, and the paragraphs, sentences, and words are the contents of your toolbox. So learn your craft and how to use your tools before starting to construct your masterpiece.

Much of this chapter is fundamental English 101—just adapted to medical writing. However, it is not a comprehensive course in composition and grammar. In fact, if my

© Springer International Publishing AG 2018
R.B. Taylor, *Medical Writing*,
https://doi.org/10.1007/978-3-319-70126-4_2

English teachers from high school and college ever read this, they might say, "Bob, is this all you remember of everything we taught you?" It is not really all I recall, but it represents the "cliff notes"—the bare bones of what the medical writer needs to know.

Idea Development

The Great Idea

A good idea is the most important thing a medical writer can have. It can come to you in a variety of ways. One might be as a result of a discussion with colleagues, as happened to me a few years ago. At that time, there had been a sudden drop in students matching in my specialty. Yet, in trying to place an unmatched student in a residency program using phone contacts, I encountered inefficiency and almost indifference—all from residency directors who had vacancies and whom I assumed really needed to recruit graduating medical students into their programs. I described this phenomenon at our department's weekly faculty meeting and reported briefly what I thought the residency directors needed to know. In my remarks to the faculty, I listed five things that residency directors should do to be receptive to unmatched students attempting find residency positions. And then I thought: Why not write it up? I returned to my office and finished the short piece by noon. It was published as an editorial a few months later [2].

A second source of ideas should be your area of interest and expertise. For example, I was once asked by a medical journal to write an editorial; almost any topic would be okay. I considered the significance of a current whooping cough scare, the health risks to travelers in the holiday season, and even the changing demographics of medical school classes. In the end, I decided to do what I should do, and that is to write about what I know. I did some research and wrote a nice, short editorial, "How Physicians Read the Medical Literature" [3]. The journal editor liked the topic and how I handled it, and no readers wrote to say that I was uninformed or misguided. Also, some of what I learned was useful in planning Chap. 5 of this book.

A third possibility is looking at clinical implications of current public issues. Here is an example: From time to time, I have taught a course in medical writing for faculty members at our medical school. This course involves 90-min sessions held once a month over 6 or 8 months. The course is for beginning medical writers, and one objective is to have each participant write a review paper and have it on its way into publication before the last session ends. In our most recent course, one faculty member with a certificate of added qualifications in geriatrics announced her plan to write an article titled "Assessing Older Persons for Their Ability to Operate a Motor Vehicle Safely." She had a very good idea, timely and clinically relevant. (I will discuss below how she developed the idea). As a course assignment, she called a review journal editor to discuss the article; the response was encouraging, with a discussion of holding a spot for the article in a future issue. A few months later, the article was in print.

The points I have tried to make in the anecdotes above are:

- When something excites you and you have, you believe, an answer to a current problem—such as residency directors needing to learn about the opportunity presented by unmatched students—think about writing it up. Then do it now, before the idea gets cold.
- Write on clinical topics in your area of expertise. In general, medical publications need articles about practical aspects of disease diagnosis and management. And, of course, research journals need reports of original research studies.
- Write on what excites you. This helps maintain your interest and also helps focus your writing on the topic that will move your career along.

Dream Catching

Thoughts will come into your head while you are in the shower or driving your car. Sometimes they occur in the middle of a meeting, when a comment creates a synapse in the writing center of your brain. Think of this process as *dream catching*. Thoughts about your writing may appear in that shadow land between wakefulness and deep sleep, when all the aspiring notions, some inspired and others fanciful, in various parts of your brain, embryonic ideas generally held in check by the oppressive distractions of the day, can emerge and express themselves. American writer Henry David Thoreau (1817–1862) wrote: "There is a moment in the dawn when the darkness of night is dissipated, and before the exhalations of the day begin to rise, when we see all things more truly than at any other time." Some Native American tribes use dream catchers—willow hoops decorated with feathers and other items—to corral good dreams. We need to learn to use our internal dream catchers to hold on to the insights that come when we are not fully awake.

Do not lose these gifts of your subconscious! (Parenthetically, this is exactly why I hate alarm clocks; you are jarred from sleep to wakefulness and lose the creative time of twilight sleep.) In these evanescent thoughts, you may have been blessed with a gift that can be the basis of a great article or that may make your article better. Whatever you do, hang on to it and don't let it get away. Many times I have left a shower or a warm bed to jot down a writing idea that I knew would escape if not captured at that moment. I like to think that one difference between a writer and a normal person is that the writer recognizes when his or her subconscious has released a good idea.

Idea Incubation

For major projects—in contrast to the short editorial about the residency "scramble" described above—you should let your idea germinate for a while. I like to think of this activity

as "free-range" accumulation of odd facts, phrases, and con-
nections. For example, the metaphor of the "free-range" accumulation of items to flesh out an idea occurred to me during
a long airplane ride; it was Thanksgiving time, and I had read
about "free-range" turkeys that sought their food in a more
or less natural way. I jotted the phrase on the blank sheet of
paper I always carry for this purpose. (Today I would be more
likely to record the thought on my smartphone.) Now here it
is in print, courtesy of United Airlines, some handy notepa-
per, and then my notebook computer. It may not be the
brightest metaphor I ever created, but at least it didn't get
away. A better example may be the analogy, described in
Chap. 1, of the three questions asked by Princess Turandot of
the prince and the three questions writers must answer about
their current work; this occurred to me while listening to a
very long aria at a performance of Puccini's opera, and I
scribbled the idea on the printed program between arias.

In preparing to write this book, I created a file of ideas for
each chapter. Under each chapter I record miscellaneous
notes, brilliant thoughts, literary allusions, and short paragraphs that seem witty. Then I go to this "Notes" file as I begin
to write each chapter.

Focusing the Topic

Most article ideas are too broad, and an early task is generally to limit the focus. Here is an example: Let's say that I
want to write an article about the diagnosis of headache. This
topic is much too broad, and so I might limit it first by focusing on the diagnosis of a type of headache, such as migraine,
tension type, or even cluster headache. But these topics are
still too broad. Let's choose migraine headache, and limit it
some more. We might discuss diagnosis of migraine headache
in women, in adolescents, or in the elderly; the implications
are clinically different in each. Another way to approach the
diagnosis of migraine is to consider when diagnostic imaging
(computed tomography or magnetic resonance imaging) is

needed. Now we are getting more specific. In the end, a good topic and title might be: "Red Flags in the Headache History: Five Reasons to Obtain Diagnostic Imaging."

The astute writer avoids telling too much. This helps prevent "overwriting"—producing an article much too long for any journal and thus in need of ruthless pruning. By this I mean that if your article is about when to seek diagnostic imaging in a headache patient, you should make it clear to your reader (and to yourself) that you will not discuss what blood tests to order, drugs and doses, or special diets. You will plan ahead and stick to your topic.

Jotting notes and focusing the topic help move you to the next step—planning the concept and structure of your article.

Article Structure

Your article or chapter is intended to provide information or answer questions for your readers. To achieve this goal, you must present your information in the best possible format. Possibilities include the review article, editorial, case report, letter to the editor, book chapter, or report of original research. Each has its own rules for structure and will be covered in chapters to come. At this time, I will use the review article format to discuss article structure. I choose this format since the review article allows the writer the greatest opportunity to express creativity in how to handle material.

Sometimes the focused topic yields the concept. In the instance of "Red Flags in the Headache History: Five Reasons to Obtain Diagnostic Imaging," the article structure is self-evident: The article will begin with an introduction stating the epidemiology and background for the problem. Next will come a five-part section on the red flags, which would include migraine associated with a neurologic abnormality on physical examination (such as unexplained unilateral deafness or weakness in an extremity), a seizure, or a trajectory of increasing pain and frequency of headaches. Last will come the summary/discussion section that pulls it all together. With this framework, the article practically writes itself.

The secret of structuring an article is the topic's component parts. An article on treating back pain may have four components: medications, physical therapy, determination of appropriate activity levels, and preventing future recurrences. If writing a piece on diagnosing depression in teenagers, I might cover the stresses teens face in life each day, symptoms of depression that teens may exhibit, and how to confirm a diagnostic hunch. I might even include a table, "High Pay-Off Questions to Help Spot the Depressed Teenager." Such a list might prove especially useful to readers.

In the end, the focused topic and presentation concept should evolve into an outline. Yes, an outline. The outline allows us to bring order to what would otherwise be an unstructured and perhaps even a messy process. In planning this book, I developed a 12-page expanded outline that gave the topics for each chapter down to the third level of topic heading. Of course, as I write each chapter, I may rearrange things a little, but the overall outline tells me where I am going and what will be presented in each chapter and under which heading. It also, I hope, helps me avoid too much repetition.

In planning the article cited above on assessing driving skills in the elderly, our faculty member decided on the following preliminary outline:

Introduction

    Background, including statistics.
    Legal aspects of the problem.

Areas to assess

    Mental competence and dementia
    Physical competence and handicaps
    Special senses
        Vision
        Hearing
    Medications

Making decisions
    Dealing with the patient
    State laws
    Family issues

Conclusion

In general there are some time-tested ways to structure articles. Of course, if you are writing a report of original research, you must, repeat *must*, use the IMRAD model, which describes Introduction, Methods, Results, And Discussion; this will be described in detail in Chap. 11. If writing a book chapter or review article on a disease such as gastroesophageal reflux disease (GERD), the headings are likely to be Background, Clinical History, Physical Examination, Laboratory Tests and Imaging, Treatment Options, and Prevention.

For other articles, general approaches might be:

The List

This is a straightforward, time-tested way to organize a review article or an editorial. Examples might be:

Three exercises that may prevent back pain
Four herbal remedies for chronic joint pain
Five ways to improve collections in your office practice.
Six questions that can help diagnose panic disorder.

What's New?

A new procedure for ventral hernia repair
A new federal regulation that will affect your practice
A review of deep brain stimulation for Parkinson disease
New drugs to treat fungal infections of the skin

Questions and Answers

What are safe antibiotics to use in pregnancy?
Who should perform head and neck surgery?
Which vaccines should be given to the international traveler?
What are the early signs of pancreatic cancer?

Current Controversies

Do statins prevent dementia in the elderly?
Should medical marijuana be part of your practice?
The current status of stem cell therapy.
The ethical issues in concierge medical practice.

Mistakes We Make in Article Structure

Beginning writers often make the following mistakes in defining the concept and structure of their articles:

- Starting to compose without a unifying concept. Having a good idea is wonderful, but you must also decide how you will handle the idea. Starting to write without a "flight plan" is the *Ulysses method of writing*—starting on a journey and hoping for the best. Such a method can lead to challenges not unlike those faced by Ulysses in his 10-year trip home from the Trojan War.
- Attempting to write without an outline. Maybe some creative and experienced writers can do so, but for the beginning medical writer, an outline is a must. A study by Kellogg found that preparing a written outline, compared with not doing so, led to higher-quality documents as indexed by ratings of judges [4]. As I work on this chapter today, my outline is located to my left on my desk.
- Having an outline with too many major headings and not enough development of each. More than five main headings in the outline is almost certainly too many for a medi-

cal article. Please notice that this chapter, which is about twice the length of a medical article, has only five main headings plus a reference list.

- Trying to cover too much ground. Focus, limit, and then narrow some more.
- Failing to introduce the purpose of the article very early in the writing. Don't make the reader wait until the third paragraph to learn the topic of your article.
- Developing a good concept and structure, and then failing to follow the blueprint. Editors—and astute readers—will quickly spot when you have left the main highway and strayed off on a side path.
- Beginning to write the manuscript without thinking the project through. This will only lead to much painful rewriting later. Clear writing comes from clear thinking. See the completed project in your mind before starting the first paragraph.

Paragraph Development

A paragraph is a collection of sentences that all relate to a common theme. In a sense, each paragraph is a small essay. This means that you should follow the basic rules for writing an essay: tell your reader what you are trying to say early, develop the theme using some concrete examples, and then conclude in a thoughtful way. In an essay, sometimes it is good to reprise the opening sentence at the end in some way, and this can also work well in a paragraph. An alternative conclusion to a paragraph may be a transition to the next paragraph. Choose your ending, and then move on.

The first sentence in a paragraph is classically the "topic sentence." The topic sentence states what the paragraph is about and is thus probably going to be somewhat general in nature. Let's look at the paragraph just before this one: The topic sentence is "A paragraph is a collection of sentences that all relate to a common theme." Then the paragraph goes on to give three steps in developing the paragraph: (1) State

the topic early; (2) use examples; and (3) conclude in a meaningful way, perhaps with a hint of transition to the next topic.
To use a sample from the literature, in a 2017 *New England
Journal of Medicine* (NEJM) article titled "The End of
Obamacare," the author's first paragraph begins: "Donald
Trump's triumph in the 2016 presidential election marks the
beginning of an uncertain and tumultuous chapter in U.S.
health policy" (Oberlander J. NEJM. 2017;376:1). This is a
classic topic sentence for both a paragraph and an essay. It
sets the stage and offers hints of what comes next.

There are occasional exceptions to the classic format, such
as when the example is stated first to get the reader's attention, followed by a general statement telling what the example means. Here is a demonstration of what I mean:

Article Title: "Over-the-counter drug availability and
unintended consequences".

Initial example to get the reader's attention:

Since H2-blockers became available over the counter (OTC) in
drugstores, Mary Smith, a public assistance patient with persistent
upper gastrointestinal distress, has ceased her use of these medications and is experiencing recurrences of symptoms. Why?

General statement explaining the significance of the
example:

Sometimes regulations that are intended to make drugs more
available to patients have a paradoxical effect of reducing their
use. [The paragraph will go on to explain why—because public
assistance patients could previously get the H2-blocker drugs at
no personal cost by prescription, but now that the drugs are available OTC, they are no longer eligible for prescription coverage
and patients must pay for the medication.]

Organizing the Paragraph

Thoughts in a paragraph must be presented in an orderly
fashion, not jumbled like a bag of toys. Sentences can be
arranged in a chronology of what happens. I used this in the
preceding paragraphs: moving from topic sentence, to examples, to conclusion. Or you may decide to order sentences by

rank of importance. In describing causes of a low back pain, you might mention lumbosacral strain (the most common cause) first, then herniated lumbar disc (less common, but very important), followed by less common causes such as spinal abscess, metastatic cancer, and so forth. An alternative method of ordering sentences within a paragraph might be a reverse ranking order: In this setting you might describe the medications currently used to treat peptic ulcer disease, briefly describing the least expensive or the least effective ones first and then spending most of the space on today's popular remedy, the protein pump inhibitors. Or sometimes the rational order is nothing more than a simple list. In this paragraph I told you about four ways to organize sentences in a paragraph, presented in no particular order, simply because there was no logical reason to present them in any special sequence.

When you have finished writing a paper, try this test to see whether you have organized your paragraphs well. Begin with a paper copy of your manuscript and some colored highlight markers. Then first highlight in yellow (or another favorite color) the key sentence in each paragraph; the sentences highlighted in yellow should, in most instances, be at the beginning of each paragraph.

Next, use another color (let's say blue) to highlight the examples that support the key general statement. Most or all paragraphs should have supporting facts, and they should generally follow the yellow-highlighted topic sentence. The exception, as noted above, will be when the example is used as the lead item—the attention-grabber—in the paragraph. In the next section, we will spend some more time considering supporting examples.

Using Concrete Examples

At times you will read an article and think, "This is dull." When this happens, ask yourself why. Often the answer is that the writer has written in broad general statements and failed to provide examples to illustrate theory. This happens especially in philosophy and sometimes in the psychological literature. Medical writers are often spared this transgression because we present specific data such as laboratory tests, drugs, and doses. In other instances, and perhaps ideally, we describe cases. In all writing, we must be vigilant about unsupported general assertions.

Why do we see writing without examples? Here is one reason: Writing general statements is easy. We all like to share our great ideas. But finding or thinking up examples to support our favorite philosophical thoughts is often a struggle. Identifying specific examples can be difficult, but concrete facts are what make writing come alive.

To illustrate the use of examples to clarify general statements, let us look at three examples:

Role of the Primary Care Physician

General statement:

The primary care physician must be the expert in the care of common illnesses and in the recognition of uncommon diseases.

Example:

The general internist or family physician should be skilled in the management of degenerative joint disease and be able to differentiate it from rheumatoid arthritis, intra-articular infection, gout, and other causes of joint pain.

Changing Our Minds About the Use of Drugs

General statement:

Sometimes we find that drugs once avoided in certain diseases actually can be helpful.

Example:

It was once axiomatic that one did not prescribe beta-blocker drugs for patients with congestive heart failure, but now we have discovered that these drugs are useful in treating some heart failure patients.

Use of Multivitamins by Healthy Individuals

General statement:

In this age of evidence-based medicine, some clinical advice seems to be based on intuition or tradition, rather than the results of scientific studies, and sometimes in the face of contradictory evidence.

Example:

Many of our patients take multivitamins daily, despite a paucity of evidence that vitamin supplements have any favorable effect on cardiovascular disease, common cancers, or overall mortality. In fact, a 2010 study conducted in Sweden suggests that multivitamin use might be associated with an increased risk of breast cancer. (Larsson et al. Am J Clin Nutr. 2010;91:1268.)

Being Considerate of Your Reader

Be considerate of your reader by making your paragraphs not too long, not too short, and not too dense. In medical writing, paragraphs often seem to go on for pages and pages; that may be a little exaggerated, but when the prose is unnecessarily burdened with complex medical words and phrases, and when there is sentence after sentence without a break, the resulting paragraph becomes just too long. Whenever you find a paragraph that continues for more than eight or ten sentences, look and see whether there is a logical break in the middle, even if you need to add a transition phrase or sentence. If a paragraph covers several topics, it almost certainly needs to be divided.

Don't make your paragraphs too short. I generally like short paragraphs. They give the reader time to breathe. That said, we must remember that a paragraph is, as noted above, a collection of sentences that relate to a common topic. One or two silver dollars do not make a collection, and most paragraphs need more than one or two sentences. Are there exceptions? Yes, the exception is when a one-sentence paragraph is used for emphasis. But, like a person who sends e-mail messages laden with exclamation points or shouts while talking, using more than the occasional one-sentence paragraph will irritate the reader.

How you construct your paragraphs affects the density of the page. We like some journals and books in part because of the information contained and in part because of their pleasant appearance. The computer screen has not yet equaled the pleasure of holding and reading something with printed pages. Part of the pleasure of the printed page is what is *not* there. By that I mean, there must be a balance of printed words and "white space"—the area of the page that has no ink. On any page there is probably an amount of white space that is just right. This is achieved by alternating paragraph length, avoiding an article with all very long paragraphs (tiresome) or all very short paragraphs (annoying), and perhaps by using tables or figures (discussed in Chap. 4).

The density of the printed page is also managed by the use of headings. I have made liberal use of headings in this book. This allows the presentation of white space to frame the paragraphs and does so in a way that I hope you find aesthetically appealing. After all, the pleasant appearance of the pages is part of the joy of reading.

Sentences

Active Versus Passive Voice

Here is a single answer quiz. Which is better? Pick one.

1. We found that…
2. It was found that…

About two decades ago, several colleagues and I submitted a paper to a prestigious academic journal. It described an innovative medical school clerkship for students. Our paper read something like this: "We identified a need in the curriculum. We developed and presented a 6-week clerkship for the students. At the end of the year, we evaluated the outcome of the program." Following appropriate peer review, the journal editor wrote to us, accepting the paper contingent on certain modifications. One of these modifications was that we authors change all statements to passive voice. And so, we laboriously revised our prose to read: "A need was identified for an addition to the curriculum. A clerkship was developed and presented. The outcomes were evaluated at the end of the year." The changes continued throughout the rest of the article. In due time, the paper was published, but what was presented in print lacked the punch of what we originally submitted and actually took more words to express the same thoughts.

If active voice has more vigor than passive, why do we use the latter? Somehow, it may seem easier to express our thoughts in passive voice, and perhaps we thereby take a little less responsibility for them when "I" or "we" is not stated. I wonder if we are more likely to use active voice when we feel confident about positive results in research and passive voice when our confidence is lacking or the results are equivocal. Another theory is proposed by Day: "Perhaps this bad habit [using passive voice] is the result of the erroneous idea that it somehow impolite to use first-person pronouns" [5]. In fact, I submit that, in contrast to being impolite, when we use the active, first-person voice, we respectfully take ownership of our words.

We are definitely moving toward using more active voice in medical writing, especially in reporting original research. Here are some representative phrases from medical journals that have crossed my desk:

From *The Lancet Infectious Diseases* (2011; doi:https://doi.org/10.1016/S1473-3099(10)70288-7):

> "We aimed to assess the efficacy and safety of triple antiretroviral compared with zidovudine and single-dose nevirapine prophylaxis in pregnant women infected with HIV."

From the *New England Journal of Medicine* (2016;375:1845):

"We report, at a median follow-up of 5.3 years, the efficacy of adjuvant therapy with ipilimumab on all survival end points in patients with high-risk state III melanoma...".

From JAMA (2016;31:1181).

"We undertook a systematic review and meta-analysis for the UK Food Standards Agency...".

There are, of course, times when the use of passive voice is best. The classical example is when who does something is less important than the recipient of the action. In this instance it may be better to say that "the patient was injected with the test drug" rather than "we injected the test drug into the patient." Or perhaps it doesn't matter who performed the action, just that it occurred. For example, in the statement "The patient was transported to the hospital by ambulance," it does not matter who drove the vehicle.

Construct Sentences with Care

Words Per Sentence

We medical writers often write jumbled and tortuous sentences. We try to put too much into them, and we forget that the best sentences generally contain one thought. When a sentence is too long, it may become barely intelligible. As an example of a barely comprehensible sentence, I am going to rewrite the last paragraph in the section above on *Being Considerate of Your Reader*, the one just before the heading SENTENCES. Here goes:

The density of the printed page is managed by how we use headings, and you will note that I have made liberal use of headings in the book, which allows the presentation of white space to frame my usually well-written paragraphs, doing so in a way that is aesthetically pleasing, which is, after all, part of the joy of reading a book.

This 63-word stinker of a sentence did not even trigger my Microsoft Word grammar and spell-checker to tell me that it is too long—but it is, even with the relatively small words it contains. Imagine how bad it could be if weighed down with long scientific terms or unfamiliar abbreviations.

If you have more than about 25 or 30 words or more than two commas in a sentence, consider breaking it into two sentences, and you will usually find that it will read better. As an example, I wrote the previous sentence—on purpose—using 34 words and combining two thoughts. Now let's rewrite it as two sentences:

> If you have more than about 25 or 30 words in a sentence, consider breaking it into two sentences. You will usually find that it will read better.

Do you agree that the rewrite is an improvement?

Words Per Verb

If a sentence seems weak, count the words per verb. Verbs, the action words, are your strong words in a sentence. More than 20 words per verb tend to create a weak sentence. Here are the thoughts in the previous three sentences, considerably rewritten into one awkward sentence with 37 words and only one verb ("makes"):

> The use of an excessive number of words in conjunction with a single verb makes for a weak sentence, deficient in strong words, often complex in structure, and very likely complicated by a number of subordinate clauses.

Using Variety in Your Sentences

To make your writing vibrant, be sure to vary your sentence beginnings, type, and length. Avoid using the same word repeatedly, especially at the beginning of the sentence. Also, try to have some simple declarative sentences, some a little complex, and some that even begin with prepositional phrases.

We have already discussed excessive sentence length, which can be tiresome to the reader. On the other hand, using too many short sentences is also poor writing. The following, not atypical for a clinical record entry, is intended to illustrate all three points—sentence beginnings, type, and length:

> The elderly patient fell on a scatter rug at home. The patient struck his shoulder when he landed. The patient sustained a fracture of the left humerus.

The three sentences all begin alike, are all simple and declarative, and are all quite short. No one of the sentences is improper in any way, but taken together, the writing is unskillful. A much better way to express the three facts would be:

> The elderly patient fell on a scatter rug at home, striking his shoulder and sustaining a fracture of the left humerus.

Sentence Density

Single sentences, like paragraphs, can be too dense for comprehension by mere mortals. Consider the following sentence from a published report with the very clear title "Effect of Improving Depression Care on Pain and Functional Outcomes Among Older Adults with Arthritis." This is a topic of interest to all of us who treat elderly patients. And so I read with great interest the first of two sentences in the Results section of the Abstract:

> In addition to reduction in depressive symptoms, the intervention group compared with the usual care group at 12 months had lower mean (SE) scores for pain intensity (5.63 [0.16] vs. 6.15 [0.16]; between-group difference, -0.53; 95% confidence interval (CI), -0.92 to -0.14; $P = 0.009$), interference with daily activities due to arthritis (4.40 [0.18] vs. 4.99 [0.17]; between-group difference, -0.59; 95% CI, -1.00 to -0.19; $P = 0.004$), and interference with daily activities due to pain (2.92 [0.07] vs. 3.17 [0.07]; between-group difference, -0.26; 95% CI, -0.41 to -0.10; $P = 0.002$).
> (Source: JAMA. 2003;290:2428).

As a practicing physician and a medical writer, what are my issues with this sentence and how could it have been improved? First, it is much too long and convoluted. I believe that it could have been divided into three or four shorter sentences to enhance clarity. Second, the abbreviation CI (for confidence interval) is explained, but SE remains a mystery and is not explained elsewhere in the Abstract. Finally, the sentence is, in my opinion, much too stuffed with data. Do I really need all of these numbers in the abstract? What has been saved for the Results section of the article?

Fortunately, the authors subsequently translate the difficult sentence for us mere mortals and do so in very clear English: "In a large and diverse population of older adults with arthritis (mostly osteoarthritis) and co-morbid depression, benefits of improved depression care extended beyond reduced depressive symptoms and included decreased pain as well as improved functional status and quality of life." Okay, even this sentence is a little long and complicated, but I can read it without difficulty. And I like that the author used simple words such as "mostly" instead of "predominantly" and "osteoarthritis" rather than "degenerative joint disease." I will present more on words in the next section.

Cadence

Sentences have a cadence that the reader can sense, much like the rhythm in a song. If a sentence is convoluted by too many clauses or if it is burdened by too many unnecessary long words, the pleasant rhythm is lost. For example, take the first sentence in this paragraph, beginning, "Sentences have a cadence…" It's not Haiku poetry, but I think the sentence has a nice rhythm. It has several short words, then a long word, and only one word with more than two syllables. Could the sentence be worse? Yes, it could. Here's how:

> Very analogous to the rhythm that may be found in a song, we are readily able to discern pleasing cadences in sentences when they are well constructed.

Ugh! The sentence is syntactically correct, but not enjoyable to read. Make your reading a pleasure for the reader, if you can. If you wonder about the cadence of your sentences, read them aloud.

Punctuation: Commas, Periods, and More

Commas, semicolons, periods, and question marks are called stops. They improve sentence cadence and clarity and thus make reading easier. According to Jordan and Shepard, "the stops should fit with the rhythm of respiration as well as with the sense of what is said" [6].

Commas

Commas, like all stops, break up the flow of words. This "pause of power" was invented by Italian printer Aldus Manutius (1449–1515), who also gave us italic type. In a series of items, a comma is correct if it could be replaced by *and* or *or*. In her charming book *Eats, Shoots and Leaves*, Lynne Truss describes commas as "separators," likening the comma to a grammatical sheepdog that "tears about on the hillside of language, endlessly organizing words into sensible groups and making them stay put: sorting and dividing; circling and herding; and of course darting off with a preemptory 'woof' to round up any wayward subordinate clause that makes a futile bolt for semantic freedom" [7]. Consider the sentence at the beginning of this paragraph and how it would read without commas:

Commas like all stops break up the flow of words.

I suspect that you would need to read it twice to discern my meaning and then would mentally insert the commas.

The placement of commas can actually change meaning. For example:

The physician thought the patient looked gravely ill.

or

The physician, thought the patient, looked gravely ill.

The presence or absence of commas changes who seemed ill.

Bernstein [8] has reported how the state of Michigan discovered that its state constitution inadvertently legalized slavery. Section 8, Article 2, read:

> Neither slavery nor involuntary servitude, unless for the punish-
> ment of a crime, shall ever be tolerated in this state.

Upon consideration, it was sagely decided to delete the comma after servitude and place it after slavery.

Semicolons

The semicolon is used when you almost need a period; yet, a period would break up linked thoughts. If I used a period to divide the previous sentence, I would have created two short sentences in sequence. It might be acceptable, but joining the two thoughts with a semicolon seems right to me. In the setting of related thoughts and phrases, the use of semicolons is often a matter of individual style.

Semicolons are very useful in a series of items when the comma is needed within items. Truss describes this role as performing "the duties of a kind of Special Policeman in the event of comma fights" [7]. For example:

> Musculoskeletal injuries may be treated with rest; analgesics or
> muscle relaxant medication; and physical therapy including heat,
> ice, and stretching exercises.

American physician Lewis Thomas (1913–1993) wrote: "Sometimes you get a glimpse of a semicolon coming, a few lines farther on, and it is like climbing a steep path through the woods and seeing a wooden bench just at the bend in the road ahead, a place where you can expect to sit for a moment, catching your breath" [9].

Periods and Question Marks

The period is the "full stop" that ends a sentence. Period. Oh, yes, there are some technical uses, such as in abbreviations (e.g., Mr., Ph.D., or Dr.), but these do not affect sentence flow.

The question mark is an interrogatory symbol that appears after a direct question. A period is used with an indirect question. For example:

- The direct question:

  The physician asked the patient, "Where is the pain located?"

- The indirect question:

  The physician asked the patient where the pain was located.

Verbosity

US Secretary of State John Kerry once said of President Barack Obama: "The President is desirous of trying to see how we can make our efforts in order to find a way to facilitate." Translation: "The President wants to help" (Money. March 2015, p. 65).

A disease that afflicts many sentences in medical writing, verbosity is simply using a long phrase to express a thought when fewer words will do nicely. A classical example is saying "fewer in number" instead of "less" or even simply "fewer." Or a careless author might write, "has the capability to" when meaning to say "can."

Table 2.1 presents a list of verbose phrases.

Of course, it is not just phrases that are afflicted with verbosity. Sometimes entire sentences are involved. Here is one:

The thesis is herein offered that woman (like man) is a biological, social and cultural creature, and as such is dependent for health on the acceptance, approval, support, and encouragement of significant individual members of the social group to which she belongs.

What the author means to say, I believe, is that a woman's health can be influenced by her peer relationships.

You can usually spot a verbose sentence before you are halfway through. How? Because it often begins with a phrase like:

- We are reminded of the necessity for the consideration of…

TABLE 2.1 Verbose phrases: why use one word when more will do?

Verbose phrase	What you mean to say
At this time	Now
At the conclusion of	After
With the exception of	Except
In only a small number of cases	Rarely
In many instances	Often
In light of the fact that	Because
More often than not	Usually
In the absence of	Without
On a daily basis	Daily
In close proximity to	Near
The great majority of	Most
With regard to	About
In the event that	If
In the not too distant future	Soon
Consensus of opinion	Consensus

- Although certainly not a new finding, it is pertinent to remind the reader that...
- At this time, it is appropriate to emphasize that...
- It is a well-recognized fact that...
- Let me make clear that...
- It is interesting to note that...

Of course, all this verbosity is really an excess of words, and often large words. So let's next consider our most basic tools—words.

Words

Words are the most basic tools we use to write. Sir Winston Churchill once wrote: "Short words are best and old words, when short, are best of all." Sir Winston's sentence has a pleasing cadence. It uses the active voice. It is not long and convoluted. Most important, it uses only short words; in fact, the sentence contains only words of one syllable. They are old-fashioned English-language words, even though, like most words, they can be traced to some language in antiquity. In a similar vein, William Faulkner once wrote of Ernest Hemingway (and claimed he was not being derisive), "He has never been known to use a word that may send the reader to a dictionary."

The preferred styles of Churchill and Hemingway may work in the writing of history and literature, but one of the inescapable difficulties in medical writing is our dependence on scientific words derived from the classical languages. Their specificity is a benefit, but their complexity can become a curse in medical writing. Let's look at a few medical words.

Understanding Medical Words

I have always been fascinated by medical words, and I try hard to know the origins of those I use. I advise medical students and residents to keep a "medical word journal" to help them learn the classical roots, and various other origins, of words we use in clinical care. I believe that knowing the etymologic derivation of words such as *acetabulum* (from the Greek word for "vinegar cup") and *Norwalk virus* (from the small town in Ohio where the microorganism was first isolated) might make me a better writer. Even if this theory is flawed, knowing how these words arose enriches my life [10].

According to Sobel, the newly minted physician has learned 55,000 new words [11]. Most of these come from Latin and Latinized Greek. The Latinization of Greek began when the Romans conquered the Greeks, and they appropriated everything, including their language. Later, in the post-Renaissance era, scholars and scientists turned to these languages as new words were needed to describe their discoveries. Why ancient Greek and Latin? The answer is that they are both "dead languages," with no capricious changes or additions. They are, metaphorically, chiseled in stone. Examples of words coming from Latin and Latinized

Greek are *dementia* (to be mad), *placenta* (a flat cake), *gingiva* (gum), *scabies* (to scratch), *rubella* (diminutive of red), and *digitalis* (from digit, meaning finger or toe, and used because the drug came from foxglove, also called "ladies' fingers").

Later, the Anglo-Saxon tongues gave us *sick*, *blood*, and *gut*. (The latter is now the name of a prestigious journal.) Middle English gave us some medical words such as *eye* and Italian contributed *belladonna* (meaning beautiful lady). Others that are borrowed from foreign languages include *beriberi* (from the Singhalese word *beri*, meaning weak; the doubling indicates extreme weakness) and *ammonia* from the Egyptian word for Jupiter (the rest of the story is that Jupiter was called Jupiter Ammon, and many persons came riding camels to worship the god at a shrine near the Libyan city of Ammonia; from the accumulated camel dung came a substance that was named ammonia). *Bezoar* came from a Persian word meaning antidote, and *quinine* arose from the Spanish spelling of the Peruvian word *kina*, meaning bark (of a tree).

Some medical words come from literature or mythology. These include *Pickwickian syndrome*, *panic*, *syphilis*, *atlas*, *Munchausen syndrome*, and *Achilles tendon*. Some more recent medical neologisms involve places: The disease name *tularemia* comes from Tulare County in California, where the disease was first described. Even universities and patients get in the game: Warfarin, first marketed as a rat poison, is named after the Wisconsin Alumni Research Foundation plus the last four letters of its chemical name; and the name *bacitracin* comes from "baci" for bacteria and "tracin" for Margaret Tracey, whose wound drainage permitted identification of the antibiotic.

Table 2.2 lists some of my favorite medical words and their origins. I hope that this section and the table inspire you to seek the sources, as well as the definitions, of unfamiliar words as you encounter them.

TABLE 2.2 The origins of selected medical words

Medical word	Origin of the word
Botulism	From German *botulismus*, meaning "sausage." in the Victorian times and later, persons sometimes contracted the disease by eating sausage
Carotid	From Greek *karotikos*, meaning "to render unconscious." the ancient Greeks noted what happened when you compressed these arteries
Clap	Although not a proper medical term, the word comes from medieval French word *clapier*, meaning "brothel"
Hysteria	In ancient Greek, the word *hystera* ("womb") evolved to *hysterikos* ("malfunctioning womb"). I will say no more about this
Influenza	Our word for flu borrowed the Italian word *influenza*, meaning "influence." they believed the disease was due to the power of the heavens
Mastoid	From Greek *mastos*, meaning "breast." this is the shape of the postauricular bony outcropping of the temporal bone
Mitral	The valve looks like a bishop's miter, his official headdress. The word comes from the Greek word *mitra*, describing a cloth headband or girdle
Penis	The word *penis* in Latin originally meant "tail"
Quarantine	From Latin *quadraginta*, meaning "forty." in medieval Venice and other ports, vessels were moored offshore for 40 days before being allowed to enter, a delay exceeding the incubation period of most infectious diseases
Thalassemia	From Greek *thalassa*, meaning "sea," and *haima*, the word for blood. The disease affected chiefly those who lived near the Mediterranean Sea
Tsutsugamushi (fever)	This is the Japanese word meaning "dangerous bug"
Vitamin	When it was noted that an amine of nicotinic acid prevented pellagra, it was called a "vital amine," shortened to "vitamine" by a polish biochemist with the euphonious name Casimir funk. The use of the word was expanded to include other compounds; some were not actually amines, and hence the final "e" was eliminated

Some Thoughts About the Types of Words We Use

We use many types of words, which include nouns and pronouns, verbs, modifiers such as adjectives and adverbs, metaphors and similes, onomatopoeic words and alliteration, literary allusions, and eponyms.

Nouns and Pronouns

Nouns are generally strong words, and short nouns make for easier reading than longer ones, but, as noted, this is sometimes not possible in medical writing, as we sacrifice readability to precision. We seldom get in trouble with nouns.

Pronouns are another story. We sometimes confuse the pronoun and its antecedent, the word the pronoun replaces, as in the following:

> A new vaccine is available to prevent the flu, and to get it you should see your doctor now.
>
> This disease stands unique as the first truly American disease, and the guiding spirit that made this accomplishment possible is….
>
> The resident anesthetized the patient as the attending surgeon waited; he then made the incision in the abdomen.

Over the past few years, we have discovered another way to introduce complexity with pronouns, namely, the use of clumsy neologisms to avoid the perception of sexist language. Newly created unisex pronouns have included "shim" and "s/he." Or, in the quest for gender-neutral writing, we have also begun to accept annoying constructions such as, "The physician should treat their patient with respect." Probably the best of the compromises is the use of plural pronouns ("they") or using both genders ("he or she," "her or him"). In this book you will not find "their" used with a single noun as an antecedent. I have tried to minimize the use of wordy phrases such as "he or she" or "him or her," but found that I could not avoid their use altogether.

Verbs

Verbs, the action words, are the strongest we have: *go*, *stop*, *admit*, *examine*, and *cut*. Every sentence needs a verb, which should be close to the subject noun in the sentence. Verbs can be expressed in active voice ("We found that…") or passive ("It was found that…").

Verbs also have tense—past, present, future, and variations thereof. There are two conventions in medical writing worth noting:

- Within a scientific article, we use past tense to describe results:

  We found that one-third of the rats survived, one-third died, and the third rat got away.

- In describing a published work, present tense is used:

  In their groundbreaking work, Smith and Jones report a 33% survival rate in the test population.

The infinitive is the basic form of a verb (e.g., "to clarify"), and in high school, we were warned to never split an infinitive. Today's custom allows a split infinitive if it will make the sentence clearer. For example:

- Clumsy:

  Splitting an infinitive might greatly serve to clarify a sentence.

- Better with a split infinitive:

  Splitting an infinitive might serve to greatly clarify a sentence.

Modifiers

Adjectives modify nouns and adverbs modify verbs, adjectives, and other adverbs. Although judicious use can enrich your writing, beware the tendency to overuse modifiers, which can produce wimpy writing. They creep into our writing easily, and beginning writers tend to overuse them. In seeking economy in our words, we use abundant modifiers when writing clinical notes ("well-developed, well-nourished, male factory worker in no acute distress"), and sometimes we carry this over into our scientific writing. Here are two examples of sentences that string several modifiers together; the sentences contain all the necessary information but lack vigor. In the sentences below, we lose the full impact of any one of the modifiers, which might benefit from more discussion:

- Multiple adjectives:

    The patient was a tall, gray-haired, anxious, marasmic, elderly man.

- Multiple adverbs:

    The neurosurgeon operated quietly, skillfully, carefully, decisively, and seemingly effortlessly.

When you find yourself stringing several modifiers together, ask if all are really desirable. Do I truly need all these adjectives or adverbs?

Peer reviewers found the article to be timely, interesting, scholarly, articulate, and comprehensive.

Metaphors and Similes

A metaphor is an implied comparison: "For the patient in the critical care unit, his wife's arrival at the bedside was always a ray of sunshine in his dull day." At the beginning of this chapter, I wrote ideas and structure as our blueprint and paragraphs, sentences, and words as our tools. The words *blueprint* and *tools* used in this way represented metaphors. In contrast, an explicit comparison is a simile: "A meal without wine is like a day without sunshine." In fact, the word *metaphor*, having evolved from Greek words meaning *between places* and *to carry*, can itself be considered a metaphor. Our struggle as writers is to create metaphors and similes that are novel, and perhaps even memorable, as when

Flannery O'Connor, in her tale "A Good Man is Hard to Find," depicts the face of the mother as "broad and innocent as a cabbage" [12].

We often use metaphors and similes in medical writing, and some are embedded in our medical terminology: "coffee-ground vomitus," "cotton-wool exudates," "leonine facies," and "spider nevi." We say that a penetrating injury "invaded the abdominal cavity." Medical similes include poorly perfused feet that are "cold as ice" and the anemic patient whose skin appears "pale as a sheet."

Pogo, from Walt Kelly's classic comic strip, said that "Words are for people who can't read pictures." But words can be used to create vivid images in our minds. Consider the following: Tobacco causes the deaths of 400,000 Americans each year. Big number. To be more specific, in the United States more than 1000 persons die each day of the effects of tobacco use. This has a little more punch. But try this word picture: The loss of life in the United States due to tobacco use is the equivalent of three jumbo jets crashing each day. For me, this image has dramatic impact!

Metaphors and similes enrich our writing, and the chief way we go wrong is mixing our images:

> Following three days of gastroenteritis, the patient was bone-dry, like an old prune.
> After a night on duty, the surgical resident was dog-tired, like a deflated inner tube.

Eponyms

Diseases, anatomical structures, remedies, and other items named for famous physicians and scientists represent eponyms. The word itself comes from the Greek word *eponymas*, meaning "named after." Some of the many eponyms we all know include Bright disease, tetralogy of Fallot, Graves disease, Raynaud syndrome, Hodgkin disease, Hippocratic facies, and Alzheimer disease. Note that the current custom is to avoid the possessive style in eponyms. For example, we now write Paget disease instead of Paget's disease.

The eponym, admittedly a handy linguistic shortcut, is falling out of favor, and today's tendency is to replace these historic names with more scientific terms. Hence, von Recklinghausen disease is now properly called neurofibromatosis, and Caffey disease is infantile cortical hyperostosis. There are some exceptions: I still find the eponyms Hansen disease and Down syndrome in common use, persisting, I suspect, for euphemistic reasons. The use of eponyms has even become entangled in world politics. It seems that Hans Reiter (Reiter syndrome) and Friedrich Wegener (Wegener granulomatosis) both had some Nazi ties, and Woywodt and Matteson have written that "the continued use of tainted eponyms is inappropriate and will not be accepted by patients, relatives, or the public" [13]. The medical writer should follow the current custom in most cases, stating the accepted Greco-Latin phrase, perhaps followed by the historic eponym in parentheses—for example: relapsing febrile nodular nonsuppurative panniculitis (Weber-Christian disease).

Choosing the Words We Use

Words must be chosen with care. You should strive to use just the right word in an exact, precise way. And you must try to avoid words that can annoy or confuse your reader.

Using Words Precisely

The following statement about a vaccine for traveler's diarrhea was published a few years ago. In my opinion, it contains an error. Can you find it?

> The new, one-dose vaccine is presently given in liquid form but could be developed in oral form.

Is not a liquid also an oral form? I think that the author means to say that the new form will be a capsule or tablet.

Here are two other examples that found their way into print:

> He complained of numbness in his feet, which was gradually speeding proximally.

I believe that the author means that the numbness was spreading, not speeding.

> The incidence of uremic pericarditis occurs in 14–20% of patients undergoing dialysis.

The sentence above is from one of America's leading medical journals. Incidence "is"; incidence does not "occur."

As you read medical journals in the months and years to come, look for small errors and imprecise word use. It will be amusing and will help make you a better writer.

Words That Might Annoy

Be alert to your readers' sensibilities. Do not call an anesthesiologist an anesthetist or refer to a family physician as a family practitioner. Never write about the orthopedic surgeon as an orthopod. Some of the words that arose as managed care jargon can irritate various clinicians, and writers should think twice before using them. Table 2.3 lists words that might grate on some readers.

One consideration under the heading of possibly annoying words is what we call those who receive medical care. Throughout my career they have been patients. Recently, however, I have heard them called "clients." The recent emergence of "client" merits scrutiny. In part, at least, the word is an outgrowth of managed care, which also helped bring us "provider" and "covered lives." It also may be the discipline-specific stylistic choice of some clinician authors. Therefore, let us try to understand "client" vs. "patient" by going to the origins of the words.

"Patient" in English comes from Latin *pati* (to suffer), then Old French *pacient*, and later Middle English *pacyent*. The words have denoted a suffering person receiving medical care and that the person endured the illness calmly and with forbearance ("patience"). "Client," on the other hand, comes from the Anglo-French word *clyent*, meaning a person who is dependent on another. The word entered the English language to describe those who depended on lawyers and later metamorphosed to include customers of other services, but

TABLE 2.3 Annoying words (and abbreviations)

Words that may annoy	Why the word annoys some readers
Provider	Our readers are physicians, nurse practitioners, physician assistants, clinical psychologists, and other health-care professionals. "Provider" is a lumping term that originated with third-party payers. Many are offended by this term, and the journal *American Family Physician* has specifically ceased its use. Goroll has called for elimination of the term primary care "provider" [14]
PCP	This is supposed to refer to "primary care provider" or "primary care physician." the abbreviation can also stand for phencyclidine (phenylcyclohexyl piperidine) also called "angel dust," pulmonary capillary pressure, prochlorperazine, and *Pneumocystis carinii* pneumonia
Covered lives	This phrase is another illegitimate spawn of the managed care payers. We treat patients or perhaps clients if that is your discipline's preference. We do not care for "covered lives," a term that only dehumanizes those persons that we serve in our practices
Mid-level provider	Nurse practitioners and physician assistants do not like this term, which is perceived as disrespectful
Case	The sick person is a patient—or perhaps a man, woman, child, or person—But not a case. Cases are what lawyers argue in court
Customer	Administrators like to talk about "customer service," as though we were selling used cars

not of physicians. When I am next ill, I wish to be considered a patient and not a client.

Misused Words

Medical writers often misuse words. Sometimes it is hospital team conversation showing up in manuscripts. It may be an attempt to be "scientific." Perhaps the author is overusing the thesaurus. Examples of misused words include using *symp-*

tomatology when we mean symptoms, using *impact* as a verb when the correct word would be *affect*, and dropping adverbs such as *hopefully* somewhere in an otherwise perfectly good sentence.

> Incorrect use: The patient hopefully will recover.
> Correct use: The clinicians and family all hope that the patient will recover.

All adverbs, most of which end in *-ly*, must modify a specific word that is not a noun. I hope that you will not allow adverbs such as *happily*, *sadly*, or *tragically* to wander about in your sentences like lost children.

Table 2.4 lists some words that, I hope, you and I will not misuse in the future.

TABLE 2.4 Some words (and phrases) we misuse

Word or phrase	How we misuse the word
Data	This is a plural word. To write that "the data shows" is incorrect. The correct phrase is: "The data show…"
Mitigate	Mitigate means "to lessen in intensity or force." thus it is wrong to say that an infusion of dextrose in water mitigated *against* the insulin-induced hypoglycemia. The addition of "against" is redundant and, in a sense, is a double negative
Parameter	An arbitrary constant in a mathematical equation is a parameter. Other uses of this statistical term in scientific writing are generally incorrect
Significant	When used in a scientific paper, this word has a statistical connotation. For this reason, other use of this word in medical writing can be confusing, even misleading
Etiology	Remember that *-ology* at the end of any word means "the study of." therefore, we should not write about *S. pneumoniae* as the "etiology" of pneumococcal pneumonia when we are really discussing the cause
Very unique	The word "unique" means that there is only one (from Latin *unus*, meaning "one"). Thus, it is one of a kind or it is not, and no modifier is appropriate
Equal halves	Halves cannot be unequal

Moving On

In this chapter, I have covered basic elements of article topic and organization, as well as issues in composing paragraphs, writing sentences, and selecting words. In the next chapter, I discuss putting it all together to create an article, with an eye to publication.

References

1. Souba C. The language of leadership. Acad Med. 2010;85(10):1069–74.
2. Taylor RB. Learning to scramble. Fam Med. 2001;33(8):629–30.
3. Taylor RB. How physicians read the medical literature. The Female Patient. 2004;29(1):8–11.
4. Kellogg RT. Attentional overload and writing performance: effects of rough draft and outline strategies. J Exp Psychol. 1988;14(2):355–65.
5. Day RA. How to write and publish a scientific paper. 7th ed. Westport, CT: Greenwood; 2011. p. 209.
6. Jordan EP, Shepard WC. Rx for medical writing. Philadelphia: WB Saunders; 1952. p. 24.
7. Truss L. Eats, shoots and leaves. New York: Gotham Books; 2003. p. 79.
8. Bernstein TM. The careful writer: a modern guide to English usage. New York: Atheneum; 1972. p. 360.
9. Thomas L. The medusa and the snail. New York: Viking Press; 1979. p. 129.
10. Taylor RB. The amazing language of medicine: understanding medical terms and their backstories. New York: Springer; 2017.
11. Sobel RK. MSL—medicine as a second language. N Engl J Med. 2005;352(19):1945–6.
12. O'Connor F. A good man is hard to find. In: The complete stories. New York: Farrar, Straus & Giroux; 1971. p. 117.
13. Woywodt A, Matteson E. Should eponyms be abandoned? Yes. BMJ. 2007;335(7617):424.
14. Goroll AH. Eliminating the term primary care "provider:" consequences of language for the future of primary care. JAMA. 2016;315(17):1833.

Chapter 3
Medical Writing: Getting Started and Getting Finished

"Begin at the beginning," the King said gravely, "and go on until you come to the end. Then stop."

—Lewis Carroll, Alice's Adventures in Wonderland. London: Macmillan; 1865

In Chap. 1, I reviewed your motivation to write, discussed how to find needed information, and enumerated the important questions that must be asked about any writing project. In Chap. 2, I discussed the blueprint for your project—the idea and structure—and the tools you will use, namely, paragraphs, sentences, and words. Now let's look at putting it all together, from page one to the end, starting with your idea and how to handle to it.

Prewriting

Medical writing actually begins with a phase called prewriting, when you think about your topic and what you want to say about it. Fowler and Hayes describe the process in this way: "Because writing as an act of thinking is messy and mysterious compared to the concrete product, we tend to leave composing up to the vagaries of chance and god-given

© Springer International Publishing AG 2018
R.B. Taylor, *Medical Writing*,
https://doi.org/10.1007/978-3-319-70126-4_3

talent to relegate it to independent warm-up exercises designated as '*pre*-writing'" [1]. Prewriting generally begins with a topic idea.

You might begin with a nice focused subject such as "the new drug that cures the common cold: indications, administration, side effects, and cost." Or perhaps you have just concluded the seminal study on whether or not eating rhubarb daily cures baldness; the medical world is awaiting the report, and it is time to write up your results. Generally, however, your idea will be something like "the office approach to" acute sinusitis or chronic pelvic pain, or perhaps pain management of the patient with terminal cancer.

With a general topic idea in mind, the next step is to limit the topic and find the best way to approach it. We discussed this briefly in Chap. 2. Because deciding on the concept and structure—how you will handle your topic—is so important, I will return to this process here, using the review article as a model.

Let us use sinusitis as an example of a general interest topic. How might we limit the topic and organize an article? Logical questions are: Shall I write on pathophysiology, diagnosis, or treatment or all three? Shall I write on acute or chronic sinusitis or both? Shall I cover adults or children or both? Is there any logic to covering women vs. men as patients? If covering treatment, should I include both medical and surgical therapy? How about herbal as well as traditional medical therapy? The following lists some of the article concepts possible with the general topic of sinusitis:

Pathophysiology:

Common precursors of acute sinusitis
Microorganisms found in acute sinusitis
Complications of bacterial sinusitis
Chronic sinusitis in men and women: is there a difference?
Causes of sinusitis in children and adolescents

Diagnosis:

Recognizing bacterial sinusitis: common signs and symptoms
Uncommon presentations of acute sinusitis
Acute vs. chronic sinusitis: how to tell the difference
When to image the patient with sinusitis
Warning signs in the patient with acute sinusitis

Treatment:

The best drugs to use in acute sinusitis
Current surgical therapy of chronic sinusitis
Herbal therapy of sinusitis
Treating chronic sinusitis: an evidence-based approach
Managing chronic sinusitis: treatments that do not work
When to refer the patient with sinusitis

Any symptom, sign, or diagnosis in medicine can yield many ideas for an article. Here is a useful exercise. Pick a general area—such as skin rash, abdominal pain, or pneumonia—that interests you, and then think of at least ten approaches to a review article about this topic.

If there is one aspect of an article you want to get just right, it is how you deal with your topic. A copy editor can correct spelling, fix grammatical errors, and untangle convoluted syntax. But a copy editor cannot fix structure. Think of a house: copy editing represents redecorating. Structural change, moving walls and raising roofs, is major reconstruction, much more ambitious. Because finding the best concept and structure for the article is so important, I will return to the topic again in Chap. 6.

After selecting a focused topic and deciding on a structural concept, the experienced writer embarks on a "gestational period" during which the idea is pondered from various viewpoints, thinking about cases, lists, headings, examples from personal experience, and what really should be shared with the reader. During the gestational time, you will collect and organize data that will be needed for your paper.

Collecting and Organizing Data

The "data phase" is important because it provides the basic facts you will present in your article. You will need these facts—for example, in a headache article I may tell that migraine headaches affect 18% of women and 6% of men during their lifetimes—when you actually begin to write. In the end, you will need to know the source of these figures. Not having necessary data at hand will break your train of creative thought, a cognitive interlude that could result in disconnected prose.

What you need before you start writing varies a little with the type of article or book chapter you are writing. I will cover the differences later as we discuss writing case reports, editorials, reports of original research, and so forth. However, for all articles you will need your basic research tools, notes, outline, and references.

Network Research

Every writer's research tools were discussed in Chap. 1, including selected books and clinically oriented web sites. Here I want to discuss one more information collection tool: network research. Let's assume that I want to learn how many parking spaces are in the parking lots at Miami International Airport. I would start by calling someone in the airport administrative offices, who will refer me to someone who knows something about parking, and then this person will know some more specifics about the various lots. I would wager that I could get the exact answer by the seventh telephone call. This is network research.

If I wanted to find out whether someone is working on the brilliant research question I just dreamed up, I would embark on some network research. I would search PubMed, BioMedLib.com, or Google Scholar to find out who is writing on the topic currently, including reviewing the references cited in recently published papers. Then I would turn to the telephone or e-mail and call these authors. My favorite question is: "Who else could I contact that might know about this topic?"

Notes

How you save and organize your notes is very personal, and your method is very likely to change over time. After all, few of us use 3- by 5-in. index cards any more.

In preparing this book, I have used a combination of paper and computer. For my research, I have photocopied article and book pages. I have also printed PubMed abstracts from computer screens. For each of these paper documents, I have been careful to include the detailed identification of the source. Published article printouts typically contain full citation information. Printouts of web pages come with the web site identified. For book pages, this is easily accomplished by creating a small piece of paper telling the source and then taping it so that it is photocopied onto each page. I believe that including the full citation on every note page is important to help avoid later confusion about the source of ideas and phrases. It is much too easy to become an accidental plagiarist if you make notes without careful attribution. (More about plagiarism in Chap. 5.)

Notes may include personal "bright ideas." These can come at any time, and getting them in your notes can be like catching a sunbeam. In 1974 economist Arthur Laffer had an idea about the relationship between tax rates and tax receipts. So as not to let it get away, he scribbled it on a napkin, and later this idea became the *Laffer Curve* that was the foundation of the supply-side economics we remember from the President Reagan era. Your "bright idea" notes can be recorded on paper or, as I have done in working on these chapters, added to a Microsoft (MS) Word document labeled "Booknotes. doc." I arrange these "bright idea" notes by chapter. Then as I begin work on a new chapter, I "cut and paste" the notes into the first draft, thereby avoiding retyping.

I suggest that you be expansive in assembling notes. What seems not pertinent today may be an idea that proves useful later. After you complete your project, what was not used can be discarded or saved for another project. It is perfectly okay that, in the end, more than half of your notes will probably not be used, at least in the current project. Assembling these thoughts helped clarify your thinking and perhaps suggested an idea for another paper.

Outline

As you have already discovered, I am an outline advocate [2]. I like to determine the topic and concept first and then think about the general structure of the article. For example, assume that you are writing an article on the general topic of edema. The concept might be "five uncommon causes of edema." Then the outline's major headings could be:

Abstract
Background
Selected causes
Clinical significance
References

From here you might expand the outline to the next level of headings:

Abstract
Background
    Epidemiology
    Definitions
    Why the issue is important

Selected Causes
    Hypothyroidism
    Sodium overload
    Hypoalbuminemia
    Cyclic edema in women
    Medication side effect

Clinical Significance
    When to consider an uncommon cause
    What is important in daily practice?

References

After taking notes and thinking about the topic, you might further expand the outline to include topics to be covered under each subheading:

Abstract

This will be a summary of the main sections: background, the five selected causes of edema, and the clinical significance of these causes.

Background

Epidemiology

How often do we see patients with unexplained edema?
    What clinicians are likely to see these patients?

Definitions: "localized" vs. "generalized" edema
Why the issue is important
    Value of early therapy
    Dangers of missed diagnoses

Selected Causes (give presentation and diagnostic features of each)

Hypothyroidism
Sodium overload
Hypoalbuminemia
    Malnutrition
    Cirrhosis of the liver
    Nephrotic syndrome
    Protein-losing enteropathy

Cyclic edema in women
Medication side effect

> Nonsteroidal antiinflammatory drug (NSAID), estrogens, corticosteroids, antihypertensives, and others

Clinical Significance
  When to consider an uncommon cause
  What is important in daily practice?

References

You can see how the expanded outline grows. It will be very useful when you write the first draft because you will already have made many of the critical decisions. My outline for this book became the Table of Contents; the outline for this chapter became the various level headings.

Yet, despite my strong advocacy for outlining, I want to say a word about flexibility. It is important that the outline does not become a straitjacket. Be willing to modify and enhance your plan. New ideas will emerge as you write and sometimes will be good enough to prompt a change in the outline. I always hope that the change is minor (redecorating) rather than major (moving a weight-bearing wall). Embarking on a structural change when halfway through the first draft is, at best, a frustrating activity.

References

Managing references during article preparation is an art. There are many ways to manage references, and the method you choose will vary with the number of references in your article or book chapter. If your article has relatively few references, fewer than 20, I think it is acceptable to use the method I have used in each of these chapters. First, remember that each page or saved document of notes should contain the full reference source. Then as I create a sentence that calls for a reference citation, I type the full source in parentheses at the end of the sentence and put it in bold font so I can find it easily later. It looks like this:

> …so I can find it easily later. It looks like this: (**Taylor RB. Medical writing: a guide for clinicians, educators, and researchers, Ed 3. New York: Springer; 2018:125.**)

Then I continue to write and revise successive drafts. At the end, when I consider the article or chapter almost done—and beyond any major changes—I substitute sequential numbers for the references, and I move the citations to the reference list using the MS Word "cut and paste" feature. In the end, the manuscript sentence will be:

> ...so I can find it easily later. It looks like this [3].

The method may seem a little primitive, but it works well for me, perhaps because my writing rarely has a large number of reference citations.

Another way to manage references is the use of EndNote software. This sophisticated program allows users to search online bibliographic databases and to keep track of their references. Once you have mastered its use, you can create and edit bibliographies readily. The disadvantages are cost—currently $249 to download the full product—although a free 30-day trial is offered. There is a steep learning curve facing the new user. The program is not "intuitive," and the online instructions are challenging. You can learn more about EndNote software by starting with www.google.com, searching "Endnote," and then following the trail. There are other reference management tools available without a fee: Mendeley and Zotero.

Reference management software is great for experienced and prolific medical authors, especially if compiling long lists of citations. However, in my opinion, beginning medical authors should use my more primitive "cut and paste" method and spend their energy learning how to be better writers.

How Much Preparation Is Enough?

It is possible to over-prepare to write. Some authors seem to become mired in the prewriting and data acquisition phases and never emerge. When you have your topic, research tools, notes, outline, and references all together, the time has come to begin the first draft.

Beginning: The First Draft

Getting Started

Finding Time to Create

There is one more thing you will need for an outstanding first draft: uninterrupted time. Collecting data, constructing an outline, and later revising are all important grunt work that can be accomplished in discontinuous periods of time. This is not true of writing the first draft, which is the truly creative part of the work. For this effort, you will need several hours of time that will be free of interruptions. (See Chap. 1 for some hints on how to find this elusive block of time.) For the average length article, and with adequate preparation, you should plan on 2–3 h to create the first draft. When writing a first draft, I have joked to my colleagues that, if interrupted, when I open the door, I expect to see flames in the hallway.

Not breaking your concentration also means not stopping to look things up. The first draft is about getting your thoughts down on paper in a logically organized way. It is not about spelling, minor grammatical errors, or perfect word choice. This is not the time to consult the thesaurus. Do not stop writing to verify details online; this can come later in the revision phase.

Where and How to Begin

When faced with an empty computer screen, what do you do next? For both beginning and experienced authors, getting the first few words in type can be the most difficult step in writing. Jordan and Shepard state, "The first few words are like a plunge into an ice cold pool. It isn't so bad after the start has been made" [4].

Here are some diverse ways to get started:

- As the King advised Alice, start at the very beginning and keep going. Some very experienced authors can do this and can intuitively control the length of the finished article.

I admire these gifted individuals and hope someday to achieve this exalted state.

- Expand the outline with chunks of words, jumping about as the spirit moves you. In the edema article outlined above, I might write a paragraph about a patient I saw with edema and then another paragraph covering how sodium overload occurs and how it may be recognized. In the end, I will fit these disparate bits and pieces together like a jigsaw puzzle, using the planned structure, to create a draft of the article.

- Create the tables and figures. This is one of my favorite methods. Many articles and book chapters are built around one or more tables. Creating these tables—making decisions on column headings and what to include—can bring clarity to the entire piece you are writing. In writing this book, I first assembled my expanded outline and notes. My next step was to create the tables for each chapter, all the way to the end of the book.

- Write the abstract. In general, I advise writing the abstract last. After all, it is a synopsis of the article, and you won't really know the full content of the article until it is done. But when at a loss for a beginning, writing a tentative synopsis can focus your thinking and get some words on paper.

- Answer the WIRMS question: *What I Really Mean to Say is…* If having trouble getting started, answer the WIRMS question in one to three sentences and see if this starts the flow of words.

Delaying Tactics

Budd Schulberg joked about the writer's uncanny ability to avoid work. His habit was, "First I clean my typewriter. Then I go through my shelves and return all borrowed books. Then I play with my three children. Then, if it's warm, I go for a swim. Then I find some friends to have a drink with. By then, it's time to clean the typewriter again."
—James Charlton, Lisbeth Mark. *The writer's home companion.* Danbury CT: Franklin Watts; 1987:105

At this point, I want to talk about delaying tactics. When it is time to sit down and write, almost any other activity seems to be more interesting or urgent. My favorite delaying tactics are getting coffee, surfing the web in search of one more nugget of information, or rearranging items on my desktop. For others, they are making a telephone call or answering e-mail messages—anything but engaging the brain and writing.

For some authors, actions such as sharpening a handful of pencils are actually rituals that signal them that it is time to write. For others the activities are impediments to writing and should be recognized for the undesirable behavior they represent.

Words One, Two, and Beyond

The actual opening sentence of a paper is important, first to get words on the screen and second to establish the direction and tone for the article. The first sentence often states the problem in very general terms. For example, "Unexplained edema can be a diagnostic challenge." Or, "Osteoporosis is a common problem of women over age 60."

An alternative opening for an article or book chapter is to present a clinical vignette: "The patient was a 32-year-old woman, in otherwise good health, with swelling of the feet and hands for more than 6 months." Such a first sentence piques the interest of most clinicians. Here is another from the literature: "A 30-year-old woman presented to the emergency department . . . with chills and a sudden worsening of abdominal pain in both lower quadrants" (Simmons LH et al. NEJM. 2016;375:1672).

Whatever the first sentence, the beginning of an article should set the stage and get the article moving. Not all articles begin with the general, unassailable statement. Table 3.1 lists examples of other ways to start an article or a chapter.

TABLE 3.1 Some ways to begin an article or chapter

The beginning	Example
Purpose of the article	This paper presents an evidence-based approach to the management of the common cold
Scope of the article	This paper discusses five causes of generalized edema
Viewpoint of the paper	Calling clinicians "providers" insults our professionalism
Quotation from a respected source	In a recent report in *Lancet*, Smith et al. report that…
Approaching a problem	What is the best way to reduce teen pregnancy?
Challenging a current opinion	Chondroitin is not helpful for pain from osteoarthritis of the knee or hip. So why do some physicians continue to recommend this substance?
Focus on action	Now is the time for physicians to speak out on the proposed changes in Medicare
Compare and contrast	Some physicians prescribe antibiotics empirically for adult patients with acute bronchitis manifested as fever and severe cough. Others do not
Beginning with a question	The next patient you see may have pertussis. Will you recognize the symptoms and signs?
The startling statistic	Up to one-third of Americans with hypertension are undiagnosed, and only about half of those known to have hypertension are adequately controlled

Getting Stuck

American newspaper writer Gene Fowler (1890–1960) once commented: "Writing is easy. All you do is stare at a sheet of blank paper until drops of blood form on your forehead" [5].

At some time while writing the early drafts, you are likely to get stuck. The words just won't come. You look out the window, go out for the mail, or play with the dog. You engage in all the delaying tactics listed above. You wonder if you are having a TIA (transient ischemic attack, a small stroke). Face it. You have writer's block, a temporary affliction that strikes every author eventually. You are waiting in vain for the muse to appear. You may be postponing writing until your ideas are absolutely, 100% perfect. Perhaps the cause relates to the fear of others criticizing your work; maybe you suffer from excessive self-criticism. Or, for the time being, you are out of words.

Here are some methods to help get unstuck:

- Brainstorm the main idea. Forget your careful outline for a while. Write down lots of new ideas about your topic. Do this as rapidly as you can. That is why they call it "brain-*storm*." Expand a few of them. Can you think of cases to use as examples?

- Revisit the outline. Go to each main heading and write down what you mean to present in each section. Expand the outline to include some phrases you will use in the actual writing.

- Review your notes. Add new ideas, maybe short paragraphs, as they occur to you. Add examples and quotes.

- Leapfrog. Stop trying to write sequentially. Jump around in your draft to the section that interests you next. Fill in the gaps later.

- Change your writing method for a while. Leave your computer and use pen and paper.

- Reread what you have done so far. As you look over what you have written, maybe new ideas will come to you.

- Change your writing time. We are almost all either morning or evening people—larks or owls—and probably write during our best time. If stuck, try writing during your "off time." That is, if you are a morning person, try writing in the evening for a while.

- Prepare a lecture. Imagine that you must present your paper to colleagues tomorrow morning. How would you organize and present the information?

- Talk to a colleague. Discussing your project with an insightful coworker can help bring out the ideas hiding just below the surface.
- Rewrite. If desperate, try restating a key section of what you have already written.
- Rest your mind. If all else fails, try delaying tactics that actually rest your mind. Take a walk, listen to classical music, watch football on television, or meditate.

Eventually you will get unstuck, and you will finish the first draft. Next comes the less creative, more tedious, but very essential task—revision.

The Middle: Revising Your Work

When I begin revising a work, I think of the words of Irish poet Oscar Wilde (1854–1900): "I was working on the proof of one of my poems all the morning, and took out a comma. In the afternoon I put it back again." If only we medical writers had the time to make such leisurely revisions. But happily, unlike writing the first draft, revisions can be made in discontinuous bits of time. That is, revising a manuscript is tuning, not creating. You can stop and start without causing damage. Yes, that is the good news.

On the other hand, revision, editing your own work, may seem like extracting your own impacted molar. It must be done, but it can be painful. The analogy of this editing and tooth extraction is appropriate because of the origins of the word *edit*. This word comes from Latin words *dare*, meaning "to give" and *e*, meaning "out." In Latin, these root words gave *editus*, meaning "to put out" [6]. Thus, the editing function is chiefly one of "putting out," and this is especially true of revising (editing your own work).

There is, however, one major difference between revising (removing your own molar) and editing (having the procedure performed by someone who probably has more skill than you). Lester King, an experienced editor, describes this difference very well: "If, when engaged in editing, you feel that major changes are in order, you cannot be sure that any alterations you propose will express what the author wanted to say. You may be distorting his meaning. In revision, however, you are in control at all times. You have complete freedom to make all the changes you want" [7].

There are probably as many ways of revising as there are writers. With that said, I wish to consider some principles. The first principle is the number of revisions. The astute reader has noted that the previous section of the chapter was titled "Beginning: The First Draft." An article should undergo at least three preliminary drafts before the final version. In performing the three pre-final drafts, you may choose to follow this pattern:

- *First revision*: In the first look at your creative first draft, look at the "wholeness" of the paper. At this stage, try not to be too focused on small spelling and grammatical misdemeanors. Instead, verify that your structure is sound and that what you say is really appropriate for your intended audience and the target journal (or the edited book, if writing a book chapter). It is okay to fix the level of a heading or two, but the emphasis must be on reviewing the organization, logic, and validity of what you have written. Does it all hang together? Have you said what you wanted to say?

- *Second revision*: The second time through the manuscript is when you verify. Look for errors in spelling, grammar, and syntax. Check carefully for factual errors. Be sure to run your Microsoft (MS) Word spelling and grammar checker, but do not rely on it to pick up every spelling error, especially when it comes to small, common words such as "one" and "on." If a sentence or paragraph is in the wrong location, now is the time to move it. If a heading is needed, insert it now. If you find superfluous phrases or wordy constructions, eliminate them.

- *Third revision*: By now you have checked for any major problems and repaired minor errors. Before undertaking the next revision, it is a good idea to put the paper away for a week or two. This cooling-off period will "disconnect" you from the writing, and when you read the paper again, you will often wonder: How could I have ever written this sentence?

In the third revision, you vigorously polish your work to make it shine. The emphasis here is on clarity and style. You will simplify words, seek the best way to express your thoughts, and eliminate unnecessary verbiage. You will also be looking for danger signs: inappropriate stance, favored but inappropriate phrases, and cuteness.

Style and Clarity

When we see a natural style, we are always astonished and delighted, for we expected to see an author, and we find a man. [Or a woman–RBT]

— French philosopher Blaise Pascal, *Pensées*, 1669

Style, in writing, describes the way ideas are expressed. It has to do with word selection, how the words are arranged into sentences, and how the sentences are linked together to create paragraphs. Whether or not quotes and borrowed material are used is an element of style. Style includes the use or absence of humor, playfulness, and even one's self in the writing. Style represents the fingerprints of the author. As an editor of multi-author reference books, I have received some chapter manuscripts created by two or three authors. If one author wrote the first half and author number two the second, I can tell when authorship changes within the chapter, even if the manuscript has the same font throughout. The shift in authorship is clear because the style abruptly changes.

Scott A. Norton states, "Remember that a straightforward and unadorned writing style has its own elegance" [8]. We should all strive for the style Norton describes, clear exposition of ideas, written in the smallest words, and cleanest sentences possible. If such writing seems a little bland, it can be flavored with some variety in word choice, alternatively constructed sentences and a few carefully selected quotations.

Clarity in writing refers to the simple, direct expression of ideas. In medical writing, clarity is often the victim of completeness. How often do we read convoluted sentences with abundant phrases strung together just so that everything is included before getting to the terminal period? Such convolution is most often seen in the results section of the abstract but can occur anywhere in a medical article. Just to illustrate what I mean, here is a sentence that is complete but is less than crystal clear:

> As they begin to study medicine, and especially the pathogenesis and early manifestations of disease, medical students are likely to be taught by lecturers that use the same notes from year to year, prompting complaints that the teaching is not responsive to advances in clinical practice, but on the other hand, delighting the students who can purchase typed notes from members of previous classes, feeling secure in the knowledge that the lecture content has not changed, and allowing them to skip classes, while studying for examinations from notes that might otherwise not be considered outdated if only the professor updated the content a little each year, a task unlikely to be seen as a high priority by a professor whose chief interest, and whose main source of salary support, is bench research.

Whew! It is okay to breathe now. My trusty MS Word spelling and grammar checker did not highlight this sentence as being too long.

Weighty Words and Sentences

Good style calls for careful word selection. During revision, you should seek all the heavyweight words in your article and, whenever possible, replace them with those that are shorter and perhaps less "Latinized." Doing so will make your article easier to read (style) and understand (clarity). Oliver Wendell Holmes (1809–1894), writing more than a century ago, remarked: "I know there are professors in this country who 'ligate' arteries. Other surgeons only tie them, and it stops the bleeding just as well" [9]. Table 3.2 lists some weighty words and good choices to replace them.

Alternative Ways to Express Your Thoughts

Experienced writers have a bank of alternative words and constructions to express their ideas. The beginning writer does also but in a different way. For the experienced author, the reservoir is in his or her head, deposited there by years of

TABLE 3.2 Selected heavyweight words and suggested replacements

Heavyweight word	Good choice as a replacement
Initiate	Start, begin
Terminate	Stop, end
Sufficient	Enough
Perform	Do
Ultimate	Last
Transpire	Happen
Individual	Person
Institution	Hospital
Predominate	Chief
Etiology	Cause
Numerous	Many
Diminutive	Small

experience. For the neophyte, the reservoir is the thesaurus, whether a printed book or as part of the MS Word program. I will first discuss alternative forms of expression and then the use and misuse of the thesaurus.

In the last paragraph, I wrote of the "beginning writer" in the second sentence and then referred to this person again in the fourth sentence. Here I used the word *neophyte* to avoid using the term *beginning writer* again. In sentences one and two, I used the word *writer*, and in sentence three, *author* was substituted. These are alternative words.

In the paragraph just above are two alternative constructions. Can you find them?

In the first sentence "wrote of" in the first part of the sentence became "referred to" in the second part. In the third sentence the active tense "I used the word" alternates with the passive "was substituted."

I must speak sternly about use and abuse of the thesaurus, the best-known version being the work of physician Peter Mark Roget, first published in 1852. Properly used, the thesaurus is an excellent source of synonyms and can give a list of alternative words when you find you have used favorite words repeatedly. For example, my MS Word thesaurus yielded the following alternatives to the word *word*:

Utterance
Sound
Statement
Expression
Speech
Remark
Declaration

Changing the search to the plural form *words* gave a very different list:

Language
Vocabulary
Terms
Expressions
Terminology
Lexis

After reviewing the lists for alternatives to *word* and *words*, I might select *statement* or *expression* from the first list and *terms* from the second list. I probably would not use *utterance*, which seems to connote verbal, not written, expression. Nor would I choose to use *lexis*, which denotes the total stock of words in a language.

On the other hand, it is possible to misuse the thesaurus. By consulting the thesaurus for synonyms for only three words, this simple sentence,

The patient had a dull pain in the low back.

might become

The patient had an uninteresting hurting in the low rear.

The opportunities for malapropisms are endless, especially when one tries to use the thesaurus to create an air of erudition. I call the act of consulting a thesaurus to find a complex word to replace a short one "thesaurus abuse." This is my term, and you read it here first. I hope that no reader of this book engages in this nefarious practice and that you resolve today to use the thesaurus only to seek the best word and appropriate alternative ways to express your ideas.

Removing Stuff

If you are like me, your first draft is chock full of stuff, bursting like an overfilled Christmas stocking. The stuff—items typed because you wisely did not stop your creative journey to ponder best words and ideal sentence structure—needs to be debrided during revision. Remember from above that much of self-editing is "taking out" stuff.

A favorite principle for writing and thinking is called *Occam's razor*. William of Occam was an English philosopher and theologian who lived in the fourteenth century and held the enviable title of Doctor Invincibilis and Venerabilis. The Occam's razor principle arose with his statement, "Entities [he was referring to assumptions used to explain things] should not be multiplied beyond what is needed" [10]. According to this dictum, you should "shave off" anything superfluous to the core message. Say only what is needed and no more. That applies to unnecessary words, paragraphs, and even sections of an article.

Removing Words

Good candidates for removal are instances of "doubling." This occurs when you use two words with virtually identical meaning to express the same thought:

This is my *last* and *final* offer.

She had a *life-threatening* and *potentially fatal* disease.

The physician was *concerned* and *worried* about the patient's progress.

Other words begging to be removed are redundant phrases. Consider how the following awkward sentence can be simplified:

The patient was admitted to the hospital for the specific, express purpose of ruling out the admittedly somewhat remote possibility that he might have pancreatic cancer.

Sometimes the words to be removed are vacuous adjectives and adverbs, such as the intensifiers *very* or *really*. American writer Mark Twain (1835–1910) is often credited with this simple solution: "Substitute *damn* every time you're inclined to write *very*; your editor will delete it and the writing will be just as it should be."

Removing Paragraphs and Sections of the Article

Sometimes you must remove entire paragraphs and sections, or perhaps move one to another location. The removal process is usually prompted by one of two events: First, you realize that the paragraph is inappropriate, irrelevant to the core message, or perhaps illogical, silly, or contradictory to something appearing elsewhere in the paper. In such instances, removal is needed. In the second instance, the journal editor mandates that your 20-page paper be shortened to 10 pages. In such instances, you are unlikely to find that half your words can be eliminated by fine-tuning sentences one by one. In such a case, major surgery is required, and you will probably need to jettison one or more parts of the article.

Danger Signs

In revising your drafts, be alert for danger signs: red-flag phrases, the statement that warms your heart, and cuteness.

Red-Flag Phrases

We all recognize a red flag as a sign of danger. Possible trouble lies ahead. A red-flag phrase is what I call a cluster of words that should warn you, during revision, that you risk getting into trouble. You may be about to write something that will undermine the credibility of your article or invite criticism by experts in the field. You may even be exposing that you could have dug more deeply during your research

Table 3.3 Red-flag phrases

Red-flag phrase	Tongue-in-cheek translation
There are no prior published studies on the topic of…	Actually, I didn't spend much time searching the literature
Authorities agree that…	We discussed this over coffee
It is well known that…	I think I am right about this
One can reasonably assume that…	I really hope that what I am about to say is true
It is interesting to note that…	At least I think it is interesting
The data clearly show that…	I don't have any numbers, but my intuition makes me believe that what I am about to write is correct
It is evident that…	Ditto above, and my statistics are shaky
In other words…	I am about to repeat myself
Based on the results presented, all practicing clinicians should…	It must be done this way! (Trial attorneys love this language)
Further studies are required to further investigate…	I need another research grant

phase or spent more time analyzing data. Or your red-flag phrase may simply annoy your educated reader. Table 3.3 lists my favorite red-flag phrases.

The Statement That Warms Your Heart

Sometimes you will find a wonderful thought, and you just must get it in. You may believe that you have found the interesting odd fact during your research, and even though it is superfluous to your hypothesis, you really want to include it somewhere in your report. This is generally a signal that you should take it out.

Someday you may even be tempted to include a phrase that, to those in the know, is a subtle personal attack on a rival. Such thoughts should never make it as far as your computer screen.

Other candidates are the instances of alliteration as discussed in Chap. 2, which sound so good in your head, and read so poorly. Also consider eliminating the tendency to "name something." As I type this, I am considering taking out the term "thesaurus abuse" above, but I decided that the invented expression has value. I hope this turns out to be a good decision.

Cuteness

I began Chap. 1 by asserting that being a good clinician or academician does not make one a capable writer. It also does not make one humorous. Most of us are not actually as funny as we think, and writing humor is especially difficult because we are not blessed with the inflections and timing that help make stories funny. Thus when you and I attempt humor, we often become "cute." Cuteness in a medical article is terrible.

"You can observe a lot by just watching." One way beginning writers introduce cuteness is by using a popular quotation—this Yogi Berra expression, for example, or a passage from the Peanuts comic strip. Sometimes using such quotations enhances your writing, especially when an Oslerian aphorism or a passage from Shakespeare is woven as a colorful thread into the fabric of the prose. Sometimes.

Of course, some levity can make reading more enjoyable. In Table 3.3 I created fanciful translations of the worrisome phrases. Did these attempts at wit work for you or not? If not, please consider them to be planned examples of what not to do.

The Colleague as a Critical Reader

When you have finished at least three revisions and are almost ready to prepare the final draft, it is time to pass the manuscript to a colleague for critical review. The process is sometimes called "informal refereeing." If your critical reader does the job you expect, you will learn at least some of the weaknesses in your paper and be able to correct them before submission to your target journal. Believe an experienced writer when I say that it is much better to find the manuscript's flaws before it leaves my office than to have the errors discovered by the journal's peer reviewers and thereby trigger rejection by the very journal that I most wanted to publish the paper.

What are the characteristics of the critical reader? This colleague must understand the science involved and know the principles of good writing. More important, the critical reader must not be intimidated or overly impressed with your writing skills. Reading the article and reporting that it is flawless has wasted everyone's time. There is always something that can be improved. You need someone who is tough, honest, and not afraid to use the red pen liberally. Among medical writers, this has been called "benign brutality." Of course, there is the understanding that, when your critical reader is writing an article sometime in the future, you will provide a reciprocal reading.

Must the critical reader be a clinician in your same specialty? No. In fact you may just want to send your manuscript to two types of readers: One would be the local expert in your field, who will point out your errors of commission and omission. The other may be the naïve reader, someone not an expert in your field. The naïve reader will be able to let you know if your article is intelligible, has too little or too much detail, and leaves too many questions unanswered. Your invited naïve reader may be someone who knows a little about your field of medicine, but not too much. I, a family physician, have served as critical reader for a gynecologic oncologist who was an international medical graduate and whose English language skills lacked some of the subtleties needed for precise written prose. A totally nonmedical person may also review the article, looking for clear English and logical development of the message. For decades, my best critical reader has been my wife, a non-physician medical educator who is a successful author in her own right.

Instructions for the critical reader are important. You are not asking for redaction—the process of word-by-word, sentence-by-sentence editing. And you do not merely wish for general comments. Being told, "This is just simply a wonderful article," is no help at all. Here are some specific questions for the critical reader:

- Can you state in one sentence what the article is trying to say?
- Is what I am saying medically (or scientifically) sound?
- Are there any errors of fact?
- Should the structure be changed in some way?
- Is my prose clear?
- How can the article be improved?

Getting Finished: The Final Draft

All writing can be criticized as too broad or narrow, too elementary or complex, and too long or too short. At only 266 words, the Gettysburg address was criticized in its day. No paper can be perfect because writers, readers, and reviewers have different ideas about content, structure, style, and occasionally even spelling (think orthopedic vs. orthopaedic).

Certainly, each of us should aim for excellence and should revise as needed—within limits. It is interesting to note that Ernest Hemingway revised the last page of *A Farewell to Arms* 39 times [11]. Rachel Carson, author of *The Sea Around Us* (1951) and *Silent Spring* (1962), said that writing is "largely a matter of application and hard work, of writing and rewriting endlessly until you are satisfied that you have said what you want to say as clearly and simply as possible." She states that for her that means "many, many revisions" [12].

On the other hand, you must eventually finish, as did Hemingway and Carson. In the quest for the final draft, do not let the perfect become the enemy of the good. There will come a time when you must say, "This is as good as I can make it."

TABLE 3.4 Excuses that have been offered for late or missing manuscripts

---

Illness or injury: A wide variety of maladies was reported in authors and their families. These included nervous breakdown, depression, cancer, auto accidents, and more

Divorce: "My wife has left me, my life has fallen apart, and I don't know what I am going to do. But I am sure I will not get the book chapter done"

Technical problems: "I was almost done and then my computer crashed, and I had not backed up the file"

An act of God: "We had a fire in our house and the manuscript burned"

Blame the other guy: "My coauthor hasn't completed his half of the manuscript yet"

Job change, especially when it was involuntary: "Dr. Smith doesn't work here anymore, and I don't know where she might be"

I have to pay the light bill: "Sorry, but I am way behind on writing grants, which I need to support my salary"

A report from the administrative assistant: "Dr. Jones is away at a conference again. I don't know anything about a manuscript"

Academy Award excuse: "The manuscript was washed away by a flood"

My favorite: "You weren't really serious about a deadline, were you?"

Completing a manuscript and letting it go is not easy for some. As a veteran editor of more than a dozen multi-author, compiled reference books, I have heard a lot of excuses for late manuscripts. Some that I have actually received are presented in Table 3.4.

There are some ways to help you finish the job. One is to establish a deadline: I will definitely finish the article and get it mailed before the end of the month. Then stick to this deadline, even if you must work evenings and weekends. Another method to reach closure is to establish a reward goal: When I finish and mail the manuscript, I will take a long weekend and go to the beach. As for me, I have a nice trip planned for just after I submit the manuscript for this third edition of the book.

References

1. Fowler LS, Hayes JR. Problem-solving strategies and the writing process. Coll Engl. 1977;39(4):449–61.

2. Taylor RB. The joys of outlining. Med Writing. 2012;21(3):1.

3. Taylor RB. Medical writing: a guide for clinicians, educators, and researchers. 3rd ed. New York: Springer; 2017. p. 125.

4. Jordan EP, Shepard WC. Rx for medical writing. Philadelphia: WB Saunders; 1952. p. 7.

5. Fowler G. Quoted in: Roberts SK. Taking a technological path to poetry prewriting. Reading Teacher. 2002;55(7):678.

6. Partridge E. Origins: a short etymological dictionary of modern English. New York: Macmillan; 1966. p. 177.

7. King LS. Why not say it clearly? A guide to scientific writing. Boston: Little, Brown; 1978. p. 97.

8. Norton SA. Read this but skip that. J Am Acad Dermatol. 2001;44(4):714–5.

9. Holmes OW. Quoted in: Strauss MB. Familiar medical quotations. Boston: Little, Brown; 1968. p. 609.

10. Benet WR. Reader's encyclopedia. 3rd ed. New York: Harper & Row; 1987. p. 706.

11. Plimpton G. Writers at work. New York: Viking Press; 1963. p. 124.

12. Brooks P. The house of life: Rachel Carson at work. Boston. Mifflin: Houghton; 1972. p. 1.

Chapter 4
Technical Issues in Medical Writing

Increasing organization in the field of medicine, as in every other field of human endeavor, has raised the level of contributions to medical literature. Far too often, however, physicians still prepare their contributions with a striving and agony and delay comparable to the delivery of human progeny by one untutored in the refinements of obstetrics.

—American physician and author Morris Fishbein (1889–1976) [1]

Some of the "striving and agony and delay" described by Fishbein can be related to the technical aspects of medical writing, including the preparation of tables and figures (aka illustrations), perseverating over borrowed materials and copyright issues, and corralling herds of reference citations. In contrast to the past three chapters, which have covered the concept and prose aspects of medical writing, this chapter addresses some nuts-and-bolts issues you will face. Do not, however, think that constructing tables and figures is any less creative than composing words and sentences; in fact, developing these supplements to the text may be the most innovative part of writing your article. Other practical issues—such as copyright, permissions, and reference citations—may become important as you seek publication of your work.

© Springer International Publishing AG 2018
R.B. Taylor, *Medical Writing*,
https://doi.org/10.1007/978-3-319-70126-4_4

Tables

Tables are lists of words and numbers; they do not contain artwork. If what you are presenting includes a drawing, photograph, or diagonal lines that connect data (such as an algorithm), it is a figure (see figures, below). Tables offer the following advantages:

- Presenting data: A table is usually the best way to arrange data sets or lists, especially long lists.
- Combining words and numbers: Tables allow the clean presentation of groups of words and numerical data.
- Avoiding unintelligible complex sentences: A table is usually better than a long string of items in a 75-word sentence.
- Breaking up the flow of text: Tables allow some variety in the appearance of your article by introducing something other than page after page of long paragraphs.

There are two types of tables—the so-called text table and the more formal table. The four-item list in the last paragraph (about the advantages of tables) is a text table. It fits nicely into the flow of prose, and it introduces some variety into how information is presented. Text tables should be logical groupings and must be relatively short. They need to be "introduced" in the text but do not require separate legends. Because they are integrated into the flow of the paragraph, generally no citations in the text are needed.

Formal tables are separated from the written paragraphs and are cited in the text. Table 4.1, which lists the characteristics of a good table, is an example of a formal table. And I just cited it in the text.

About Tables

In many articles, the table is the key feature you want to present. For example, if you wished to describe the presenting symptoms and signs of meningococcal infection, a table

TABLE 4.1 Characteristics of a good table

Characteristic	What I mean to say is...
Not too long or wide	The ideal table fits on a single journal or book page. Tables that run over to a second or even third printed page are difficult to fit into the publication and for the reader to follow
Clearly written title	The title should make sense without referring back to the text
Not too much text	If you are inserting long paragraphs into a table, maybe the information should be in the text and you don't need a table at all
Not too many columns	Probably the ideal table has three to five columns. More than five columns may be needed but sometimes at the expense of easy reading
Not too many abbreviations	Excessive use of abbreviations can compromise readability; this is especially true in a table
Not too many footnotes	As a reader, I don't like jumping from table to footnotes and back

would be an economical way to do so. In this instance, I would construct the table before beginning to write the prose.

Do not use too many tables in your article, because this may cause difficulty in page layout. I recently reviewed an article with nine manuscript pages and ten tables. I advised the author to find a way to do without at least half the tables.

Every table must have a title (caption) that describes its content, and the table with its title should be able to stand alone. Here is what I mean: A lecturer speaking on your topic, such as childhood infections or backache, should be able to transpose your table directly into a PowerPoint slide and have it make sense. Thus, all abbreviations used must be explained in the table, either in a footnote or in the table itself.

Tables should not duplicate what is written in the text. Choose one site to present your information—such as the characteristics of a good table (above)—but don't repeat what you want to say in both text and table.

When it comes to borrowing items from existing publications, tables are like artwork. If you wish to borrow someone else's table for use in your article, even a short list from a PowerPoint presentation, you need written permission. You also need permission if you "adapt" a published table, or even an unpublished table that a colleague has created, perhaps for a lecture presentation. For these reasons, I advise authors to create their own tables whenever possible. In this book, there are no borrowed tables.

In editing book chapters, I find that tables are especially prone to errors during production. One reason that tables are error magnets lies in the difficulty of constructing a table and communicating this through the editing and production process. Columns especially tend to become jumbled. I have found many errors introduced at the hands of copy editors who, understandably, do not know the medical meaning of what is in the table. Then things continue during proofreading. When reading proofs, we authors seem to focus on the prose and glance carelessly at the tables, allowing errors to slip through. The more complex and data laden the table, the more the author seems reluctant to proofread it carefully.

Here, in another text table, are some technical tipson constructing tables for medical articles:

- Be sure that it is clear at first glance what your table is intended to tell.
- Keep your column headings concise.
- Include units of measurement in table headings.
- Strive for readability. The stub, a term describing heading and line captions that are listed at the left side of a table, describes each row of items in the field. The column to the right of the stub is often used to present normal values, for the benefit of the reader who might not be familiar with the range of data being presented.
- Do your best to use round numbers or at least numbers that are not too long. Tables are generally not the place to list numbers to the fourth decimal place.
- Align decimal points vertically.
- Be consistent in your tables, using similar titles and headings throughout your article or chapter.

What Journal Editors Want

The *Journal of the American Medical Association* (JAMA) instructs authors to use the Table menu (e.g., under the "Insert" tab in Microsoft Word) in the software program used to prepare the table [2]. The publisher of this book, Springer, likewise instructs authors, and all of the tables in this book were created in this manner. Each table must have a legend (caption), and each column must have a short heading. If the table is borrowed, the source should be identified in the table footnote according to the style of the journal. Tables must be numbered in the order in which they are cited in the text. Instructions for preparing tables can differ from one journal to the next, and the International Committee of Medical Journal Editors (ICMJE) advises preparing tables according to the specific journal's requirements [3].

Footnotes in Tables

Sometimes a footnote is needed, perhaps to explain the presence of an empty cell or to tell why your percentage numbers add up to 100.8%. If you must use footnotes, consult the journal's instructions for authors to find the journal's preferred footnote symbols (*, †, ‡, §, ||, ¶, **, ††, ‡‡, §§, ||||, ¶¶, etc.) and required sequence [3].

Submitting Tables

Like most journals today, JAMA requests that authors include the tables at the end of the text document for electronic submissions. These instructions also require that you do not embed tables as images in the manuscript file or upload tables in image formats [2].

Sometimes, in a large clinical trial, there are backup data too extensive to be included in the print version of the paper but which may be included in the electronic version of the journal and deposited in an archive accessible to readers.

Figures

For medical authors, figures are an integral part of writing. Some classic and popular writers include illustrations in their work, but for the most part, writers such as Sir Arthur Conan Doyle, Jane Austen, and James Baldwin were not concerned with figures. Nor are Stephen King and Zadie Smith. One interesting exception was Lewis Carroll, who illustrated the original version of *Through the Looking Glass* with figures that he drew himself. The medical historians among us may be interested to know that Carroll was a migraineur, and some have speculated that his line drawings represented visual distortions experienced during his migraine auras, a phenomenon called metamorphopsia. Science writers, however, going back to Galileo and Copernicus and beyond, rely on figures to communicate their ideas to their contemporaries and later generations alike.

Figures contain art and look more or less like a picture. This is a broad definition because figures include photographs and shaded drawings, line drawings, graphs, and algorithms. I prefer the term *figures* to *illustrations* because all are cited in the text using the word *Figure*, as shown below when I cite the figures in this chapter. Including figures enhances most medical review articles, research reports, and book chapters.

About Figures

One or more carefully selected and meticulously constructed figures can turn an average article into a great one. Some articles you decide to write will be clearly deficient without a figure or two. For example, let's imagine that over the past year I have encountered three instances of sixth cranial nerve paralysis presenting as the initial manifestation of a pituitary tumor, and I wish to report these cases. Such a case report will be greatly enhanced by the addition of magnetic resonance images and perhaps by a photograph of one of the patients.

One illustration may be just right and two or three too many. The reader needs to see only one photo of a patient with ocular esotropia. Presenting illustrations showing the identical physical finding in two more patients adds nothing.

As with tables, each figure must have a descriptive legend (caption) that allows the illustration to make sense on its own. Many published illustrations will be used directly by lecturers in slide presentations.

Displaying photographs or even drawings in which the person is recognizable presents special issues. Subjects must not be identifiable, or their pictures must be accompanied by written permission for use. A parent or guardian's signature will be required for a child. Some journals provide model permission forms for patients or their "agents" to sign.

Here are some technical tips on constructing figures for medical articles:

- Assure that the reader can easily discern what the figure is all about without referring back to the text.
- Identify each figure by Arabic number with a corresponding citation in the text.
- Create and submit the figure legend (caption) separately from the figure itself.
- Describe all digital modifications or enhancements of photographic images.
- Indicate any magnification in photographs by using a scale bar within the figure.
- Do not use faint lines in drawings.
- Use consistent lettering throughout your figures.

Types of Figures

Photographic Images

Photographic images submitted to biomedical journals must be of high quality, with good resolution. Halftone art, defined as photographs, drawings, or paintings with fine shading, should have a minimum resolution of 300 dots per inch (dpi).

According to the Instructions for Authors of the *Journal of Neurology*, which I have chosen as a representative specialty-oriented clinical journal, all figures should be supplied electronically [4]. JAMA Instructions for Authors states, "Images created digitally (by digital camera or electronically created illustrations) must meet the minimum resolution requirements at the time of creation. Electronically increasing the resolution of an image after creation causes a breakdown of detail and will result in an unacceptable poor-quality image" [2].

For color art, you should consult the journal as to specific requirements such as color prints, positive transparencies, or color negatives. Also determine if there will be a cost to you to include color images. The *Journal of Neurology* states that color figures are published at no cost to the author. In some cases, the print version of your paper may present black and white images, with color images used online. Some colors look alike when converted to halftones, so in such an instance you must check to see if your color image converts clearly to black and white. You can get a good idea how the conversion will look by simply using your office photocopy machine to print a black and white copy of the color image.

According to the NEJM Instructions for Authors, "Acceptable formats for pictures, photos, and figures are PDF, DOC, PPT, JPG, GIF, TIF" [5].

X-rays, which are actually photographic images, often lack good contrast, a problem that is magnified if the image must be enlarged. Figure 4.1 combines a good-quality photograph and an X-ray that clearly shows the fracture.

Line Drawings

Sometimes line drawings, defined as black and white art with no shadings, can illustrate what you want to show better than a photograph. This is especially true in illustrating body anatomy. These drawings can sometimes be done by you and used directly in the article or book. Figure 4.2 is an illustration of a line drawing done by the chapter author and included in a clinical reference book. In other instances you

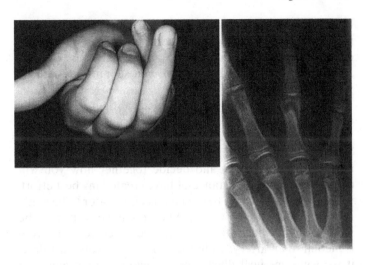

FIG. 4.1 High-quality halftones with good contrast showing the consequences of a fracture (from Taylor [6], with permission)

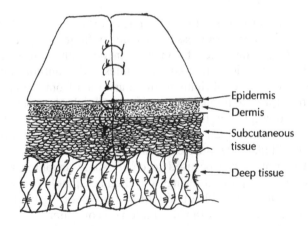

FIG. 4.2 An illustration hand-drawn by the author to illustrate a laceration repair (from Taylor [6], with permission)

may draw a rough draft, which is then converted into the final artwork by a professional artist. For example, the *New England Journal of Medicine* (NEJM) states: "Medical and scientific illustrations will be created or redrawn in-house.

If an outside illustrator has created a figure, the Journal reserves the right to modify or redraw it to meet our specifications" [5]. Most journals, however, lack the resources of JAMA and NEJM, and the figure you submit may well be what ends up in print.

Today it is customary to have medical figures, especially drawings, prepared by a professional medical illustrator. Working with a medical illustrator can be an art in itself. When your illustration involves a professional, it is ideal to make personal contact and decide together how you will collaborate. In most instances, I have created my best effort, with labels, and given it to the medical illustrator to be made into professional-quality art. When doing so, you must be sure that your illustration is anatomically correct. If a vein is medial to an artery (as in the groin), then you must draw it so. Some medical illustrators know more anatomy than the average medical student; some do not. What is certain, however, is that it is expensive to alter completed line drawings.

When a professional medical illustrator creates art, there are special permission issues, including future use of the work. In the instance of "outside" medical illustrators, the NEJM Instructions for Authors states: "The author must explicitly acquire all rights to the illustration from the artist in order for us to publish the illustration" [5]. In the terminology of copyright law, this means that the author must pay for *exclusive* rather than *non-exclusive* use of the illustration, which will likely be more expensive.

A computer can be used to create some uncomplicated drawings. Computer drawings are often acceptable provided they are of comparable quality to line drawings. Figure 4.3 is an example of a line drawing created on computer.

Sometimes very simple drawings can be added to your electronic manuscript using a conventional office scanner, set at a minimum of 600 dpi (dots per inch). Drawings in shades of gray need 1200 dpi or greater, which may not be available on your office scanner.

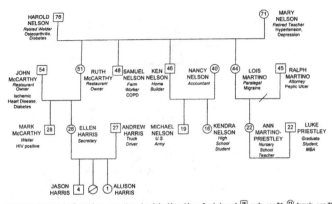

Nelson family genogram: family members, occupations, chronic health problems. Symbols used: [76], male, age 76; (71), female, age 71; □—○, marriage; □—⁄—○, divorce; ∅, deceased.

FIG. 4.3 A line drawing created on computer showing a family genogram (from Taylor [6], with permission)

Graphs

There are four basic types of graphs: line graphs, bar charts, pie charts, and complex graphs. Line graphs are often the best choice when showing what happens over time (Fig. 4.4). A bar chart can also show trends over time, or it can be used to compare relative amounts such as the incomes or work hours of various medical specialties. You may choose a pie chart to show proportions such as how many of your clinic's patients have private insurance, Medicare, Medicaid, or no insurance at all. The JAMA Instructions for Authors, however, states: "Do not use pie charts, 3-D graphs, and stacked bar charts as these are not appropriate for accurate statistical presentation of data and should be revised to another figure type or converted to a table" [2].

Computers have made graph creation quite easy. Several software options are available and can sometimes be as simple as using the Chart Wizard feature on your computer's Microsoft Excel program. I found a good tutorial at http://www.internet4classrooms.com/excel_create_chart.htm [7].

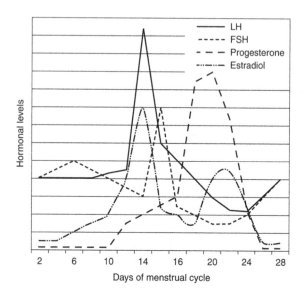

F ${}$ IG. 4.4 A line graph that illustrates hormone changes through the menstrual cycle (from Taylor [6], with permission)

Keep in mind that various publications have different requirements for graphs and charts.

Algorithms

Algorithms are combinations of graph and table. The word *algorithm* comes from the name of a ninth-century Persian mathematician and astronomer, al-Khwarizmi, whose writings also gave us the decimal-based number system we use today. The algorithm is an excellent way to show a decision tree, as shown in Fig. 4.5. I like to use an algorithm to illustrate specific steps in clinical reasoning: If the patient has this symptom, do this and not that. If there is this physical sign, obtain this laboratory test, but that one is not needed.

On the negative side, I find algorithms a little difficult to construct both clinically and technically. On the medical side,

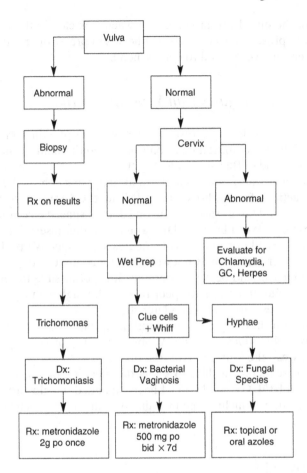

Fig. 4.5 An algorithm that illustrates a decision tree for vaginitis symptoms (from Taylor [6], with permission)

decisions often depend on more than one variable, and the algorithm may not allow presentation of all the possible influences on a diagnostic or therapeutic decision. Technically, algorithms generally call for diagonal lines or even lines that bend around boxes; I find these difficult to create on a computer, and errors can occur in production.

In the end, I use an algorithm when it is clearly the best way to present a decision tree. Otherwise I prefer figures that are easier to draw and to comprehend.

Submitting Figures with Your Manuscript

Your figures, like the rest of your manuscript, will almost certainly be submitted electronically, a requirement of most journals today. Be sure to identify the graphics program used to create the graphs, charts, and diagrams. The NEJM Instructions for Authors states: "All text, references, figure legends, and tables should be in one double-spaced electronic document (Word Doc or PDF). You may either insert figures in the text file or upload your figures separately. We prefer the former, but this may not work well for complicated graphics, which should be sent separately. It is permissible to send low-resolution images for peer review, although we may ask for high-resolution files at a later stage" [5].

If you have questions about adapting your favorite PowerPoint slides or using Adobe Illustrator or other programs, call the journal's editorial office.

For readers who like to know the meaning of acronyms such as DOI, GIF, and RPG, I have expanded the glossary of this edition to include the meaning of some arcane technical terms.

Copyright

Do not worry too much about copyright. The law and the ethics of medical publishing protect us quite well. And the protection extends beyond the printed word. If you create a PowerPoint slide, write an unpublished thesis, or even draw a clever diagram, you own the rights to your intellectual product.

Copyright is a form of protection provided by US law to authors of "original works of authorship," including literary, dramatic, musical, artistic, and certain other intellectual works. Section 106 of the 1976 Copyright Act generally gives the owner of copyright the exclusive right to do and to authorize others to do the following:

- Reproduce the work in copies or phonorecords.
- Prepare derivative works based on the work.
- Perform the work publicly in the case of performance art.
- Display the copyrighted work publicly [8].

As broad as copyright protection seems to be, it does not extend to ideas, concepts, principles, systems, or factual information described in the work. Nor is an improvised speech protected by copyright—unless and until you write it down somewhere [8].

The Copyright Act holds that copyright in the work of authorship immediately becomes the property of the author who created the work as soon as it is in some fixed form, such as a book or article [8]. In fact, you hold copyright to your work as soon as the pen leaves the paper, or perhaps even when your fingers leave the keyboard, although ownership of online work may seem a little murky. The Copyright Act states: "Copyright protects 'original works of authorship' that are fixed in a tangible form of expression. The fixation need not be directly perceptible so long as it may be communicated with the aid of a machine or device" [8]. For this reason, we medical writers should afford online creative works the same copyright respect as printed material.

The intellectual property rights of the author are separate from the publication of the work, a fact that the new medical writer discovers shortly after receiving the first "We would like to publish your article" letter. Upon acceptance of an article by a print-based medical journal, you will be asked to sign a "release of copyright," assigning rights to the journal. This often does not hold for open-access journals, described in Chap. 12.

There is one more important exception to the "author holds the copyright" principle: the "work made for hire." This includes a work prepared by an employee within the scope of employment and a work ordered or commissioned, such as an instructional text or a translation. There may or may not be a written agreement that a work is considered a work made for hire [8]. In addition, many books are, by contract between author and publisher, works made for hire.

In fact, with a work made for hire or, for that matter, with any published medical article or book, copyright rarely becomes an issue, even though medical publishers insist that copyright be assigned to them, in writing, as a condition of publishing the work. That means that of all the books and articles I have published, I currently hold the copyrights to only a few of them. The few exceptions are old books that are out of print; the publishers have, as a courtesy, reverted all rights to me, which means that I can exercise those rights as I wish.

In all other instances, the publisher of scientific journals and books holds the copyright. As I type these words, I own the copyright to them; by the time you read this, the publisher, Springer New York, will hold copyright. And the rights to the article I wrote a few months ago are held by the journal that published it.

What is the significance of not holding the copyright to my articles and books? Not much, and it is largely administrative. I can think of two items to mention. One is that I must seek permission for use from Springer Publishers if I wish to use big chunks of text, tables, or figures from my Springer books in writing for any other publisher. The same holds true if I want to reuse a table or figure in one of my articles previously published in various medical journals. Getting such permission involves sending a request (see below), and this has not been a problem. The second time copyright ownership comes to my attention is when other authors request permission to use something published in my books. The publisher now often charges a fee for this permission and shares the revenue with me; on royalty statements I occasionally find a (very small) payment for "permissions granted." Parenthetically, I always wonder what small part of my work someone felt moved to borrow, who borrowed it, and where was it subsequently printed. Although I never find out, I remain grateful to the anonymous person who seemed to value something I created.

Inexperienced authors sometime wonder whether someone will steal their great idea if they submit a proposal to a journal or book publisher. I am happy to report that medical editors have much higher moral standards than most politicians or chief executive officers of large corporations—and they are well-schooled regarding the perils of plagiarism. Also, there really are very few article or book ideas that are revolutionary and worth pilfering. You are quite safe in sending proposals and article ideas.

Borrowed Materials and Permissions

I wrote above that you should not worry excessively about the copyright to your work. In contrast, you should be very concerned about permissions if you intend to borrow words, tables, art, or anything else from previously published work, even your own. In Chap. 5, I discuss plagiarism. Here I discuss the situations in which you need permission to use borrowed material and how to get the documents you need.

Let's first look at what's free: All government publications may be used without seeking permission. For example, in the previous section I listed the rights protected by the 1976 Copyright Act. What appears on the page is taken almost word for word from the US Copyright Office web site. I did not use quotations around the material because I edited out some discussion about sound recording, pantomimes, and choreographic work, which we are unlikely to encounter in medical writing. I did, however, give attribution by citing the web site, because that allows the reader to seek more in-depth information and because it is the ethical thing to do. However, if I had not attributed the words by citing the US Copyright Office as the source, I would have technically been within my legal rights.

Items not protected by copyright include slogans, short phrases, and data that are considered common and authorless property such as standard calendars, height and weight charts, and tape measures and rulers [8]. Also considered fair game are works in the "public domain." This can actually be a confusing area, especially with the estates of long-dead authors still holding rights. I suppose that public domain would include the sonnets of Shakespeare and Elizabeth Barrett Browning, but the dialogues of Plato, which are much older, may not be in the public domain if the translation I am using is still protected by copyright. Recently, when seeking images for my book *White Coat Tales*, I visited the web site of the National Library of Medicine (NLM) [9]. Here I found an image of a bust of Hippocrates, ideal for my purpose. The NLM web site stated: "The National Library of Medicine believes this item to be in the public domain." I felt safe in using this image in my work, with attribution to the source.

When Do I Need to Seek Permission for Use of Borrowed Material?

Part of the answer is easy. You need permission to reproduce any previously published table or figure that is not in the public domain. You also need permission to "adapt" any table or figure. If you use data from four studies to create your own table or figure, I think that the creation is yours and no permission is needed; but you should identify your data sources in the table or figure legend. Some editors may disagree with my opinion about tables or figures based on multiple published studies and will require that you seek permissions from all sources.

The next gray issue is the use of text (phrases, sentences, and paragraphs) from published sources. All borrowed work, even a few words, should be attributed to the source. This may be done in a number of ways, attributed in the text as I did with the Pogo quotation in a previous chapter or cited as a formal reference. This protects you from allegations of theft. You borrowed the words and told where you got them.

What about a few sentences or more? When do you need to seek permission for use? This is a bit of a legal neverland, and the answer is not nearly as clear as with tables and figures. The doctrine involves "fair use," and you will see allusions to needing permission to borrow *lengthy quotations*. What constitutes fair use and how long is a "lengthy quotation?" Section 107 of the Copyright Act lists four factors considered in fair-use issues [10]:

- The purpose of the use, including whether it is for commercial or nonprofit educational use
- The nature of the copyrighted work
- How much of the work is used in relation to the whole copyrighted work
- The possible effect on the potential market and value of the copyrighted work [10]

It is very rare that a legal issue arises when credit is given for reasonable use of borrowed words. Allegations of plagiarism are one thing; legal complaints are quite another and are unlikely when the author has used a quotation with careful attribution to the source. I don't think anyone has provided chiseled-in-stone definitions of *fair use* and *lengthy quotation*, since all legal issues are ultimately settled by trial or negotiated agreement. Court decisions have described fair use of scholarly or technical work as including short passages to illustrate or clarify the author's thoughts and reproduction by a teacher or student of a section a work to facilitate learning. I will go out on a limb and state that you should seek permission if you are quoting more than 100 words, even with attribution.

Obtaining Permission to Use Borrowed Material

Who Must I Contact to Obtain Permission?

I always start with the publisher, and I include in my letter (Fig. 4.6) a question about anyone else that must be contacted. Since publishers almost always hold copyright to published

---

Letterhead

Date:

Dear:

In the forthcoming book, ***Medical Writing: A Guide for Clinicians, Educators, and Researchers***, to be published by Springer-Verlag – New York Publishers, I request permission to reprint the following material:

Author(s):

Book/Journal/Article Title:

Specific Material:

I request your permission to reprint the material specified, with nonexclusive world rights in the forthcoming book and all future editions, translations and revisions, including electronic media. If you agree, please indicate by signing and returning this letter. Full credit will be given to the author and publisher. If you do not control these rights in their entirety, please let me know with whom I should communicate and kindly provide me with an address.

Consideration of this request at your earliest convenience will be greatly appreciated.

Thank you,

Robert B. Taylor, MD

Please return to:

> Robert B. Taylor, MD
> Oregon Health & Science University, Mail Code FM
> 3181 SW Sam Jackson Park Road
> Portland, Oregon 97239-3098

....

We grant the permission requested on the terms stated in this letter

By: ....   Date: ....

FIG. 4.6 Sample permission letter. This letter should be modified by substituting your article or book name, identifying the requested material, and adding your name as the requester. Then print on your own letterhead or submit online

articles and books, their permission for borrowed use should be sufficient. Nevertheless, some permissions editors (yes, such persons exist) insist that you also seek permission from authors; some do not.

Who Is Responsible for Getting Permissions?

The answer is short and direct: You are. The author is responsible for getting acceptable permissions and submitting them with the manuscript. I have reprinted in this book two borrowed illustrations (from the same journal). I sent a request for permission as soon as the book contract was signed, long before I began working on the chapter containing the figures.

There is one very good reason to seek permissions early. The article or book cannot be published until all permissions have been submitted and approved. When you consider the difficulty you may encounter in finding the person or persons who can actually sign your form, it pays to get moving on this task.

One of the surprises in medical writing may be the cost of permissions. A typical fee is $100–300 per table or figure used. In updating Chap. 7 of this book, I sought to use a 12-word short poem published in a specialty journal. The fee to use this three-line work? $100 or $8.33 per word. Be prepared.

The news, however, is not all bad. Many science, technical, and medical (STM) publishers have signed an agreement whereby reasonable amounts of previously published material can be borrowed and used among member publishers without cost as long as the use is properly cited and reported according to the various publishers' protocols. If you are writing for an STM journal or book publisher, check with your editor about whether they participate in this agreement. You can learn more about this initiative at the following web site: http://www.stm-assoc.org/copyright-legal-affairs/permissions/permissions-guidelines/.

How Do I Obtain Permission?

Today, most permissions are requested online. Publishers' web sites can almost always be found in a Google search. You will be asked to describe the material you wish to borrow and where it will be printed. Sometimes this system works smoothly.

In other instances, you may wish to use an old-fashioned request letter. In my experience, no publisher has ever questioned my standard permission request, as shown in Fig. 4.6, although some have qualified their responses and others respond by sending their own form.

My chief problem arises when publishers qualify their permissions. These qualifications include limitations such as: "valid for only one edition of the book"; "not to include electronic media"; or "for English-language publication only." I wish publishers would not do this, especially when they are charging me. But they do. These issues are important—your publisher will require, for example, permission to use the borrowed material in e-books as well as print books—so if you encounter such limits, contact the permissions editor and ask what needs to be done.

One special problem may be medical illustrations created by a professional illustrator. The artist may have contracted with the author and publisher for "one-time" use of the figure you wish to use. In this instance, you will need to track down the artist, an often-difficult quest, and obtain written permission. You will also almost certainly be asked to pay a fee. Here is an example of the exasperation that can occur: A few years ago I sought permission to borrow a brilliant and complex figure that had been previously published in a specialty-oriented medical magazine. The magazine happily offered permission (for a fee), on the condition that I also obtained the artist's permission. Try as I might, I could not locate the artist, and thus my book chapter lacked a helpful illustration.

I hope that all the above has persuaded you to create your own tables and figures whenever possible. It is usually easier than getting (and paying for) permission, and you will have added something new to the medical literature.

Finding Illustrations in the Public Domain

In many instances, it is possible to find high-quality illustrations that are in the public domain—no permissions needed. Many are historic images, such as those depicting the great giants of medicine, such as Edward Jenner, Sigmund Freud, and Sir William Osler. But also available are illustrations that were published by government employees or that are free to use simply because the copyright protection has expired. Others yet are images that the author has placed online for others to use, provided the person who created the figure is credited.

There are several sites where you may find images in the public domain: The web site https://99designs.com/blog/resources/public-domain-image-resources/ lists 30 free public domain image web sites. These include free stock photos, the British Library, and the Public Domain Review. My favorite is Wikimedia Commons [11], "a database of 34,817,187 freely usable media files to which anyone can contribute." I have used this source heavily in several books over the past few years and found it a gold mine of possibilities. A surprising number of these images come from published scientific papers.

There are some caveats with the use of public domain image sources. First of all, many of the historic images lack the crispness of today's photographic images and may be rejected by journal and book editors—or else the images are accepted as "historic" and therefore are a little fuzzy. The other warning is that each image has some sort of description of its conditions for use: Even someone taking a photo of an old statue (e.g., of Hippocrates) in a museum may have attached some sort of qualification for use. So user, beware!

Reference Citations

Virtually all medical writing contains references, and I am happy to report that most follow the model of the ICMJE. In fact, the instructions for JAMA, NEJM, and ICMJE all differ

TABLE 4.2 Examples of the three most common types of references

1. *Article citation*: If six authors or fewer, list all; if seven or more authors, list the first three and then add "et al.": Kaddourah A, Basu RK, Bagshaw SM, Goldstein SL. Epidemiology of acute kidney injury in critically ill children and young adults. N Engl J Med. 2017;376(1):11–20.
2. *Book citation, noting chapter, and authors*: Massart MB. Genetic disorders. In: Paulman P, Taylor RB, editors. Family medicine: principles and practice. 7th ed. New York: Springer; 2017. p. 205–15.
3. *Electronic source*: Journal of the American Medical Association. Instructions for authors. Available at: http://jamanetwork.com/journals/jama/pages/instructions-for-authors#. Accessed 5 Jan 2017.

very slightly, notably in how they choose to cite books as sources. Do not worry about this. The differences are minor, usually regarding punctuation or how to list terminal page numbers. The information needed is virtually the same for all, and if your style is not exactly what the journal uses, the copy editor will make the small changes in periods, commas, and semicolons. In my opinion, this issue will not cause rejection of a good paper. Table 4.2 lists examples of the three most common types of citations. I suggest that you copy this table and tape it to your computer.

Number references in the order that they appear in the text. Do not alphabetize your reference list unless this is the style of your journal. Citation numbers in the text should follow the journal's style, which may be superscript or in parentheses or square brackets. I believe that the way you present your text citations, just like how you punctuate your reference list, is not a deal-breaker. Just be sure all the information is included and is presented clearly and consistently.

Do not "borrow" someone else's list of citations. It is perfectly permissible to use a published list as the basis for your research, just as you would use PubMed to review current research on your topic. But then you must seek out and review the original publications, reading each paper cited carefully to be sure that the source says what you say it does. If you do not do this, someone knowledgeable in the field will surely spot the "cognitive dissonance" and correct you in a letter to the editor.

Here are some more tips regarding the correct use of references:

- Have the right number of references, not too many and not too few.
- Avoid using citations from the so-called gray literature, such as abstracts from scientific congresses, as references.
- Do not cite a "personal communication" as a reference, except in extraordinary circumstances in which vital information is unavailable from a public source.
- If you really must cite a paper known to be accepted but not yet published, you should first obtain written permission of authors to cite their paper. Such articles are then typically designated as "in press." Many such designations are then updated later in proofs.
- Verify all reference citations against an online bibliographic source such as PubMed.

When you are finished with the paper, keep all your copies of reference files you reviewed, permission letters received, and perhaps even brilliant tables and figures that were not just right for the current article. They may be useful in future writing.

Acknowledgment Figures 4.1, 4.2, 4.3, 4.4, and 4.5 are from Taylor RB. Family medicine: principles and practice. 6th ed. New York: Springer; 2003. I am indebted to the contributing authors who created these figures.

References

1. Fishbein M. Introduction. In: Medical writing. 3rd ed. Philadelphia: Blakiston; 1955.
2. Journal of the American Medical Association. Instructions for authors. http://jamanetwork.com/journals/jama/pages/instructions-for-authors#. Accessed 28 Feb 2017.

3. International Committee of Medical Journal Editors. Recommendations for the conduct, reporting, editing, and publication of scholarly work in medical journals. http://icmje.org/recommendations/. Accessed 28 Feb 2017.

4. Journal of Neurology. Instructions to authors. http://www.springer.com/medicine/neurology/journal/415. Accessed 28 Feb 2017.

5. New England Journal of Medicine. Author Center: new manuscripts. http://www.nejm.org/page/author-center/manuscript-submission. Accessed 28 Feb 2017.

6. Taylor RB. Family medicine: principles and practice. 6th ed. New York: Springer; 2003.

7. Internet4Classrooms: Excel-create a chart/graph. http://www.internet4classrooms.com/excel_create_chart.htm. Accessed 28 Feb 2017.

8. U.S. Copyright Office. Copyright basics. https://www.copyright.gov/circs/circ01.pdf. Accessed 4 Mar 2017.

9. National Library of Medicine. Images from the history of medicine. https://collections.nlm.nih.gov/?f%5bdrep2.isMemberOfCollection%5d%5b%5d=DREPIHM. Accessed 28 Feb 2017.

10. United States Copyright Office. Chapter 1: subject matter and scope of copyright. https://www.copyright.gov/title17/92chap1.html. Accessed 28 Feb 2017.

11. Wikimedia Commons Images. https://commons.wikimedia.org/wiki/Category:Images. Accessed 28 Feb 2017.

Chapter 5
What's Special About Medical Writing?

Writing is a historical act. The role of written communication has been to document human history; our knowledge of human culture and values exist because someone has written about it.

American physician and educator John J. Frey [1]

There are written works—such as the *Bible* and the *Quran*, the *United States Declaration of Independence*, and *Quotations From Chairman Mao Tse-Tung*, the latter known to many of us as *The Little Red Book*—that have changed the world. There is also writing that is lost or has not been deciphered yet. We know little about early central African cultures because no one recorded what happened at the time. Our knowledge of Mayan and Inca cultures is deficient because most of their writing was destroyed by zealous Christian conquerors. Native American languages were first written (in contrast to being spoken) in 1921, when a phonetic alphabet of 86 symbols was developed by a Cherokee named Sequoyah; this feat was honored when the redwood tree was named *Sequoia* [2]. It was in 1952 when we began to decipher the written language of ancient Crete [3].

In the sciences, writing records the evolution of ideas, sometimes even the journey from wrongheadedness to wisdom. In the middle ages, influenza was considered to be caused by celestial

© Springer International Publishing AG 2018
R.B. Taylor, *Medical Writing*,
https://doi.org/10.1007/978-3-319-70126-4_5

"influence," although we now know that the cause is a virus. We once treated a variety of illnesses by bleeding the patient; now this therapy is reserved for the management of polycythemia. One of the joys of writing over a lifetime is to read your own past published works, just to see how prescient (or how short-sighted) you were.

Poetry, short stories, mystery novels, historical documents, and other types of writing all have their peculiarities and conventions. Medical writing is, first of all, factual. It is expository. Opinions must be clearly stated as such. Values, when offered, are typically implied, rather than stated. Credibility often rests on evidence cited. The chief virtue is knowledge, especially new knowledge.

In a sense, the peculiarities of medical writing are what make it special: These include the imperative that what is printed is as accurate as current knowledge allows. We strive to state things correctly and precisely. We should avoid jargon, be exact in what we say, and be careful with abbreviations and acronyms. Perhaps I use the "we" pronoun here because, in contrast to our colleagues who write fiction, there is the tendency of medical authors to write as groups. Finally, we medical writers face a minefield of ethical issues that can impair our credibility or worse.

About Medical Journals

Types of Journals

Medical journals are not all alike. Although many journals do not fit into the categorization I am about to use, I think of medical journals in a hierarchy consisting of very broad types. I hope you see the merits of this hierarchy; you will certainly sense its lack of specificity.

Broad-Based Peer-Reviewed Journals

A peer-reviewed journal is one that submits most of its published articles for review by experts who are not part of the editorial staff [4]. These journals are at the top of the scholarly food chain. Most of their content is composed of reports of original research. They contain advertising but also have a large base of paid subscriber support.

Many hold that there is a "big four" of peer-reviewed journals that are read and respected internationally: the *New England Journal of Medicine* (NEJM), *The Lancet*, the *British Medical Journal* (BMJ), and the *Journal of the American Medical Association* (JAMA). For example, the *British Medical Journal*, published by the BMJ Publishing Group, "aims to publish rigorous, accessible and entertaining material that will help doctors and medical students in their daily practice, lifelong learning and career development." The BMJ has a weekly circulation of more than 120,000. The Massachusetts Medical Society publishes the NEJM, although its circulation far exceeds the number of physicians in the state. *The Lancet* is published weekly by Elsevier Publishers and can be accessed on line at http://www.thelancet.com. JAMA is published by the American Medical Association, and members receive the journal as a membership benefit; many non-AMA members subscribe.

Most of the more than 4000 scientific and medical journals published in the world are peer reviewed. Few have strong support from paid subscribers.

Specialty Oriented Peer-Reviewed Journals

Because it pulls no punches in its name, leaving no doubt as to its specialty orientation, *Gut* is one of my favorite journal names. *Gut* is the official journal of the British Society of Gastroenterology and is edited by the BMJ journals department. Membership in the Aerospace Medical Association includes a subscription to the peer-reviewed monthly journal, *Aviation, Space, and Environmental Medicine*. The *American Journal of Surgery*, published by Elsevier Publishers, is the official publication for six different surgical societies. There is also the *Journal of the American College of Surgeons*. Some of these publications are owned by specialty organizations and are heavily subsidized by dues. Others are more dependent on advertiser support.

Not all of these journals publish reports of original research. *American Family Physician*, published by the American Academy of Family Physicians, publishes peer-reviewed review articles and virtually no original research. Its total circulation exceeds 180,000.

Controlled-Circulation Journals

Controlled-circulation publications are almost entirely dependent on advertising for survival. They are sometimes called "throwaways," but I have always considered the epithet to be unfair and elitist. The truth is that practicing physicians read journals such as *Postgraduate Medicine*, *Consultant*, and *Medical Economics*. Years ago, I had the experience of publishing an article titled "How to See Patients More Efficiently in Your Office" in one of these journals, *Physicians' Management*. In the same month, I published a scholarly article in a peer-reviewed research journal. Several of my colleagues in community practice congratulated me on the practice-based article; none mentioned the research report.

Most of the controlled-circulation publications specialize in some way. There is *The New Physician*, published by the American Medical Student Association, with articles about education and health policy issues pertinent to medical students; *Cutis*, covering diseases of the skin; *Hospital Practice*, presenting topics related to inpatient care; and *Family Practice Management*, an online journal with articles about economic issues in family medicine.

Indexing and the Impact Factor

Most medical journals are "indexed" although some are not; those that are not would like to be. A medical journal such as *Gut* can be—and is—"indexed" in three ways: Index Medicus, the Excerpta Medica Database (EMBASE), and the Institute for Scientific Information (ISI). What does this all mean, and why might it be important for the medical writer?

Briefly stated, indexing means that the publications in a journal are listed in one of the three databases noted above. Publishing your article in an indexed journal means that when an author or a scientist consults PubMed or another reference site on your topic, your article will appear on the list. Without indexing, your article is not likely to be found by others, and, although brilliant and groundbreaking, it may languish in obscurity.

Note that whether or not your article is indexed is determined not by the excellence of your article but by the journal in which it is published. Each of the index organizations makes ongoing decisions as to which journals are indexed and which requests are denied. Index Medicus/MEDLINE makes its decisions based on:

Scientific merit of a journal's content: validity, importance, originality, and contribution to the field
The objectivity, credibility, and quality of its contents
Production quality
An audience of health professionals
Types of content, consisting of one or more of:

Reports of original research
Original clinical observations with analysis
Analysis of philosophical, ethical, or social aspects of medicine
Critical reviews
Statistical compilations
Descriptions or evaluations of methods or procedures
Case reports with discussions

The report of original research is not the only type of article included in Index Medicus. Review article journals may be indexed.

The Three Index Databases

Index Medicus and its online counterpart, MEDLINE, are used internationally to provide access to the world's biomedical literature. Both are part of the National Library of

Medicine. *Index Medicus* currently contains more than 5500 titles. For more information, go to http://www.nlm.nih.gov/tsd/serials/lji.html.

EMBASE, the *Excerpta Medica* database, is a biomedical and pharmaceutical database that gives information to medical and drug-related subjects. EMBASE contains approximately 23 million indexed items and more than 7500 current, mostly peer-reviewed journals. It is especially good for drug-related searches. Access EMBASE at http://www.embase.com.

The Institute for Scientific Information (ISI) publishes the *Science Citations Index* and *Journal Citation Reports* (JCR). The JCR annually publishes information about 11,000+ journals in the medical and social sciences, including the impact factor. Learn about the JCR at http://scientific.thomsonreuters.com/imgblast/JCRFullCovlist-2016.pdf.

The Journal Impact Factor

In the 1960s, ISI developed the journal "impact factor." What is the impact factor and how does it relate to my favorite journals? First proposed by Eugene Garfield [5], the impact factor is a method of rating the influence of a journal on the scientific community and comparing this numerically to a large number of other journals. It does so by measuring the number of citations to articles published in a journal averaged over 2 years; then this number is divided by the total number of articles published in the journal over the same period. Citable articles can include review articles and editorials, as well as reports of clinical trials, a fact which can influence editorial decisions as journal editors scramble to achieve the highest impact factors possible. On the other side of the coin, scientists often consider a journal's impact factor when deciding where to submit their research reports.

As an example to illustrate the importance some attach to the impact factor, I recently received an unsolicited e-mail from *The Lancet*: "Have you heard? *The Lancet's* impact factor has recently gone up to 30.76—just one more reason why you should read the independent and authoritative voice in global medicine." A month later I received another message reporting that the *Irish Journal of Medical Science* has nearly doubled its impact factor to 0.696. In fact, this latter numerical rating is typical of most medical journals, two-thirds of which have an impact factor of less than 1.

In an effort to protest the impact factor process (and incidentally raise its lagging rating), one journal published a single editorial that cited a year's worth of papers that had been published in that journal [6]. More recently, editors of four Brazilian medical journals published articles with hundreds of citations to each other's journals, hoping that not citing their own reports would escape detection. The ruse—called "citation stacking"—failed, and penalties followed [7].

Table 5.1 lists the current impact factor for some selected journals; the higher the number, the greater the presumed "impact" of the journal. Just for the record, the impact factor of the protesting journal described above was 0.66 before the citation-laden editorial, a figure that was subsequently increased to 1.44 by the maneuver.

As might be expected, some researchers are critical of the impact factor. Ojasoo et al. observe: "The choice of citations is subjective and the non-pertinence of the citations is well known. Several variables may intervene, such as the type of journal and its size, domain concerned, language of the publication, self-citations, coding of the articles depending on their nature, and the choice of the manuscripts published ('hot papers')" [8].

TABLE 5.1 Impact factors of some leading medical journals

Journal	Impact factor
New England Journal of Medicine	59.558
Journal of the American Medical Association	37.684
Annals of Internal Medicine	16.593
Circulation	14.430
British Medical Journal	19.967
Archives of Surgery	2.191

The current impact factor for your favorite journal is available on Google. Type "impact factor" followed by the name of the journal

The impact factor is an indicator of citation numbers and not of their quality and can certainly not be used to assess an author's work [8]. Some journals post their current impact factor on their web sites; some do not. In an ideal world, your article will be published in the journal with the highest possible impact factor, but without making a special effort, you may never learn the number and its comparators. Although the impact factor is seldom of great importance to the beginning medical writer, you will encounter the term and should know what it means. I will return to the impact factor in Chap. 12, when I discuss getting your work in print.

Altmetrics

Altmetrics are tools to measure the "real-time reach and influence of an academic article" [9]. In contrast to the traditional citation scores, altmetrics measures online views of an article on social media, mainstream media, and other sites outside the familiar academic arena. The web site *Altemetric* publishes a yearly list of the 100 articles that received the most online attention during the year. For 2015, Warren points out that the journals whose articles were most often represented were *Nature* (14 articles), *Science* (13 articles), and *Plos One* (6 articles) [9]. Being online, *Altmetric* gives us the results much more rapidly than the citation scoring systems we have used to date. The *Altmetric* web site is https://www.altmetric.com/. This is a new metric to watch as the history of medical writing evolves.

How Clinicians Read Medical Journals

As a medical writer, you should pause to consider how clinicians read the medical literature, which is important in how you construct your articles. Do clinicians read each journal cover to cover, beginning with page one, studying all sections of each article? No, they don't. In practice, I propose three ways in which clinicians read journals: They graze, hunt, and gorge.

Grazing

Clinicians are most likely to *graze* the paper journals that cross their desk, and they do so when they have "spare time." There are just too many publications to read each in depth. For example, I receive JAMA and NEJM, several monthly journals in my specialty, and about four controlled-circulation publications. In fact, as a subscriber I increasingly receive previews of these publications online. The only way to handle the volume is to graze. By this I mean that I read the table of contents carefully. If I see a title that looks interesting, I will turn to the first page of the article and read the abstract. If I am very interested in the method and results of the study, I will read those sections and the summary. I estimate that I read the abstract of every third or fourth article, and then I read about one-fourth of these in depth.

In fact, several journals include a synopsis of major articles. One of these is the NEJM, which publishes "This Week in the Journal," a section early in each weekly issue that presents a brief synopsis of each major article. JAMA summarizes the issue's articles in "In This Issue of JAMA." These short summaries may be all that many busy clinicians read.

The grazing habits of readers have implications for medical writers: First, compose your title with great care, because this is likely to be the only part of the article read by most of your intended audience. Then, devote the same care to the abstract; of those who turn to your article, most readers will stop here. Of course, I tend to pay more attention to my two "major," broad-based journals—JAMA and the NEJM—and to the leading journal in my specialty. This means that less prestigious publications get less attention.

Do I have data to support the grazing assertions above? Not really. If your reading habits are different, I would be pleased to hear from you.

Hunting

When clinicians need information about a specific problem, we *hunt* for answers. Years ago, I would hunt in my file of journal clippings or go to the library. Now hunting is done online. Seldom do I go to a paper journal to hunt for a clinical fact. My file of journal clippings, already a historical curiosity when I wrote the first edition of this book, is now in recycling heaven.

The tendency to hunt makes it vital that your important studies are published in indexed journals. Those who read your work are likely never to hold the actual journal in their hands; but by locating your work online and citing it in future scientific articles, these writers disseminate your findings and advance medical knowledge.

Gorging

We writers would like to think that each reader ponders every word we write. To do so would be to *gorge*—to take in way too much. Perhaps the most sedentary, semiretired, literarily omnivorous emeritus professor has the time to read every golden word of every article in every journal. Few of us have this luxury.

Getting It Right

In a speech in the US Senate in 1850, Henry Clay stated, "I would rather be right than be president." I hope that he was right, because he never became president.

For the medical writer, being "right" is paramount. More than probably any other discipline, medical science is unforgiving about errors. Printer's ink is indelible, and the requirement to present truthful information is one of the special aspects of medical writing. Your data must be factual, your conclusions justified, your recommendations based on the best evidence available, your opinions unbiased, and your writing "right."

Medical Jargon and Slang

We clinicians love medical jargon: We turn nouns into verbs, such as "to scope" or "to surgerize" a patient. We use cute phrases such as "gas passers" in reference to anesthesiologists. We "turf" a patient when making a transfer of care. Not surprisingly, much medical jargon originates with young clinicians, sometimes sleep-deprived, as they busily care for patients. The terms are often shorthand, sometimes intended to speak to one another in code without the patient understanding (e.g., "lues" used to refer to syphilis), and may be derogatory ("circling the drain" or CTD, for short, used to describe someone in whom death is imminent).

Jordan and Shepard propose a nicely written definition of jargon: "Jargon refers to technical expressions used by a profession or cult which by no stretch of the imagination can be considered good English and which are often confusing, not only to those outside the fold, but often also to those within it" [10]. American medical jargon can be especially bewildering to physicians for whom English is not their first language. How would such a physician interpret the slang terms *bounce back*, *crump*, and *frequent flier*, terms actually unlikely to confuse any American clinician? Table 5.2 lists some examples of medical jargon and slang. The careful medical writer uses such terms rarely, if at all. If jargon or slang is used in your writing for some special reason, be sure your purpose is clear and provide your reader with the meaning of the word used.

Accuracy and Precision

When I am frantically searching for the treatment of a disease, it helps me little to read that the patient should receive, "a first- or second-generation cephalosporin, 250–500 mg every 8 to 12 hours." Might the writer have identified one or two preferred drugs in this crowded pharmaceutical category? Could there have been a little more specificity in the dose and frequency of administration? And what might be the recommended duration of therapy? It is even more frustrating if a drug is mentioned without a recommended dose. Worst of all, by far, would be a wrong dose.

In my files is an Errata Notice, received from a major medical publisher and referring to what was a newly published major medical reference book. I can happily report

TABLE 5.2 Medical jargon and slang: some selected examples

Jargon or slang	What you probably mean to say
Digitalize	To initiate therapy with a digitalis derivative or perhaps to perform a digital rectal examination
Train wreck	When one thing after another has gone wrong
Prepped	Prepared for surgery
Acute abdomen	Acute disease affecting an abdominal organ, often requiring surgery
Negative	Absence of abnormalities
Gland	Lymph node
To appendectomize	To perform an appendectomy
To buff (a chart)	To be sure the medical record is complete, accurate, and defensible
Antibiotic deficiency	Indicating that the patient has an infection that warrants antibiotic use
To turf (a patient)	The act of referring a patient to another clinician or institution
FLK (pronounced "flik")	A term that clinicians really should not use, meaning "funny-looking kid"
Shotgunning	Ordering a wide range of tests, hoping to hit upon a diagnosis

that I was not the author or editor of the potentially fatal error that prompted the following notice:

> Table 116–1 on page 880 and the bottom line in the left-hand column on page 881 erroneously indicate that the dilution of epinephrine to be used for intracardiac injection in cases of cardiac arrest is 1:1000. The correct dilution is *1:10,000.*

An issue of NEJM contained an error notice as follows:

> Emergence of Multidrug-Resistant Pandemic Influenza A (H1N1) Virus (Correspondence, N Engl J Med 2010;363:1381-1382). In the figure (page 1381) the term "275 Histamine" should have been "275 Histidine." We regret the error.

"Reading maketh a full man; conference a ready man; and writing an exact man," wrote Francis Bacon (1561–1626). The value of months of research and writing can be undermined by a single factual error in a published paper. If you have published a book with an error, a reviewer will unfailingly discover this mistake and report to the world when writing the critical review. In the many stages between your keystroke and the printed page—copyediting, typesetting, and correcting proofs—there are ample opportunities for errors. The careful author will pay close attention at each stage.

Abbreviations and Acronyms as Sometimes Misleading Shortcuts

Among the items that can cloud meaning and introduce errors are abbreviations and acronyms (AA). They can also annoy readers and cause eyes to glaze over.

Abbreviations

As a reader, I wish that writers would use fewer abbreviations. The rule is that you can create any abbreviation you wish as long as you identify it with first use. For example, I created an abbreviation—AA—for the phrase *abbreviations and acronyms.* From now on in this chapter, I am free to use either the phrase or the abbreviation. The problem is that I may not use the abbreviation again for another six pages, and the reader using this book as a reference source and encountering this abbreviation later on must search this entire chapter to discover that, on these pages, AA does not mean Alcoholics Anonymous, aplastic anemia, or Australia antigen.

Here are some of my guidelines for the use of abbreviations:

* Don't use more than one abbreviation in a sentence. Think twice if you are tempted to write something like "The patient who has IUGR or PPROM has an increased risk of PTL and PTB." (Translation for those who don't do maternity care: The patient who has intrauterine growth retardation or preterm premature rupture of the membranes has an increased risk of preterm labor and preterm birth.)

- Do not use an abbreviation in an article title. Sure, there will be exceptions such as "... prevalence in the U.S." However, generally you should spell out all words in the title. Remember that you should explain an abbreviation with first use, and the title is not the place to do this.
- Try to avoid abbreviations in the abstract. Here it will be possible to explain the abbreviation, but since most of your readers won't read the body of your paper anyhow, why break the flow by introducing your abbreviation meaning here?
- Be wary of "standard" abbreviations. What is standard today can change. Do you remember when "mg%" was the standard?

When properly selected, abbreviations can be a space-saving convenience. If used improperly, they can introduce confusion. Table 5.3 lists some examples of abbreviations that

TABLE 5.3 Examples of abbreviations that may mislead readers

Abbreviation	What the abbreviation might mean
BP	This abbreviation means blood pressure, doesn't it? Not always. BP may also indicate bedpan, bathroom privileges, bullous pemphigoid, or even British Pharmacopoeia
DI	When you see DI, think of diabetes insipidus—or perhaps diagnostic imaging, detrusor instability, drug interaction, or date of injury
ID	When you ponder this abbreviation, choose from among identification, infectious disease, intradermal, or initial dose
IT	Possibilities include intensive therapy, inhalation therapy, or even incentive therapy. Confusion between intrathecal and intratracheal when administering medication could be harmful
MI	MI might mean myocardial infarction or mitral insufficiency
ROM	This might stand for range of motion, right otitis media, or rupture of membranes
TD	Think of test dose, tardive dyskinesia, transverse diameter, tetanus–diphtheria toxoid, temporary disability, or traveler's diarrhea. But, in a medical setting, not touchdown

can be misunderstood. In addition, at the end of this book, I have included in Appendix C a handy list of commonly used abbreviations.

Acronyms

Acronyms are words made up of initial letters or syllables or a group of words. An acronym usually is typed in all capital letters. For example, SCUBA is an acronym for "self-contained underwater breathing apparatus." World War II gave us a rich trove of acronyms: AWOL (absent without leave), SONAR (sound navigation ranging), and CINCUS (commander in chief of the United States/navy). Some acronymns, including SCUBA and SONAR, have evolved into legitimate words (scuba and sonar are now the dictionary terms), but that is an honor reserved for only a few.

We pronounce the acronym as a word; CINCUS is pronounced "sink us" (and, because of that pronunciation, the acronym ceased to be used after Pearl Harbor). TURP, representing transurethral resection of the prostate, is pronounced as "turp," rhyming with "burp." In contrast, abbreviations are pronounced letter by letter; human immunodeficiency virus infection is pronounced as "H-I-V," sounding out all the letters. But acquired immunodeficiency syndrome has become the acronym AIDS. Some day we may, in fact, have forgotten what the four letters once stood for, just as most persons today know of sonar but don't recall the origin of the word.

Here are some examples of medical acronyms:

- ACE inhibitors: angiotensin-converting enzyme inhibitors are used to treat hypertension and other illnesses.
- CABG: pronounced as "cabbage," the acronym stands for coronary artery bypass graft.
- CREST syndrome: a cluster of limited scleroderma skin manifestations and late visceral involvement that includes calcinosis, Raynaud's phenomenon, esophageal dysmotility, sclerodactyly, and telangiectasia.
- ELISA: with the enzyme-linked immunosorbent assay, the addition of "test" is redundant.

- GOMER: from "get outta my emergency room," refer-ring to an ER patient who does not need emergency services. The somewhat cynical psychiatrist/novelist Samuel Shem describes the GOMER as "a human being who has lost—often through age—what goes into being a human being" [11].
- RICE: rest, ice, compression, and elevation are all used to treat acute injuries.

Problems with Stance

Both beginning and experienced medical authors can have problems with stance. By this I mean overstating or under-stating your conclusions, especially in research reports.

Overstatement and Hubris

Hubris is excessive self-confidence. It represents pride that may approach arrogance. It can take several forms. The clini-cian who holds fast to a shaky diagnosis, refusing to seek consultation, is exhibiting hubris. What about hubris in medi-cal writing? One manifestation of hubris is attempting to write far beyond your professional experience and available data. Here is a fanciful example: "Based upon our study of 5 subjects who developed fatigue following use of the drug placebomycin, we recommend that clinicians use great cau-tion in prescribing this medication." Well, that would be an extreme example of hubris, but you get the idea. Editors can quickly sniff out when they are being shoveled a load of bad-smelling stuff. Another hubristic act is making confident statements about what the future holds, which you should not do in any medium that might be read a decade later.

In medical writing, the most common manifestation of overstatement and hubris occurs in presumptuous phrases, such as "Clinicians should always..." and "It should be appar-ent at this point that...."

Table 5.4 lists more of such words that should give you pause if you use them in your conclusions.

Table 5.4 Hubristic words and phrases

Meaningful
Important
Key
Landmark
Foremost
Groundbreaking
Consequential
Central
Essential
Substantial
Major finding
Paradigm changing
It is certainly true that…
One must conclude that…
We can all agree that…

Understatement and Waffling

Just as bad as overstatement is understatement. By understating perfectly good work, you undermine your valid findings and your own credibility. Table 5.5 lists some words that should alert you that you might be understating your conclusions.

Writing as a Team Sport

Medical writing is often done in teams. In research, teams are important because various people can bring different abilities: expertise in research methods, access to subjects, grant-writing experience, personal contacts in grant-funding agencies, and statistical skills. Writing groups may be clinicians with similar abilities and experience or may include the young person with ambition and energy, the mid-level professional who knows how to get the job done, and the senior person whose participation helps assure eventual publication.

TABLE 5.5 Waffle words and phrases

Possibly
Probably
Potentially
Perhaps
Maybe
Might
May
Apparently
It appears that…
It is conceivable that…
It is very possible that…

Writing as a team has other advantages: If I have a good writing or research idea and share it with others on a team, at a later time, one of them is likely to have his or her own good idea, and I might be included. In this way we all gain writing experience and entries on our curriculum vitae (CV). And, very important, our publication successes help advance medical knowledge and understanding.

Working as part of a team can help get the job done in a practical way. When everyone on the team has a task vital to the success of the project, no one is going to want to let the group down. In my college sociology class, the professor called this a "group effect." It certainly helps to keep the writing project moving.

Guidelines for the Writing Team

Every writing team has implicit rules for how each person will behave and contribute. Some groups have more explicit rules. The following are my suggested guidelines for the writing team:

- Choose a leader. The leader is usually the one with the "good idea" and the one who calls the meetings. The person who leads need not be the most senior person, but the leader must have a strong commitment to the project.

- Agree to regular meetings of the writing team. These meetings may be monthly or every 2 weeks. The frequency is not as important as the fact that the meetings are accorded priority on everyone's schedule. Also, all team members must show up or at least send a progress report. If someone misses several meetings, the group must question that person's commitment to the project.
- Decide on the role of each member of the team. The key person is the one who will lead the writing. In most cases, this person will compose the first draft, based on contributions from all. Then all team members will submit revision suggestions. In an efficient team, the lead writer has discretion to accept or reject revision suggestions.
- Establish deadlines and then stick to them. Breaking any writing project into achievable deadlines makes it seem much more manageable. An example of admittedly tight schedule for a review article might look something like:

    - Data collected by end of month 1
    - Outline completed by the end of month 2
    - First draft completed by the end of month 3
    - Second draft completed by end of month 4
    - Third revised draft finished and read by peer reviewers by end of month 5
    - Final draft completed and in the mail in month 6

- Decide early on the order of authorship. The person who has done most of the writing should usually be the first author, but not always.

Why Problems Develop in Writing Teams

Problems can develop in writing teams for a number of reasons:

- Confusion about leadership. In this instance, the team member who agreed to be in charge is not leading. One person should be tasked with the job of taking charge, assigning roles, setting agendas, and keeping the group moving.

- Disagreements about how authors will be listed. Teams have been known to dissolve in anger over this issue. Consider the intrigue that surrounded the authorship of the original Gray's Anatomy, published in 1858. It seems that the book was a collaborative effort of surgeon and anatomist Henry Gray and Henry Vandyke, at that time a surgeon apothecary who would later become a physician. In her book *The Making of Mr. Gray's Anatomy*, Ruth Richardson describes the political shenanigans that led to Gray's enduring fame and Vandyke's obscurity (at least in regard to the book Gray's Anatomy) [12]. In short, every person who contributes to the work should be considered for authorship, and every person whose name is listed at the top of a paper as author should qualify for authorship [13].

- There is a slacker in the group. Someone is not getting the job done, and the problem is especially onerous if the slacker has a vital responsibility, such as seeking funding or performing statistical analysis. When this occurs, members of the writing team need an "intervention," with a gentle but firm confrontation.

- Group wordsmithing. Wordsmithing by two people is tedious. Attempting wordsmithing by more than two people can be like fingernails on a chalkboard. Wordsmithing is and should be a solitary activity, based on written, repeat written, suggestions from others on the team.

- The power play. Someone in the group is exerting undue force. The power play may be a challenge to the leader, or it might be an attempted veto: "I won't let this paper be submitted with my name on it unless this sentence is omitted." When this happens, the whole team must be involved in negotiating a satisfactory solution without caving in to power.

Ethical Issues

There are ethical issues involved in all types of writing. Medical writing has more than any other kind, many of these related to the rules of the road for conducting and reporting research.

Conflict of Interest

A conflict of interest occurs when a medical author has some tie to activities that could be perceived as influencing objectivity or veracity. A conflict of interest may be financial, as in receiving funding support for a project or accepting honoraria as a speaker for a pharmaceutical company whose product is recommended in the article or lecture. It may also include being a consultant, providing expert testimony, owning stock in a company, or actually being employed by a company that makes a product mentioned in an article. Conflicts may even involve family members, academic competition, and personal relationships. Because I write on medical topics, I do not serve on the speaker panels for any pharmaceutical companies, and I do not buy individual stocks of drug companies or surgical supply manufacturers.

The conflict-of-interest problem is pervasive. In a survey of orthopedic surgeons presenting or serving in another role at a 2008 annual meeting of the American Academy of Orthopaedic Surgeons, 79.3% reported directly related payments, and 50.0% reported indirectly related payments from manufacturers of joint prostheses [14]. In 2004, the prestigious National Cholesterol Education Program of the National Institutes of Health (NIH) released new stricter guidelines for serum cholesterol levels. Subsequently we learned that most members of the panel had conflicts of interest described as "financial ties to the pharmaceutical companies that stood to gain enormously from increased use of statins" [15].

There is a fundamental way to deal with possible conflict of interest: disclosure. If you find yourself faced with a gray area, full disclosure of the possible conflict will be a strong defense against later criticism.

Not only authors can have conflicts of interest. Peer reviewers and editors may also have ethical dilemmas; I discuss this in Chap. 12.

Project-Specific Industry Financial and Material Support

While surfing the web, I came across a report describing a trial involving 32 healthy young adults who experienced "robust working memory enhancement following administration of American ginseng." For the convenience of the article's audience, the article identifies the drug by both generic name (*Panax quinquefolius*) and brand name (Cereboost) [16]. I was intrigued by this seemingly safe way to boost cognitive function, until I noted that the "work was supported by a grant from Naturex, Inc, maker of Cereboost," a notation that undermined the report's credibility, for me, at least, as well as tempering my urge to recommend the product to my patients or rush to the pharmacy to purchase the drug for personal use.

In discussions of conflict of interest, project-specific industry support for research may even seem to affect outcomes. A survey of randomized clinical trials conducted over a decade reveals that "trials funded by for-profit organizations were more likely to report positive findings than those funded by not-for-profit organizations. As a group, these surveys raised questions regarding the design and conduct of industry-funded clinical trials, as well as ethical concerns about potential violations of clinical equipoise" [17]. As a physician, I value this study for the perspective provided, and as a writer, I admire the finely crafted phase "potential violations of clinical equipoise."

The JAMA Instruction For Authors states "A conflict of interest may exist when an author (or the author's institution or employer) has financial or personal relationships or affiliations that could influence (or bias) the author's decisions, work, or manuscript. All authors are required to report potential conflicts of interest including specific financial interests relevant to the subject of their manuscript in the Acknowledgment section of the manuscript…" [13].

Plagiarism

I was in a writing workshop in which someone asked a medical book editor what he thought was the biggest problem he faced. His answer surprised me: plagiarism.

Inappropriate use of the words of another may start early. A study by Segal et al. found evidence of plagiarism in 5.2% of application essays to residency programs at a single large academic medical center [18]. No one is immune from the accusation: Even American author Helen Keller (1880–1968) was once accused of plagiarism, nor are those of high rank immune. In 2008, the Harvard Crimson Newspaper carried a headline: "Harvard Medical School Professor Caught Plagiarizing" [19].

The clinician with a good article idea should write it up. Let's look at the sentence I just wrote. In the long history of literature, I believe that it is mathematically possible that I am the first person to put those 11 words together in exactly this way. On balance, my 11-word sentence does not describe a brilliantly inventive thought, and a claim to being the first to write this sentence must remain a presumptive guess. However, and modesty aside, if you or any other author wishes to use my sentence, you should make clear that it is a quotation from this book and give full credit to the source.

And just to show how readily an editor can detect plagiarism, I ask you to type my sentence "The clinician with a good article idea…" into Google, and then click "Search." The first item you see is the second edition of this book. If tempted to plagiarize, beware.

Not all accused of plagiarism are truly guilty. I have faith in the goodness of my fellow humans, and I choose to believe that some errors arise from doing research without noting carefully what were personal thoughts and what were someone else's words. I think of this as "accidental plagiarism." Yes, such plagiarism is unacceptable, but you can see what happened. I suspect that accidental plagiarism is most likely to occur when authors depend on others (students or research assistants) to do their research for them.

The rules of using borrowed material and how to obtain permission are covered in Chap. 4. If the little voice in your subconscious whispers that you may be using someone else's work inappropriately, listen carefully to the message.

Ghost and Honorary Authors

Flanagin et al. did a study of 809 corresponding authors (the author who was self-identified as the one to contact about an article) of articles published in JAMA, NEJM, and *Annals of Internal Medicine* plus three other peer-reviewed, smaller-circulation journals that publish supplements (*American Journal of Cardiology, American Journal of Medicine,* and *American Journal of Obstetrics and Gynecology*). Flanagin et al. found that 19% of articles had evidence of honorary authors, 11% had evidence of ghost authors, and 2% had evidence of both. Honorary authors were more prevalent in review articles than in research reports. The journals in the study described are among those considered to be some of our best [20]. The suspected prevalence of honorary and ghost authors is appalling, especially since authors published in these prestigious journals are generally respected academicians.

A furor, and litigation, arose a few years ago regarding the drug rofecoxib, marketed by Merck and Company. Ross et al. reviewed documents pertinent to the issue. They concluded:

> This case-review of industry documents demonstrates that clinical trial manuscripts related to rofecoxib were authored by sponsor employees but often attributed first authorship to academically affiliated investigators who did not always disclose industry financial support. Review manuscripts were often prepared by unacknowledged authors and subsequently attributed authorship to academically affiliated investigators who often did not disclose industry financial support [21].

Nor are medical reference books exempt from ghost authorship. As part of a 2010 legal discovery in lawsuits against the drug company now known as GlaxoSmithKline (GSK), documents showed that, to use the *New York Times* headline, the "Drug Maker Wrote Book Under 2 Doctors' Names" [22]. In their report, the *Times* goes on to state "The 269-page book, *Recognition and Treatment of Psychiatric Disorders: A Psychopharmacology Handbook for Primary Care*, is so far the first book among publications, namely medical journal articles, that have been criticized in recent years for hidden drug industry influence, colloquially known as ghostwriting." The book, listing as coauthors two prominent academic psychiatrists, has been considered by some to be especially favorable to an antidepressant manufactured by GSK. In the *Times* article, Dr. David A. Kessler, former commissioner of the US Food and Drug Administration, was quoted as follows: "To ghostwrite an entire textbook is a new level of chutzpah" [22].

Ghost writing—putting your name on something someone else wrote—is a form of plagiarism. In commenting on these reports, I can only say if you wrote it or otherwise contributed substantially, put your name on it. If not, do not allow yourself to be listed as an author.

Who Ethically Qualifies as an Author?

Certainly neither you nor I would allow ourselves to be listed as an author—and especially a lead author—on a paper written by someone in a pharmaceutical company when we had no hand in the writing process, nor would we want to suffer the fate of several of the coauthors of a paper by Sudbo et al. (Sudbo J, et al. Lancet. 2005;366(9494):1359). According to Swedberg, "several of the 13 co-authors claimed they were not aware of the submission or the full result" [23]. But not all questions of authorship are quite as clear.

Perhaps it will be helpful to identify what does not constitute authorship: Collecting data, acquiring funding, and providing administrative supervision do not constitute authorship, neither does being the department head who is aware of the study but takes no active role in the investigation or actual preparation of the report.

And so who is an author? The ICMJE recommends that authorship be based on the following criteria:

- Substantial contributions to the conception or design of the work; or the acquisition, analysis, or interpretation of data for the work; AND
- Drafting the work or revising it critically for important intellectual content; AND
- Final approval of the version to be published; AND
- Agreement to be accountable for all aspects of the work in ensuring that questions related to the accuracy or integrity of any part of the work are appropriately investigated and resolved [4].

Richard Smith, former editor of the *British Medical Journal*, offers us a practical concept of what constitutes authorship, citing that each author must assume *full intellectual accountability*. "If your paper is about to be presented at a big conference in Acapulco and suddenly the lead author is taken ill or drops down dead, could you get on a plane and go to Acapulco, make a presentation and answer all the questions? If you couldn't you are not intellectually accountable." Donning his editorial hat, Smith goes on to opine, "About half of authors don't meet those criteria" [24].

Duplicate Publication

The editors of the *Journal of General Internal Medicine* (JGIM) describe the following series of circumstances: "Recently it came to the attention of JGIM's editors that a manuscript just published online in another journal (Article B) bore a clear resemblance to a manuscript published in JGIM approximately six months earlier (Article A). On closer inspection, there was a reason for concern. Both papers reported on a quasi-experimental evaluation of a quality improvement intervention. The titles, by-lines, and abstracts were similar and the methods sections almost identical. Moreover, entire paragraphs of the introduction and discussion sections were almost the same" [25]. The authors go on to ask: "Had an editorial crime been committed? And if so, was this a felony, a misdemeanor or merely a technical breech akin to jaywalking?" [25].

Duplicate publication is publishing the same material two or more times, and this can include both print and electronic media. Catherine DeAngelis, MD, MPH, former editor in chief of JAMA, states that "duplicate publication is dishonorable—in whatever way it is couched" [26].

Spin

Spin is reporting research in a way that could distort the interpretation of results and mislead readers. Boutron et al. studied 72 reports of randomized clinical trials. They identified spin in the titles of 13 articles and in the Results and Conclusion sections of the abstracts of 27 and 42 reports, respectively. In the main text, spin was found in many instances: Results (21 reports), Discussion (31 reports), and Conclusions (36 reports). The authors found spin in at least two of these sections of the main text in more than 40% of reports [27].

Spin may occur in an effort to find something "significant" to report. Spin may also occur in the setting of industry-sponsored trials, when the industry sponsor has a financial interest in a positive result in the trial of their new antidepressant or antibiotic. In an editorial with the foreboding title "Spin Kills Science," Lisa Anne Harvey writes:

> Have you ever wondered why so much published research in the area of spinal cord injuries (SCI) has positive conclusions? Simple probability tells us that these results are not reflective of the full truth. Researchers can't possibly be picking winners every time they tackle a question. So what is going on here? The most likely explanation for the high proportion of positive conclusions is that many researchers are putting a positive spin on the conclusions of their negative research. Spin is rampant in all areas of medical research and SCI research is no exception [28].

Bouton et al. suggest, "The use of spin in scientific writing can result from ignorance of the scientific issue, unconscious bias, or willful intent to deceive" [27]. I suspect spin when I read language such as "non-inferior" or "nearly attained statistical significance."

What Makes Great Medical Writing?

Chapters 6–11 discuss the various types of medical articles, chapters, and books. First, let's review what is common to all great medical writing.

- A topic of general interest. The general medical reader is probably not interested in a rare tropical disease never seen in the United States or Europe but may be interested if you can tell something new about problems in daily practice, especially if you have data to share.
- Meaningful information about the topic. I use the "Monday morning" question. If I read this article over the weekend, might it possibly be of help to me in the hospital or office on Monday morning?
- Objectives clearly stated. Tell your reader early in the article what to expect. This is especially important in a research report, in which the research question should be clearly articulated in the introduction.
- A structure that presents information clearly. Don't start writing until you have the structural concept clearly in mind. The structure tells you and the reader where you are going. Of all components of medical writing, this is the most difficult to repair later.
- Articulate and authoritative prose. Good data presented in bad prose may be rejected by a journal. Lester King has summarized the requirements for good expository writing in a single sentence: "Know what you want to say, say it clearly, and then stop" [29]. Be very selective in your use of long sentences, big words, and AAs.
- Tables and figures that complement the text. Used judiciously, they can be the most important part of your article.
- A descriptive, concise title. Label your work clearly and in a way that readers may recall later.

References

1. Frey JJ. Elements of composition. In: Taylor RB, Munning KA, editors. Written communication in family medicine. New York: Springer; 1984. p. 4.

2. Wallechinsky D, Wallace I. The people's almanac. Garden City, NY: Doubleday; 1975. p. 746.

3. Highet G. Explorations. New York: Oxford University Press; 1971. p. 99.

4. International Committee of Medical Journal Editors. Recommendations for the conduct, reporting, editing, and publication of scholarly work in medical journals. http://icmje.org/recommendations/.

5. Garfield E. The history and meaning of the journal impact factor. JAMA. 2006;295(1):90–2.

6. Schutte HK, Svec JG. Reaction of Folia Phoniatrica et Logopaedica on the current trend of impact factor measures. Folia Phoniatr Logop. 2007;59(6):281–6.

7. Van Noorden R. Brazilian citation scheme outed: Thomson Reuters suspends journals from its rankings for 'citation stacking'. Nature. 2013;500(7464):510–1.

8. Ojasoo T, Maisonneuve H, Matillon Y. The impact factor of medical journals, a biometric indicator to be handled with care (in French). Presse Med. 2002;31(17):775–81.

9. Warren HR. The rise of Altmetrics. JAMA. 2017;317(2):131–2.

10. Jordan EP, Shepard WC. Rx for medical writing. Philadelphia: WB Saunders; 1952. p. 14.

11. Shem S. The house of God. New York: Dell; 1978.

12. Richardson R. The making of Mr. Gray's Anatomy: bodies, books, fortune, fame. New York: Oxford University Press; 2008.

13. Journal of the American Medical Association. Instructions for authors. http://jamanetwork.com/journals/jama/pages/instructions-for-authors.

14. Okike K, Kocher MS, Wei EX, et al. Accuracy of conflict-of-interest disclosures reported by physicians. N Engl J Med. 2009;361:1466.

15. Kassirer JP. Why should we swallow what these studies say? Adv Stud Med. 2004;4(8):397–8.

16. Scholey A, Ossoukhova A, Owen L, et al. Effects of American ginseng (Panax quinquefolius) on neurocognitive function: an acute, randomized, double-blind, placebo-controlled, crossover study. Psychopharmacology. 2010;212(3):345–56.

17. Ridker PM, Torres J. Reported outcomes in major cardiovascular clinical trials funded by for-profit and not-for-profit organizations—2000-2005. JAMA. 2006;295(19):2270–4.
18. Segal S, Gelfand BJ, Hurwitz S, et al. Plagiarism in residency application essays. Ann Intern Med. 2010;153(2):128–9.
19. Harvard Medical School Professor Caught Plagiarizing. The Harvard Crimson. Accessed 1 Feb 2008.
20. Flanagin A, Carey LA, Fontanarosa PG, et al. Prevalence of articles with honorary authors and ghost writers in peer-reviewed medical journals. JAMA. 1998;280(3):222–4.
21. Ross JS, Hill KP, Egilman DS, et al. Guest authorship and ghostwriting in publications related to rofecoxib. JAMA. 2008;299(15):1800–12.
22. Wilson D. Drug maker wrote book under 2 doctors' names, documents say. *The New York Times*. http://www.nytimes.com/2010/11/30/business/30drug.html. Accessed 29 Nov 2010.
23. Swedberg K. Who is an author? Eur J Heart Fail. 2008;10(6):523–4.
24. Smith RS. The trouble with medical journals. Medico-Legal J. 2008;76:79.
25. Kravitz RL, Feldman MD. From the editors' desk: self-plagiarism and other editorial crimes and misdemeanors. J Gen Intern Med. 2011;26(1):1–2.
26. DeAngelis CD. Commentary: the Roman article: read it again—in the same journal. JAMA. 2009;301(13):1382–3.
27. Boutron I, Dutton S, Ravaud P, Altman DG. Reporting and interpretation of randomized controlled trials with statistically nonsignificant results for primary outcomes. JAMA. 2010;303(20):2058–64.
28. Harvey LA. Spin kills science. Spinal Cord. 2015;53(6):417.
29. King LS. Why not say it clearly? Boston: Little, Brown; 1978. p. 109.

Chapter 6
How to Write a Review Article

To write an article of any sort is, to some extent, to reveal ourselves. Hence, even a medical article is, in a sense, something of an autobiography.

American surgeon J. Chalmers DaCosta (1863–1938) [1]

Many respected academicians write review articles, for both subscriber-based and controlled-circulation journals. Why do they do so? The answer is that most academic clinicians focus on one disease, such as Parkinson disease or heart failure, and by writing review articles, they assert their claims—mark their territory—on topics such as renin levels in hypertension or advances in prostate cancer surgery.

In addition to the fact that many review articles are written by experienced authors, they are also usually very well written. When presenting a new way of organizing known data or discussing how to manage a perplexing clinical problem, the article must be skillfully composed if it is to hold the reader's attention. The reader must find the content worth the effort to read. For this reason, most review articles are both peer reviewed for medical content and carefully edited to make them comprehensible [2].

This will not be a long chapter because, by using the review article as an example of how to approach concept and structure,

© Springer International Publishing AG 2018
R.B. Taylor, *Medical Writing*,
https://doi.org/10.1007/978-3-319-70126-4_6

I have already covered several of the most important topics. In Chap. 2, I discussed general ways to develop an idea into the structure of an article, and in Chap. 3, I discussed how the idea and structural concept could be developed into an expanded outline. Chapter 4 covered how to construct tables, figures, and reference lists. Nevertheless, there are still some things to discuss about writing review articles.

About the Review Article

What Is a Review Article?

Fundamentally, the review paper is an essay. It has similarities to the essays you and I have been writing since junior high school: It has a topic, a beginning, development of the theme in a logical manner, and an ending. Some may say that the review paper is not an original publication and that it is merely a reorganization of known facts and hence is not new knowledge. I understand the "not-original" viewpoint, especially if held by a research scientist. It is true that review papers add no new data to the literature. However, I believe that review articles are original in that they bring innovative thinking to the readers. They provide us with practical insights and offer new approaches to old problems. In this way they are innovative, and they expand medical understanding.

There are various types of review articles. We are all familiar with the traditional types. Sometimes called clinical updates, traditional review articles bring together known facts in a meaningful, ideally evidence-based, way [2]. Examples include:

- How to approach a clinical problem: "Failure To Thrive: A Practical Guide" (Homan GJ. Am Fam Phys. 2016;94:295)
- How to improve clinical care: "Adding Value By Talking More" (Kaplan RS et al. NEJM. 2016;375:1918)
- How we did it: "Three Innovative Curricula for Addressing Medical Students' Career Development" (Navarro AM et al. Academic Med. 2011;86:72)

- How it's done today: "In-Flight Medical Emergencies during Commercial Flight," which includes a table listing the contents of in-flight emergency kits, as required by the Federal Aviation Administration (Nable JV et al. NEJM. 2015;373;939)

Taking a closer look, we find that the prototypical clinical review article will present material along the lines of: This is how it's done today. Disease-related topics tend to fall into a few sometimes overlapping categories, three of which are diagnosis, treatment, and prevention. An example of a review article about diagnosis is "Acute monoarthritis: diagnosis in adults" (Becker JA et al. Am Fam Phys. 2016;94:810). The second of these is the management category: This is how we treat it. The September 2013 online issue of the *Journal of General Internal Medicine* (JGIM) has an article titled "Preventive Pharmacologic Treatments For Episodic Migraine In Adults." Another category is prevention: an example is the opinion article titled "Preventing Mitochondrial DNA Diseases: One Step Forward, Two Steps Back" (Cohen IG et al. JAMA. 2016;316:273). Others are simply a review of a clinical entity such as "Hepatic Encephalopathy" (Wijdicks EFM. NEJM. 2016;375:1660). And some are about what's new, such as "Asthma In 2016: Reassured About The Old, Excited About The New" (Sood S et al. The Lancet. 2016;4:937).

Some review articles are based not on a disease but upon a clinical presentation. Recently I met with one of our faculty who had accepted an invitation to write an article on the approach to the patient with dyspnea. This type of review article—the diagnostic approach to a symptom such as acute chest pain or a clinical sign such as splenomegaly—is an especially difficult challenge, simply because the path to diagnosis is likely to meander into the turf of several specialties. Yet another type of review article has to do with "current status" reports such as "Cellulitis: a Review," published in a recent issue of the *Journal of the American Medical Association* (Raff AB et al. JAMA. 2016;316:325). And some review articles combine categories. An example is the article "Venous Ulcer: Diagnosis, Treatment, and Prevention of Recurrences," published in the *Journal of Vascular Surgery* (Gillespie DL. J Vasc Surg. 2010;52:8S).

In addition to the traditional types, there are specialized review articles, which are discussed later in the chapter. These are the literature review discussing the state of the art, the systemic review, the meta-analysis, and the evidence-based clinical review.

Who Publishes Review Articles and Who Reads Them?

Who Publishes Review Articles?

Not all review articles are published in controlled-circulation journals—the "throwaways." Many journals, even some of the most prestigious ones, publish review articles regularly. They may carry a general label, such as "Review Article" as in the *New England Journal of Medicine* (NEJM) or "Review(s)" as in the *British Medical Journal for the American Physician* (BMJ-USA). Another site is the "Clinical Review and Education" section in the *Journal of the American Medical Association*, where there was a recent review article from the Medical Letter on Drugs and Therapeutics titled "Buprenorphine implants (Probuphine) for opioid dependence" (JAMA. 2016;316:1820).

The fact that virtually all journals publish review articles is favorable for the new author. If you write a thoughtful, well-organized article in competent prose, you should eventually see it in print if you are persistent in seeking publication. Realistically, your chances of success with the international "big four"—*The Lancet*, NEJM, JAMA, and BMJ—are not promising, for the very good reason that these leading publications seek contributions from the world's leaders in each area.

Do not despair. The many refereed journals in your specialty and the dozens of broad-based controlled-circulation journals need a constant supply of review papers, and because of the ongoing need for good articles, they cannot wait until the world authority in the field decides to submit a review article. In the less "prestigious" journals, those with the lower impact factors (see Chap. 5), your chances of publication are good.

I recommend contacting the journal editor first. An early discussion with the editor about your article idea can help avoid disappointment. It also establishes a personal relationship and may help lead to an eventual favorable decision. Try for telephone contact whenever possible; an e-mail is a more impersonal second choice. Table 6.1 lists some journals that may be appropriate targets for your article. Some of these journals publish only online. In addition, *MedReviews* publishes journals in the following areas: urology, cardiovascular medicine, neurological diseases, obstetrics and gynecology, gastrointestinal disorders, and primary care. *MedReviews* can be contacted at http://www.medreviews.com. The contact information listed in Table 6.1 may be different by the time you read this book: editors, telephone numbers, and e-mail addresses change. Try the listed contact information as a

TABLE 6.1 Selected journals that publish review articles

American Family Physician
    American Academy of Family Physicians
    http://www.aafp.org/afp
Patient Care
    UBM Media, LLC
    http://www.patientcareonline.com/
Journal of General Internal Medicine
    The Society of General Internal Medicine and Springer
    http://link.springer.com/journal/11606
Postgraduate Medical Journal
    The Fellowship of Postgraduate Medicine and BMJ
    http://pmj.bmj.com/
Primary Psychiatry
    Primary Psychiatry, New York, NY
    http://www.primarypsychiatry.com/

---

beginning, and then use "network research," as described in Chap. 3, to reach the correct person. If this fails, use Google to search for the journal name, and then seek the editor's contact information. Later in this chapter, I will discuss how to structure your initial approach to the editor.

Who Reads Review Articles?

The quick answer is almost all clinicians. This includes not only physicians, physician assistants, and nurse practitioners but also medical students, residents, and fellows. Other readers may be health policy experts and even attorneys. My review articles on headaches have prompted calls from attorneys across America, asking me to review records in professional liability cases involving patients who presented with headaches.

As I noted in Chap. 5, readers tend to "graze" review articles, actually reading only those whose titles seem compelling. Some busy physicians save these articles to read as relaxation in the evening. Others take a pile of review article tear-outs to read at the hospital cafeteria lunch table, on long plane rides, or—not recommended—at the poolside on vacation.

Referring physicians also read review articles, and the names of authors who write often on a topic become familiar. Many nationally known specialists in narrow fields attribute some patient referrals to review articles that they have published in medical journals.

Planning a Review Article

First Steps

Let us begin with the premise that you would like to write a review article as a way of getting started in medical writing. What should you do next? Begin with the work you do each day, which may be seeing patients in the office, serving as a hospitalist for inpatients, performing surgery, or caring for elderly individuals in a nursing home. Within the scope of your work, find what intrigues you, and ask yourself, what have I learned in my years of practice that I would like to share with my colleagues?

Along with being a bit of an autobiography, as DaCosta observed above, writing a review article soon becomes a learning exercise for the author. There are two phases. First, you must learn whether anyone else has recently published the article you are planning to write. Do this by searching PubMed, BioMedLib, Google Scholar, or your own favorite web-searching site. Be cautious with any conclusion that you have happened upon virgin territory—a topic that no one has written about yet. There are two reasons to question such a conclusion: First, there is a lag between publication and when you will find the report on the web site, and second, some controlled-circulation journals are not indexed at all. A thorough search is useful early, even at the stage of deciding whether to write the article at all. It can avoid disappointment later.

Next comes thinking about how to handle your chosen topic.

How to Approach Your Topic

As you think about how to organize your article, it is often helpful to scan your target journal and look at how authors there have organized what they wanted to say. Let us now look at some published review articles to see how the authors dealt with their material (Table 6.2).

I did not need to search very far to find the examples in Table 6.2. Publications containing traditional review articles such as the ones listed cross our desks every day. Let's look at the ways the listed examples approached their subjects: The article in JAMA about chronic pain management discusses some consequences of the mandated transition to limit the use of opioids. The article on pet infections tells of dermatophytosis, scabies, toxoplasmosis, and more. In the article titled

TABLE 6.2 Structure of selected review articles

Article title	Article concept and structure
Opioids out, cannabis in: negotiating the unknowns in patient care for chronic pain (JAMA. 2016;316:1763)	About changes in our thinking regarding pain management
Pet infections (Am Fam Phys. 2016;94:794)	An overview of diseases we share with animals
Just a cut (NEJM. 2016;375:1780)	A case-based look at a common problem that took a bad turn
The health of prisoners (The Lancet. Published online November 19, 2010. doi:10.1016/ S0140-6736(10)61053-7)	Describes various aspects of the health of prisoners, including mental illness, infectious diseases, and cancer, including a discussion of medical services provided
How to assess and treat erectile dysfunction (Emerg Med. 2004;36:28)	Uses traditional review article headings of "pathophysiology," "causes," "diagnosis," and "therapy"

"Just a cut," the authors describe a seemingly trivial finger laceration that led to a mid-forearm amputation. The article on prisoners' health includes tables on the prevalence of mental disorders, seroprevalence of markers for hepatitis B virus, and the rates of tuberculosis in prisoners in low-income countries. The erectile dysfunction article presents a textbook overview of the problem.

In each instance, the authors were writing on areas in which they worked each day. They believed that they had something to say that might help colleagues in their daily practices, and they organized their articles in ways that may enable us to remember the points made.

Many review articles are organized using one of the time-tested models. Here are three of them:

- *The approach-to-disease article.* This type of article tells how to diagnose, treat, and/or prevent a disease, such as stroke or gastric cancer.

- *The clinical manifestation/diagnosis article.* Here the author begins with a presenting symptom or clinical sign—such as backache or diplopia—and describes the path to diagnosis.
- *The organized-by-list article.* A favorite of mine, this type of article might have one of the following titles: "Five Indications for Imaging in Patients with Headache," "Seven Ways to Improve Efficiency in Your Office," or "Ten Uncommon Side Effects of Commonly Used Drugs."

Consulting with the Journal Editor

As I mentioned briefly above, I urge that you contact the journal editor, preferably by telephone. This call can help you better understand the editorial process. Making personal contact with a journal editor might not only help with the current article; it may be the beginning of a relationship that can be rewarding in the future. Medical journalism is a relatively small community, and medical editors often change jobs from one publisher to another.

Contacting the editor can also save you hours of wasted effort. It is not a good idea to prepare a review article for a favorite journal and submit the manuscript, only to have the editor reply that they have a very similar article scheduled for publication next month.

When you call the editor you should be prepared to discuss the following:

- The topic and how you will handle the subject matter
- Why you are qualified to write on this topic
- How many tables or figures you plan for the article
- When the manuscript will be completed
- If you have any possible conflict of interest

Most editors are able to give you an encouraging or dissuading answer over the telephone, which is all they can do at this time. Even if the editor likes your idea, he or she usually cannot promise acceptance without seeing the completed article. As an interim step, the editor may request to see an outline showing a draft abstract and major headings. If you submit an outline, I suggest adding a copy of your abbreviated curriculum vitae.

Special Types of Review Articles

In addition to the general categories described above, there are three special types of review articles: the literature review, the systematic review/meta-analysis, and the evidence-based clinical review. The literature review is usually recognizable, but not always. The boundaries between the systematic review and the evidence-based clinical review are often not clear.

Literature Review

The literature review is written to present the state of the art. Sometimes the authors use the phrases *literature review* or *state of the art* in the title. If not, you can usually recognize a literature review by the general title and the absence of the words such as *study of*, *clinical trial*, or *effects of*. Another tip-off that you are looking at a literature review is a long list of references, in the general range of 100, perhaps more.

In the world of medical writing, literature reviews serve several useful purposes:

- To summarize research on a topic as a bridge to applied use, that is, to present data for those who are not actively involved in the field but who need to know the latest information to provide good patient care
- To synthesize knowledge as a springboard for future research
- To support academic rigor in a field
- To serve as a database for health policy decisions

An example of literature reviews is a recent article titled "Medical Progress: Hemodialysis," presenting a discussion of "the medical, social, and economic evolution of hemodialysis therapy." The article has 95 reference citations (Himmelfarb J et al. NEJM. 2010;363:1833). Another example, conveniently labeled as a literature review, is titled "Breast Cancer During Pregnancy: A Literature Review" (Deckers S et al. Minerva Gynecol. 2010;62:585).

In the *Journal of General Internal Medicine* (JGIM) is an article titled, "Detection, Evaluation, and Treatment of Eating Disorders: The Role of the Primary Care Physician." What brought this article to my attention was the structured abstract with the headings: Objective, Design, Measurements and Main Results, and Conclusion. So far the abstract could be summarizing a research article. The tip-off that this is a review article is that, in the body of the abstract, the design is described as "A review of the literature from … ," and the conclusion is a single sentence: "Primary care providers have an important role in detecting and managing eating disorders" (Walsh JME et al. JGIM. 2000;15:577).

Another example of the state-of-the-art literature review is a thoughtful article titled "Defining and Measuring Interpersonal Continuity of Care" (Saultz JW. Ann Fam Med. 2003;1:134). This is a literature review of 146 reports on the topic of continuity of care in the clinical setting. The author provides analysis based on the commonality of findings in various diverse articles. And so the question arises: Is this article best described as a literature review or a systematic review, discussed next?

The literature review is not very difficult to write. Modern computer technology makes assembling 100 papers on a topic merely a morning's work. In this and earlier chapters, I have told you how to develop a concept and convert it into an outline. There is no reason why the beginning writer cannot create a credible state-of-the-art literature review.

There is, however, another difficulty that must be faced. A leading expert in the field usually is the person invited to write the state-of-the-art literature review on a clinical topic. Add to this fact the reality that literature reviews are often long articles—by this I mean more than 20 double-spaced manuscript pages. It takes a lot of space to catalog and discuss a hundred-plus articles on any topic. And so, when presented with a long article by an unknown author, the journal editor will look carefully to see if the author is qualified to present the state of the art to the journal's readers.

I do not wish to discourage you from writing literature reviews, but I suggest that such an effort should be done under the tutelage of an experienced and respected mentor, or perhaps postponed until you are a recognized authority on your career topic.

The Systematic Review and Meta-Analysis

Systematic reviews are actually a type of scientific investigation. What's different from clinical trials is that the "subjects" are a cluster of previous published studies that meet strict criteria. Thus, in a systematic review, the investigators cast a wide net in the ocean of bibliographic databases and then throw overboard studies that do not meet the criteria such as sufficient sample size or appropriate randomization. The process is called "systematic" because studies examined are subject to a reproducible search strategy, in contrast to a "convenience sample" of papers I happen to have in my file drawer. The chief value of systematic reviews is that they provide insights into clinical events based on data from a variety of sources, settings, and investigative approaches.

Terry and Joubert have summarized the key components of a systematic review:

- Starts with a clearly articulated question
- Uses explicit, rigorous methods to identify, critically appraise, and synthesize relevant studies
- Appraises relevant published and unpublished evidence for validity before combining and analyzing data
- Reports methodology, studies included in the review, and conclusions
- Should be reproducible [3]

Sometimes the primary studies are reviewed and summarized without attempts at statistical analysis. The product of this effort is called a qualitative systematic review. In contrast, when statistical methods are used, the result is a quantitative systematic review, or meta-analysis.

Meta-analysis is a method of combining the results of several studies into a summary conclusion, using rigorous pooling methods and quantitative strategies that will allow consideration of data found in diverse research reports. In a sense, meta-analysis is a data-oriented, statistically grounded research study *about* research studies. One source distinguishes between the systemic review and meta-analysis as follows: "A systemic review answers a defined research question by collecting and summarizing all empirical evidence that fits a pre-specified eligibility criteria. A meta-analysis is the use of statistical methods to summarize the results of these studies" [4].

Writing a meta-analysis review paper calls for a knowledge of statistical methods that is outside the scope of this book, and that is beyond the skill set of most clinician authors. This means that, if you are as statistically challenged as most of us, you should not undertake a meta-analysis without a close collaborative relationship with a coauthor who is well trained in statistical analysis.

As mentioned above, the boundaries between state-of-the-art reviews and the meta-analysis can sometimes be fuzzy. The paper titled "Parental Feeding and Childhood Obesity in Preschool-age Children: Recent Findings from the Literature" (Thompson ME et al. Issues Compr Pediatr Nurs. 2010;33:205) describes findings in 18 articles, some qualitative and some descriptive cross-sectional studies, but provides little in the way of quantitative data. Thus, this paper might be best described as a systematic review, but not a meta-analysis.

Most easily recognizable are the systematic reviews and meta-analyses that are so identified in the title. For example, consider the helpful title, "Synbiotics For Prevention And Treatment Of Atopic Dermatitis: A Meta-Analysis Of Randomized Clinical Trials" (Chang YS et al. JAMA Pediatr. 2016;170:236). The authors are very clear on what you will find in the article. In the *Clinical Psychology Review* is a report titled "Mindfulness Therapy—A Comprehensive Meta-Analysis," reporting on 209 studies enrolling 12,145 subjects (Khoury B et al. Clin Psychol Rev. 2013;33:763). A paper in the *Annals of Internal Medicine* combines the models "Calcium Intake and Cardiovascular Disease: An Updated Systematic Review and Meta-analysis" (Chung M et al. Ann Intern Med. 2016. Oct 25. doi: 10.7326/M16-1165).

The examples listed above and other similar systematic reviews often cite relative risk, odds ratios, confidence intervals, and data that are very reminiscent of reports of clinical trial research. The JAMA Instructions for Authors [5] tell that manuscripts reporting results of meta-analyses should include an abstract of no more than 350 words using the following headings: Importance, Objective, Data Sources, Study Selection, Data Extraction and Synthesis, Main Outcome(s) and Measure(s), Results, and Conclusions and Relevance. Explanations of what to include in each category are on the web site.

The tendency to consider the systematic review as a type of research places special burdens on authors. By this I mean that conclusions must be supported clearly by data and not by opinion. An article in the *Archives of Surgery* titled "Laparoscopic Surgery: An Excellent Approach In Elderly Patients" sets out to explore the following hypothesis: "A review of the literature will show that laparoscopy is safe and effective for the treatment of surgical diseases in elderly patients" (Weber DM et al. Arch Surg. 2003;138:1083). The authors selected "all relevant studies that could be obtained." Their search covered three procedures: laparoscopic cholecystectomy (16 studies), laparoscopic antireflux surgery (four studies), and laparoscopic colon resection (ten reports). Okay so far, even if the review curiously included some surgical textbooks. Their conclusions, however, seem to me to move beyond the data: "Despite underlying comorbidities, individuals older than 65 years tolerate laparoscopic procedures extremely well. Complications and hospitalization are lower than in open procedures. Surgeons need to inform primary care physicians of the excellent result of laparoscopic procedures in the elderly to encourage early referrals." Can we generalize from three procedures to *all* laparoscopic procedures in the elderly? Maybe yes, maybe no. The articles studied addressed surgical outcomes such as return of bowel function and cardiopulmonary morbidity. Did the 30 studies have anything to do with informing primary physicians? Also, even though according to the authors' criteria laparoscopic procedures had generally better surgical outcomes compared with open surgery, did the 30 studies show that *early* referrals are beneficial to the patient? A review regarding safety and efficacy of a procedure seems to have evolved to conclusions that might strike some readers as marketing. This study—which began as more or less systematic review—just might be an example of hubris, discussed in Chap. 5.

Evidence-Based Clinical Review

The evidence-based clinical review is a special type of systematic review that is focused on a clinically relevant question [2]. The emphasis is on evidence-based medicine (EBM) studies, which can be found through sites such as those listed in Table 6.3. Here is an example—Question: "Which drugs are best when aggressive Alzheimer's patients need medication?" Answer: "Atypical antipsychotics are effective; so are selective serotonin reuptake inhibitors (SSRIs), and they may be safer (Strength of recommendation [SOR]: A, multiple randomized controlled trials [RCTs])" (J Fam Pract. 2010;59(10):595–596).

Evidence-based clinical reviews pay special attention to the quality of the studies included for analysis. The US Preventive Services Task Force has been a leader in pointing out that study quality matters and that the internal validity of a study is an important consideration as well as looking at whether the authors reported a randomized clinical trial, cohort, or case-control study [6].

The journal *American Family Physician* has been a leader in advocating for the evidence-based clinical review article.

TABLE 6.3 Evidence-based medicine (EBM) sources on the web

Resource	Web site
Agency for Healthcare Research and Quality (AHRQ) is a good source for clinical guidelines and evidence reports	http://www.ahrq.gov/clinic
Bandolier contains summaries of articles on EBM	http://www.medicine.ox.ac.uk/bandolier/
Clinical Evidence, BMJ Publishing Group, presents general EBM information, EBM tools, and summaries of evidence; registration is required	http://www.clinicalevidence.com
Cochrane Database Of Systematic Review contains systematic reviews from the Cochrane Collaboration	http://www.cochrane.org
Institute for Clinical Systems Improvement (ICSI): a good site for disease management and prevention guidelines	http://www.ICSI.org
US Preventive Services Task Force presents up-to-date preventive services clinical recommendations, based on systematic reviews	http://www.ahrq.gov/professionals/clinicians-providers/guidelines-recommendations/uspstf/index.html

This journal asks authors of evidence-based clinical review articles to "rate the level of evidence for key recommendations according to the following scale: Level A (randomized controlled trial [RCT], meta-analysis), level B (other evidence), and level C (consensus/expert opinion)." Siwek et al. have written an excellent paper that I recommend to anyone planning to write an evidence-based clinical review article [2]. A more recent paper presents strength of recommendation taxonomy (SORT)to grade evidence in the medical literature [7].

Mistakes We Make When Writing Review Articles

We go wrong writing review articles in predictable ways. Since the review article is the first project many beginning medical writers undertake, I think it is useful to summarize some of the mistakes we make as neophytes. In thinking about it, some of us more experienced authors continue to make some of these errors:

- *Unimportant topic*: Do not waste effort writing a review article on a topic that no one cares about. Field-test your idea with colleagues in the office or hospital. If you are planning to write a *How to do it* article on a new way to recognize borderline personality disorder or a procedure to trim hypertrophic toenails, ask several colleagues whether they might be interested in reading such an article.
- *Stale rehash*: Be sure that you are saying something new about the topic. Step 1 is a literature search. Step 2 is a talk with a few experienceed clinicians, asking if what you propose to write about is new to them. Step 3 is a call to a journal editor. Take these steps to avoid writing an article that is not publishable because it tells nothing new.
- *A timely topic but already perhaps too timely*: As you do your literature search, you come across an article on your topic that uses the approach you planned. You may change your approach or pick another topic. Certainly you have gained useful information.
- *Getting lost along the way*: Make an outline with major headings, and stick to it. Don't wander off the path into irrelevant territory.
- *Article too long*: Some editors say that this is one of the most common problems in medical writing. Why is it, with writing being such hard work, that we often overwrite? Review articles should generally be about 16–20 double-spaced manuscript pages, including references. State-of-the-art literature reviews are the exception and may be longer.

- *Too many or too few references*: Avoid this mistake by studying similar articles published in your target journal.
- *Submission to the wrong journal:* Don't waste your time — and compromise the timeliness of your article — by submitting to journals that don't publish review articles or that are likely to accept only articles written by the internationally known expert in the field.

Summary

This chapter has been much like a review article; it had an introduction, topic development using four major headings, a summary, and a few references. In fact, this chapter could, with very little modification, be published as a journal article. The point is that classic review articles and book chapters are much alike.

There are also similarities among review articles and case reports, editorials, letters, and book reviews. On the other hand, there are important differences among these article types. In the next chapter, I discuss four more writing models.

References

1. DaCosta JC. The trials and triumphs of the surgeon. Philadelphia: Dorrance; 1944. Chapter 2.
2. Siwek J, Gourlay ML, Slawson DC, Shaughnessy AF. How to write an evidence-based clinical review article. Am Fam Phys. 2002;65(2):251–8.
3. Terry N, Joubert D. Undertaking a systematic review: what you need to know. National Institutes of Health. http://nihlibrary. campusguides.com/ld.php?content_id=1380821. Accessed 23 Mar 2017.
4. Systematic reviews and meta-analyses: a step-by-step guide. University of Edinburgh Centre for Cognitive Ageing and Cognitive Epidemiology. http://www.ccace.ed.ac.uk/research/ software-resources/systematic-reviews-and-meta-analyses. Accessed 23 Mar 2017.

5. Journal of the American Medical Association. Instructions for authors. http://jamanetwork.com/journals/jama/pages/instructions-for-authors. Accessed 23 Mar 2017.
6. US Preventive Medicine Task Force. Methods and Processes. https://www.uspreventiveservicestaskforce.org/Page/Name/methods-and-processes. Accessed 23 Mar 2017.
7. SORT: The strength-of-recommendation taxonomy. Am Fam Phys. 2016;93(8):696–7.

Chapter 7
Case Reports, Editorials, Letters to the Editor, Book Reviews, and Other Publication Models

You must be interested in writing, or you would not be here, but are you interested enough to put in some practice? What fun it can be to make a medical letter or report read well, or a case history glow like a gem. I find reviewing books, whether for a medical journal or exclusively for myself, to be fine practice. So are medical reports.

British pediatrician John Apley: "Pleasures of Medical Writing" [1]

Several writing models yield products with fewer pages than the typical review article. This does not mean that they are any easier to write or to get published. All submissions will be reviewed, either by peers or a knowledgeable editor, and there is the inevitable competition for space in every journal. However, for many clinicians and academicians, the case report, book review, or practice tip may turn out to be the pathway to an early taste of printer's ink and an entry on their curriculum vitae. Each of the models described has different characteristics, requirements, and opportunities to triumph or flounder.

© Springer International Publishing AG 2018
R.B. Taylor, *Medical Writing*,
https://doi.org/10.1007/978-3-319-70126-4_7

Case Report

The case report, sometimes called the clinical vignette, is probably the oldest model of written medical communication. As described by Jordan and Shepard, "The case report occupies a peculiar and deserved role among medical articles. Many worthwhile clinical observations do not lend themselves to controlled or scientific study but deserve recording and contribute to medical advance" [2]. For most of us, the urge to report a case occurs when we encounter a disease manifestation, therapeutic outcome, or cluster of oddities that lies so far outside our familiar realm of experience that we feel compelled to share the observation with others.

One cannot set out today to write a case report without a case. I might decide this weekend to write a review article about unusual types of primary headaches or an editorial about why we clinicians should receive more pay for what we do. But to write a case report, I need a patient with a disease, and then I must sense that there is something unusual about what I have observed or perhaps done to the patient.

When considering writing a case report, your first task is to do a literature review. You may discover that what you have found is not nearly as uncommon as you originally believed. Just because you have had your first encounter with an unexpected side effect of a drug, for example, does not mean that this side effect has not been seen and reported by several others. Even so, prior reporting validating your observation need not prevent you from writing the report. What makes a great case report is the case-related analysis that advances our collective medical knowledge.

In a sense, the case report is a focused review article. What is different is the emphasis on one or more actual cases, with a rationale for why the findings are being reported, and an evidence-based analysis of what has been found. Or there may be an unusual twist to the story. For example, one case report describes a 47-year-old Mexican woman with Huntingdon disease misdiagnosed by a *curandaro* (a Mexican folk healer) as being the victim of a magic spell. The report begins with the patient's chief complaint: "*No puedo quedarme quieta,*" which means "I can't stay still" (Penaranda EK et al. J Am Board Fam Med. 2011;24:115). Makwana et al. report an instance of a husband and his pregnant wife who were bitten by the same snake, and contrary to popular belief, the second person bit—the husband—was the more seriously affected (Makwana H et al. Int J Res Med Sci. 2015;3:3435).

Some case reports combine the clinical vignette with a literature review. One example is the report by de Gusmao et al. titled "Cerebrospinal fluid shunt-induced chorea: case report and review of the literature on shunt-related movement disorders" (de Gusmao CM et al. Pract Neuro. 2015;15:42). The case description is accompanied by 22 reference citations.

I think that the highest accolades go to those case reports that change what we do in practice. For example, Muench and Carey reported a case of a 38-year-old patient with schizophrenia who suddenly developed diabetes mellitus and ketoacidosis 12 months after starting the atypical antipsychotic medication olanzapine. The authors note that, including their case, there have been 30 such reports in the literature. What is noteworthy, in my opinion, is that on November 10, 2003, 2 years after the case report was published, my clinician colleagues and I received a "Dear Healthcare Provider" letter from a pharmaceutical manufacturer stating that "The Food and Drug Administration (FDA) has requested all manufacturers of atypical antipsychotics to include a warning regarding hyperglycemia and diabetes mellitus in their product labeling" (Muench J et al. J Am Board Fam Pract. 2001;14:278; and Letter from Janssen Pharmaceutica, Inc., dated November 10, 2003). This report and others on this topic appear to have prompted the FDA's action.

Some case reports are published as letters to the editor. Shortly I will discuss letters to the editor as a model of medical writing. Here I will offer one example of a letter-style case report: In the correspondence section of the *New England Journal of Medicine* (NEJM), Gordon et al. describe a case in which acetazolamide was used to treat lithium-induced diabetes insipidus (Gordon CE et al. NEJM. 2016;375:2008).

Types of Case Report

There are fundamentally two types of case report. The first is the observation of some unusual disease manifestation occurring in a single patient. For most clinicians, this is your most likely pathway to a published case report. One example is a report of an unusual lesion of the finger in a 53-year-old man, with some excellent color photos of a superficial acral fibromyxoma of the index finger (Meyerle JH et al. J Am Acad Dermatol. 2004;50:134). Diagnostic images or photographs greatly enhance the "single-patient" case report. In the end, this type of report must derive its value from the novelty of the finding and the perception that other physicians should be aware of your case.

Another example of the single-patient case report, bolstered by a catchy, but descriptive, title and a literature review, is the article by Cumberledge et al. titled "Risking life and limb: a case of spontaneous muscle infarction (diabetic myonecrosis)" (Cumberledge J et al. JGIM. 2016;31:696).

The second type of case report includes more than one observation. It may be several patients with an uncommon disease, such as an increased incidence of leukemia in a single neighborhood. Or perhaps you have recently encountered three young adult patients with argyria (silver poisoning). An example from the literature describes a cluster of blastomycosis victims in a rural community (Proctor ME et al. Mycopathologia. 2002;153:113).

Format for the Case Report

Itskowitz and Lebovitz report a case of a 77-year-old woman who was not taking antibiotics and who nevertheless developed pseudomembranous colitis (PMC) (Itskowitz MS et al. Adv Stud Med. 2003;3:571). In their article the authors present the classic format for a case report:

- *Introduction*: The first paragraph discusses why the case is unusual: "Almost all cases of PMC reported during the past three decades have been associated with antimicrobial use." This seems to be a valid justification for the report. As a practicing clinician, I need to know that non-antibiotic-associated PMC can occur.

- *Case description*: The authors present the relevant data, including medical history, physical findings, results of tests and procedures, and treatment received.
- *Literature review*: Nine instances of non-antibiotic-related PMC were found in the literature.
- *Discussion*: Here the authors discuss microflora of the intestine and other possible causes of PMC.
- *Conclusion*: What it all means is this: "When more common causes of acute enteritis and colitis have been ruled out, PMC should be considered in patients who develop persistent diarrhea, even without a history of antibiotic use."
- *References*: Sixteen references are listed. I think this number is about right. The case report is not intended to be a state-of-the-art literature review.

The case report should not be too long. If your case report exceeds 12 double-spaced manuscript pages, consider cutting.

What about the "first ever" report? Mukherjee and Shivakumar report a case of sensorineural hearing loss following ingestion of sildenafil (Viagra). These authors write: "We could not find any previously reported cases of sildenafil induced hearing loss and to the best of our knowledge, this is the first case report of sildenafil induced sensorineural hearing loss in the world literature" (Mukherjee B et al. J Laryngol Otol. 2007;121:395). This is a bold assertion, somehow especially since I now note that hearing loss is currently reported as a concern on television commercials for popular drugs for erectile dysfunction. Just to check, I searched two of my favorite sites—PubMed and Google Scholar—and could not find an earlier report. It seems that Mukherjee and Shivakumar may be justified in their "first ever" assertion.

The sildenafil/deafness connection represented a new and unexpected side effect of a popular drug. Such instances are not extremely rare, and the subsequent case reports are valuable additions to the literature. Newly discovered syndromes can be another thing altogether. I suggest that you think twice before you claim to have elucidated a new syndrome. Such hubris may be severely criticized. If you have, in fact, found the first case ever of jejunal pregnancy, your colleagues—not you—should record your primacy.

Then there is the topic apparently not previously studied. In a 2016 Research Letter in JAMA, there is a report titled "Association between In-Hospital Critical Illness Events and Outcomes in Patients on the Same Ward." The authors state, "To our knowledge, no study has quantified the risk to ward occupants associated with patients on the same ward experiencing critical illness" (Volchenboum SL et al. JAMA. 2016;316:2674).

Editorial

Editorials are fun to write. They are generally short and thus do not take weeks of labor. They rely on your experience and intuition and thereby don't always call for a major research effort. And they allow you to express your opinion. Unfortunately, not too many beginning writers have the chance to write and publish editorials. But some are successful.

The term *editorial* comes from the word *editor*. The connotation is that the writing is by the publisher, the editor, or a designated authority. The topic usually reflects the individual's opinion, and you may see the term *op-ed*, short for opinion-editorial. Today, journal editors are busy producing budgets and correcting errors of careless authors, and they often lack the specialized knowledge to produce the expert content needed, so they do not write all editorials.

There are fundamentally two types of editorial not authored by the editors themselves: those invited by the editor or publisher and those that are volunteered. Invited editorials may be focused, as in an invitation to comment on a specific research study being published, or the invitation may be open-ended: "Would you care to write an editorial for a coming issue of the journal?" Such an invitation is sometimes related to an upcoming theme issue of the journal, perhaps on a topic such as advances in robotic surgery or issues in medical student education. These open-ended invitations usually are extended to prestigious experts in their fields or members of the journal's editorial board.

Most journals publish editorials; the September 8, 2016, issue of the *New England Journal of Medicine* has two articles under the heading "Editorials" and four other items under the heading "Perspective" that also seem to me to be op-ed pieces. The November 14, 2016, issue of *British Medical Journal* (BMJ)-USA has 10—count' em, 10—articles that qualify as editorials. In fact, it seems to me that journals today are publishing more editorials, and less research reports, than ever.

Your best chance of having an editorial published is to submit a brilliantly written opinion piece on a topic about which you have special knowledge. For example, those who practice in Oregon have enjoyed a unique opportunity with the Oregon Health Plan. This innovative plan "provides health-care coverage for low-income Oregonians from all walks of life" [3] by explicitly rationing health care according to "the list"—a catalog of diagnosis–treatment pairs laboriously negotiated with attention to fairness and to efficacy of interventions. A number of Oregon physicians have written editorials about this plan, with their chief authority being that they practice in the state of Oregon.

Some Types of Editorials

The Salesmanship Editorial

Such editorials are really prefaces to an issue of the journal. They usually begin, "In this issue of the journal, we present...." Then the editor goes on to tell why they chose to publish the five studies on amino acids in rat livers that occupy the pages that follow.

The Editor's Opinion

In the April 11, 2015, issue of *The Lancet*, editor in chief Richard Horton makes a startling statement. He opines, "The case against science is straightforward: much of the scientific literature, perhaps half, may simply be untrue. Afflicted by studies with small sample sizes, tiny effects, invalid exploratory analyses, and flagrant conflicts of interest, together with an obsession for pursuing fashionable trends of dubious importance, science has taken a turn toward darkness" (Horton R. The Lancet. 2015;385:1380). Wow! This is an editorial sure to spark controversy. But it would only have credibility if authored by someone with highly respected qualifications.

Editorial Comment Accompanying a Published Study

"It is easy to imagine why children who are raised on farms might grow up healthy: There is plenty of fresh air, exercise and exposure to sunlight.... Surprisingly, according to the findings of Ege and colleagues in this issue of the Journal, the mechanism responsible for these health effects appears not to be related to clean living but instead to bacteria and fungi from the barnyard...." So begins an invited editorial (Gern JE. N Engl J Med. 2011;364:769) commenting on a research report titled "Exposure to Environmental Microorganisms and Childhood Asthma," published in the same issue of the NEJM.

The *Journal of the American Medical Association* (JAMA) published a research report on the effect of cranberry capsules on bacteria plus pyuria among older women in nursing homes (Juthani-Mehta et al. JAMA. 2016;316:1839). I am sad to report that the berries were no more effective than placebo. The research report is accompanied by an editorial authored by an internist who, after some paragraphs discussing the study, concludes, "It is time to move on from cranberries" (Colaizy TT. JAMA. 2016;316:1873).

As mentioned above, this type of editorial is an opportunity for the clinician to offer a "frontline" viewpoint. I suggest that practicing clinicians write to the editors of their favorite journals, offering to submit "invited commentary" related to research articles accepted for publication. Be sure that your letter is very well written, since this and the curriculum vitae that you include are the evidence the editor considers in deciding whether or not to invite you to contribute.

Sharing Special Insight

In the *Journal of General Internal Medicine* (JGIM), an editorial considers homelessness as a health hazard. The author, unknown to me, lists his name and affiliation as Jeff Singer, MSW, Health Care for the Homeless, Inc., Baltimore, MD. I strongly suspect that Mr. Singer has firsthand knowledge of the problems described in his editorial (Singer J. JGIM. 2003;18:964).

Sometimes a journal editor requests an editorial from an individual known to have a special viewpoint on a controversial topic. The journal can then publish the editorial, with the disclaimer that the opinion expressed is that of the author and does not necessarily reflect the opinion of the journal or publisher. Nevertheless, the journal editor got what was wanted in print.

Special insight editorials often concern health policy. I especially enjoyed the title of an editorial discussing uncertainty about the constitutionality of the Affordable Care Act (ACA): "Can Congress Make You Buy Broccoli? And Why That's A Hard Question" (Mariner et al. NEJM. 2011:364:201).

And then sometimes an author just can't take it anymore. I think this sort of frustration must have been behind a wonderful editorial in *The Pharos* titled, "Information And Cognitive Overload: How Much Is Too Much?" (Byyny RL. The Pharos. August 2016:2).

Writing an Editorial

Classically, an editorial is a critical argument, expressing an opinion without being opinionated. As such it should develop the thesis in a logical manner:

- *Present the problem.* Begin by telling your reader the issue you are addressing. The first sentence is a good place to do this, though it may require the entire opening paragraph: "Cardiac arrest is a leading cause of death in the developed world. In the US, more than 500,000 patients die from a cardiac arrest every year. The public health impact of cardiac arrest in the UK is also quite substantial. While mortality is high, even those who survive a cardiac arrest are at a significant risk of permanent neurological damage. Thus, improving survival and reducing neurological disability is a fundamental goal of patient care and a priority for public health" (Girotra S. Critical Care. 2016;20:304).

  Another way to introduce the problem is to use a vignette, sometimes called "the hook" in nonmedical writing. For example, the editorial on homelessness as a health hazard (mentioned above) begins, "Jim, a Korean War veteran in his seventies, lives in a '79 Cadillac. Unable to afford housing, his hygiene is quite poor; access to water is limited to restaurant bathrooms…."

- *Provide an early clue as to where you are headed.* The ACA/broccoli editorial begins as follows: "The continuing uncertainty over the constitutionality of the Affordable Care Act (ACA), illustrated by conflicting trial court rulings and scholarly commentaries, raises the question of why this constitutional question is so hard to answer. There are at least four reasons."

  Here the authors have provided a clear indication of what will follow, that is, a four-part discussion.

- *Offer evidence to support your opinions.* Here is where you should visit the literature and offer an evidence-based argument. Select your references carefully, to avoid allowing your editorial to become a review article.

- *Describe your personal insight.* What you are writing is, after all, your own opinion. It is okay to say what you think. It is even better to back up this opinion with a personal anecdote—the concrete example that breathes life into your general statements.

- *Offer counterevidence.* Not everyone will agree with you. Present the other side of the issue in an unbiased and respectful manner, and then say why you are not convinced.
- *Provide a summary.* A single closing paragraph is usually all that is needed at this point. Describe your conclusion, ideally linking what you write here to what you said in paragraph one. Perhaps include the implications of your conclusion to practice or to society. Then stop.
- *List your reference sources.* I rarely write an editorial without references, but I only include a few.
- *Include headings, sometimes.* Your editorial may include headings to break up the flow of prose and to help the reader remember the structure of your article. Headings are especially useful for long editorials.
- *Avoid overused terms and phrases.* The executive editor of JAMA, in a 2014 editorial in his own journal, advises against using shopworn terms such as "paradigm shift," "call to action," "dramatically increased," and any form of the word "impact," whether as a verb, noun, or modifier (impactful) [4].

Letter to the Editor

In 1904, more than 100 years ago, a reader identified only as E.G. wrote to the JAMA editor, "Your editorial Jan. 9, 1904, discussing why scientists are poor writers, aroused my spirit of refutation, because I think your point is not well taken..." (E.G. Why Are Scientists Poor Writers? (letter). JAMA. 1904;42:470, 477). Today, letters to the editor are very popular, with both readers and publishers.

Most journals publish letters to the editor, and journal editors are pleased when there is lively discussion in the "Letters" column, as readers indulge their spirit of refutation and debate the merits of published articles. Sometimes they share new ideas. Some journals such as the BMJ and the *Journal of the American Board of Family Practice*

(JABFP) post letters and comments online, allowing a "rapid response" by readers. In fact, as I discuss in Chap. 12, I think this interactive modality is a key to the future of medical publishing.

Letters to the editor offer a wonderful opportunity for the aspiring medical writer. There is no requirement that the author is a distinguished professor, no randomized clinical trial is needed, and there is a reasonable chance of publication, at least in the journals that have limited readership. LaVigne advocates for this type of writing model: "Letters to the editor merit your consideration as a publication option: first, because letters and short pieces stand a better chance of being published than longer articles, and second, because published letters to the editor generally are titled and indexed, thus making them retrievable as articles in the journal" [5].

The academic clinician will note that, even though letters are not always refereed, published letters, being indexed, are legitimate entries on a curriculum vitae. Whether or not one should list "rapid responses" on one's curriculum vitae is a gray area.

Types of Letters

There are many types of letter to the editor. Here are some of them:

Attaboy

Three Stanford University School of Medicine professors wrote commenting on a "perspective" paper published in the NEJM on teaching medical students about cost consciousness in patient care (Cooke M. NEJM. 2010;362:1253). The letter begins, "We commend Cooke's efforts in her Perspective article to increase readers' awareness of the near-universal ignorance of actual costs associated with the delivery of medical care" (Rivas M et al. NEJM. 2010;363:888).

Note the prestigious academic affiliation of the letter writers. In my opinion, such a letter written by the average clinician has little chance of being published. In fact, I really don't think that the authors added anything to our fund of medical knowledge regarding an important topic, and probably the journal space could have been better used in some other way.

Something to Add

As a practicing clinician, you may have a thought that expands the knowledge presented in an article. Perhaps you have seen an illustrative case, and your fellow clinicians would benefit from the knowledge. In response to an article in *American Family Physician* (AFP) about management of diabetic foot ulcers, two readers wrote to add the following: "An effective adjunctive therapy for wound debridement that was not mentioned is maggot therapy" (Summers JB et al. AFP. 2003;68:2327). They support their addition with a clear discussion and six references.

Responding to an article about doctors rushing patients through the office, a reader offers, "The recent editorial in *The Pharos* 'Time matters in caring for patients', a concise summary of the evolution of medical practice compensation, prompted me to consider my own experience with health care." He goes on to describe indifferent providers, inadequate physical examinations, and more, supporting the thesis of the original editorial (Lorenz R. The Pharos. Summer, 2016).

Differing Perspective

In August 2010, the NEJM published an article describing the risk of suicide-related events in depressed patients treated with antiepileptic drugs (Arana A et al. NEJM. 2010;363(6):542–551).

Offering another viewpoint, Zebley and Ferrando write, "We would be cautious in interpreting these findings, since antiepileptic drugs are rarely used in the management of depression, except among a subgroup of patients with a particularly high risk of suicide" (Zebley M et al. NEJM. 2010;363:1873).

Disagreement

Sometimes one just disagrees with something written in an article. An editorial in *The Lancet* criticizes United Kingdom Health Secretary Andrew Lansley for inviting soft drink, fast food, and adult beverage manufacturers to submit suggestions as to how to deal with issues of obesity, alcohol misuse, and diet-related diseases. Lansley fires back: "The accusation in your editorial of Nov 27 (p 1800) that I am 'putting the interests of big business at the heart of public-health policy' is quite simply wrong. Setting the agenda on public health is and will always remain the responsibility of government" (Lansley A. The Lancet. 2011;377:121).

A letter writer may also put forward another opinion. Writing to comment on a JAMA Clinical Challenge article, three letter writers take issue with an article in which "Dr. Ardalan and colleagues described a patient with arthralgia and fevers accompanied by a papulonodular rash, which was diagnosed as erythema nodosum and an adverse reaction to azathioprine... We have some skepticism about the diagnosis of erythema nodosum and believe neutrophilic dermatosis should be considered" (Sarantopoulos A et al. JAMA. 2016;316:1827).

Statement of Concern

In 2010 the NEJM published a report on the use of an oral spleen tyrosine kinase inhibitor in the treatment of rheumatoid arthritis. A letter from a reader questions the study's inclusion criteria: "Since the cornerstone of the treatment of rheumatoid arthritis is the optimal use of methotrexate, with a progressive increase of the dose up to 20–25 mg per week, we find it quite surprising that the inclusion criteria allowed the enrollment of patients with a suboptimal response to just 7.5 mg per week of methotrexate" (Otón T et al. NEJM. 2011;364:83).

Something That Must Be Shared

This type of letter is really a short editorial. Without reference to any published article, a reader wrote to discuss the issue of standard of care. "Medicine is not exact, and bad outcomes happen. The notion that physicians can follow a formula and avoid successful litigation is false" (Grant DC. Ann Emerg Med. 2004;43:139).

Another writer describes "Music of the Heart," in a letter that begins: "The mysterious power that music wields over many people has long been linked to its resonance with biological rhythms such as the heartbeat, and to its parallels with the intonations and cadences of spoken language." He goes on to discuss the specific role of music in diagnosis and treatment (Field MJ. The Lancet. 2010;376:2074).

Uninvited "Sounding Off" letters must be timely, pertinent, and very well written if they are to be published.

Gotcha

In the December 1, 2016, issue of the *New England Journal of Medicine*, we find: "Pocock and Stone provide an excellent primer on evaluations of clinical trials and their applications to practice. However, early on in their article they make a common but erroneous statement regarding the nature of the P value: 'A P of 0.05 carries a 5% risk of a false positive result.' This misconception is found throughout statistical and medical literature and was recently addressed ... by the American Statistical Association." (Hu D. NEJM 2016;375:2205). Gotcha!

Transformed Review Article

Whenever I read a case report or an account of original research presented as a letter to the editor, I often pause to reflect that the letter probably began life in a more robust form.

As a full article, it was submitted and peer reviewed—several times. The authors endured a few rejections by prestigious journals, until a sympathetic editor suggested that, if the findings could be shortened to 500–600 words, the work could be published as a letter. In football, this is the equivalent of an 85-yard drive with multiple first downs and then settling for a field goal. With understandable ambivalence, the authors cut the article mercilessly and accepted publication of their case or research report as a letter to the editor. I recently walked this path with an article on "imprecision" in pharmaceutical advertisements published in otherwise respectable medical journals. The article, titled "Pharmaceutical Advertisements, Citations, and Trust," ended up published as a letter to the editor (Taylor RB. Fam Med. 2010;42:744). The good news: The article—correction, letter—is off my desk, the citation to the letter is online, and I can move on.

Research Letter

Sometimes a research study is published as a letter, with headings just like those in a formal research report: Introduction, Methods, Results, and so forth. An example is the research letter published in the September 13, 2016, issue of JAMA titled "Five-Year Survival After Endosonography vs Mediastinoscopy Nodal Staging of Lung Cancer" (Kuijvenhoven JC et al. JAMA 2016;316:1110).

Writing the Letter

The successful letter to the editor is often more the result of inspiration than persistence. The urge to write a letter will often strike you when reading a journal article, and you think: I know something special about this topic or have an opinion that is important. You then do some research, and the letter, which should be fairly short, will seem to write itself. Of course, as mentioned above, some letters do not comment on published articles.

Think of the letter to the editor as a tightly packaged combination of an editorial and a focused literature review. Limit yourself to making a single point. Do not try to combine two or more ideas into a short letter. In writing, you should select each word with care to stay within tight limits imposed by most journals. Even though you are likely to be acting upon an inspirational urge, you must craft your letter skillfully if it is to be accepted for publication.

Most letters to the editor comment on published articles, and, in these instances, there is a general structure that the letter should follow:

- *Identify the paper.* In the first sentence, cite the paper that is the subject of your comments. This becomes your Reference 1.
- *State why you are writing.* State your agreement, disagreement, concern, or other reason for writing.
- *Give evidence.* The evidence may be from the literature or from personal experience. Literature-based evidence is better.
- *Provide a summary statement.* Conclude by tying all the above together.
- *Cite references.* A letter to the editor will generally have a few reference citations, especially if offering new or contrary evidence.

Do not begin writing without reading the instructions to authors for the journal. Most instructions list requirements for submitted letters, which include a deadline for receipt. The *Journal of the American Medical Association*, for example, states, "Letters discussing a recent article in this journal should be submitted within 4 weeks of publication of the article in a formal print/online issue. Letters received after 4 weeks will rarely be considered. Letters should not exceed 400 words of text and 5 references, 1 of which should be to the recent article. Letters may have no more than 3 authors" [6].

The letter to the editor should be submitted online—just as you would a review article. The letter manuscript should then be sent with a cover message indicating that you are submitting the letter for publication and not merely to communicate with the editor. You should mention any special attributes that qualify you to write on the topic and reveal any potential conflicts of interest.

Two final cautions: First, if you are personally acquainted with the author of the article you plan to discuss in your letter, you may not want to write at all. If you applaud the study, your praise may be suspect. Worse, if you criticize even some small part of the study, your comments may be interpreted as a personal attack.

And second, not every letter to the editor you write should be mailed. If you have composed a letter that might be perceived as mean-spirited or even excessively clever, put it aside for a few days. After the cooling-off period, you may decide to keep the letter in your files, saving yourself some embarrassment while unintentionally doing the journal editor and your potential readers a favor.

Book Review

Laura Hole, pediatric registrar in Bristol, UK, wrote a review of a book by Gardner M et al. titled *Training in Paediatrics* (London: Oxford; 2009). Her review begins with this engaging first paragraph: "I was thrilled to commence my first book review. The opportunity to condemn the hard work of a faceless colleague with my carefully selected witty words of deprecation seemed irresistible. Sadly, this was not to be as I'm sorry to say *Training in Paediatrics* is rather good" (Hole L. Arch Dis Child. 2009;95:659).

In 2010, Lee et al. published a guide to writing scholarly book reviews for publication in peer-reviewed journals, describing book reviewing as a "fine art," and presenting a recommended strategy and a book appraisal worksheet [7].

Salager-Meyer offers insight into the evolution of the tone and language of medical book reviews over the years, first describing the mid-twentieth century, when reviews were often laced with "face-threat intensity" and language that was "emotional, devastating, and even down-grading." She cites published comments such as "blatant attack on intellectual inquiry" and "The advice to the would-be buyer is simple: Don't (buy the book)." Today's reviews, in contrast, tend to be more civil and matter-of-fact, a welcome change for us all [8]. Thus Dr. Hole, mentioned above, did not take her opportunity to pen "selected witty words of deprecation."

Some, but not all, journals publish book reviews. Such reviews are found in the *Journal of the American Osteopathic Association*, *The Lancet*, *The Pharos*, and *Family Medicine*. Not all reviews are of medical reference and textbooks. A few journals discuss movies (see below), and reviews of medical software are now sometimes seen.

I am sorry to report that many journals, such as the *New England Journal of Medicine* and *American Family Physician*, once published book reviews but no longer do so. I consider this a loss to aspiring authors, potential reviewers, and clinician readers.

The journal editor or the journal's book review editor almost always invites book reviews. Occasionally an eager writer submits an unsolicited book review, but I doubt that many are published. Unsolicited reviews are suspect and editors need not take chances.

On the other hand, you can offer to become a book reviewer. Any literate clinician can volunteer. Do so by identifying your one or two chief areas of clinical expertise, and then write to the journal editor offering your services. If selected to write a review, you will receive a copy of the book, which is yours to keep as payment for your contribution.

Published book reviews are appropriate entries on your academic curriculum vitae.

Types of Book Review

Technically speaking, there are not different types of book reviews, but there are various approaches to the task. They are not mutually exclusive and more than one can be used in a single review. Whatever your approach, construct your book review with the same care and economy of words that you would devote to a review paper or research report.

Review in Relationship to the Author's Stated Purpose

I believe that all reviews should follow this approach, at least at the outset. I am a book author and editor, and I always begin my preface with a description of the intent of the book. For example, the Preface to this book begins with this statement: "This book is intended to make you a better medical writer." I begin my prefaces in this fashion for the reviewer, as well as the reader. I earnestly hope that the reviewer will judge my work against my intention and not against the book the reviewer *wishes* I had written. Also, as a reviewer, please do not review the book in comparison with the book that you wish *you* had written.

The reviewer who described *Atlas of Clinical Sleep Medicine* (Kryger MH. Philadelphia: Saunders/Elsevier; 2010) provides a good example critiquing the book in context of the author or editor's stated intent: "The editor of the *Atlas of Clinical Sleep Medicine* states in the preface that his aim was to create a resource that would transmit state-of-the-art knowledge about sleep medicine not just with words but also through images and sound. The result is a lavishly illustrated and well-written textbook that does exactly what it set out to do" (Rosen D. JAMA. 2010;304:2069).

Comparison to a Classic or Standard in the Field

Every field in medicine has two or three standard reference books, such as Harrison's *Principles of Internal Medicine* or Nelson's *Textbook of Pediatrics*. If and when a new book is published to challenge the champion, it is only fair that the reviewer make a comparison with the traditional front-runner.

The Biopsy of Favorite Topics

One approach to assessing the value of a book is to look up your favorite topic—for example, myocarditis, breast cancer, or myositis ossificans—in the index. Is the topic covered in the book? If so, is the information complete and timely? In your review, tell the reader what you found.

An example, perhaps an extreme example, of the biopsy approach appears in the *Croatian Medical Journal*. The review discusses one of my favorite books, a catalog of etymologic origins of medical words (Haubrich WS. *Medical meanings: a glossary of word origins*. Philadelphia: American College of Physicians, 1997). The review says a little about the book and then goes on to discuss an example for each letter of the alphabet from "A" ("ARTERY is a derivation of a Greek word for an air duct") to Z ("ZYGOMATIC was taken from the Greek *zygon*, 'a yoke or crossbar by which two draft animals can be hitched to a plow or wagon'") (Marusiae A. Croat Med J. 1999;40:38).

On a more practical level, if I were reviewing a comprehensive reference on obstetrics, I might check how the author handles specific topics such as placenta previa or antibiotic use during pregnancy. In a pediatrics text, I might check current immunization recommendations, since they change a little from year to year.

Overview with Criticism: Balancing Good Features with Problems

In assessing a 219-page book about breast cancer (Walker RA. *Prognostic and predictive factors in breast cancer*. New York: Martin Dunitz; 2003), the reviewer states, "*Prognostic and Predictive Factors in Breast Cancer* is a well-written, compact reference book." On balance, he goes on to observe, "The biggest problem with a book that attempts to review fast-moving fields such as breast cancer is that by the time it is published, some material is obsolete and the newest areas are not covered. For instance, this book has no discussion of sentinel-node analysis and clinical trials of trastuzumab, which were still in progress when it was written" (Rimm D. N Engl J Med. 2004;350:200).

A book review always has more credibility when the reviewer offers some suggestion for improvement. Can you trust a uniformly laudatory review? As an example, a review of Stuart and Lieberman's *The Fifteen Minute Hour: Therapeutic Talk In Primary Care, Fifth Edition* (London/ New York: Radcliff; 2015) describes the work as "a wonderful book for anyone working in primary care, and this new fifth edition raises the bar one step higher" (Schneiderhan J. Fam Med. 2016;48:741). Try as I might, I could not find a hint of criticism. I am sure this review warmed the hearts of the authors and publisher, but it offered no hints as to how the sixth edition could be even better.

How to Write the Book Review

In broad terms, the approach varies with the type of book reviewed. If the book is a text, intended for students, clarity is most important, and the occasional minor spelling error is less egregious. What is crucial is the book's ability to provide the student with concepts and templates that can aid in future learning.

The medical reference book is a different story. Here the book reviewer must assess the factual accuracy of the book. As Day states, "Any professional librarian will tell you that an inaccurate reference book is worse than none at all" [9]. Clinical decisions will be made based on what is in the pages. It seems melodramatic to say that a factual error on the page could kill a patient, but conceivably this could happen. (I will say more about errors in Chap. 12).

Book reviews follow a pattern: They begin by identifying the topic of the book being reviewed, often with a verbal image that draws us in to read further. Then comes the analysis of the work, including good points and any deficiencies. Finally there is the summary, including who might want to read this book. An online tutorial on writing book reviews advises: "There is, of course, no set formula, but a general rule of thumb is that the first one-half to two-thirds of the review should summarize the author's main ideas and at least one-third should evaluate the book" [10].

Beginning the Review

Since book reviews should not be too long, it is a good idea to start the first paragraph by giving a strong hint of your overall assessment. Here is a classic example, describing the Silberman's *NeuroTribes: The Legacy of Autism and The Future of Neurodiversity* (New York: Avery. 2015): "This is a remarkable book by a journalist who has done rigorous research and writes with consummate skill to help the reader understand the enigma of the modern epidemic of autism" (reviewed by Bennahum DA. The Pharos. Summer 2016;53).

With a little more flair: "*Black Lung* is a scholarly work, a grim story, grimly told" (Cameron IA. Review of: Derickson A. Black lung: anatomy of a public health disaster [Ithaca, NY: Cornell Univ Press, 1998]. The Pharos 2002;65:50).

One enthusiastic reader begins by stating, "I really liked this book" (Neelon FA. Review of: Bittersweet: diabetes, insulin and the transformation of illness. [Chapel Hill, NC: University of North Carolina Press; 2003.] JAMA 2004;291:745).

Good Points and Bad

Here is one example of the counterpoint of good versus not so good. In discussing a book about "giving news" in both everyday talk and clinical settings, the reviewer offers praise: "Readers will come to understand the sequential steps that make up 'giving news,' just what makes information into news, and the different sequences we use to deliver good news and bad." On balance the reviewer continues, "However, the reader not already familiar with linguistic terms may find the book's terminology a bit over-technical" (Platt FW. Review of: Bad news, good news: conversational order in everyday talk and clinical settings [Chicago: University of Chicago Press; 2003]. JAMA. 2003;290:3256).

One more example of the balanced approach, from a review on American colonial medicine: On the plus side, the reviewer states, "*Medicine in Colonial America* is chocka-block with detail presented in a clear writing style, covering a large territory in easy fashion—a good introduction to the novice." And yet, on the other hand, "There are a few errors. Samuel Johnson is misidentified as Ben Johnson" (Murray TJ. Review of: Reiss O. Medicine in colonial America [Lanham, MD: University Press of America; 2000]. The Pharos 2002;65(2):41).

I have been blessed with some kind, yet balanced, reviews of the first two editions of this book on medical writing. One reviewer failed to resonate with some of my humor. Another pointed out that my discussion of packing a manuscript for mailing was anachronistic. Yet another review suggested a need for increased discussion of tables and figures. These and a few other criticisms—obviously intended to balance lavish praise—were instrumental in the decision to prepare a second, and now a third edition of the book, with errors, over-sights, and anachronisms corrected.

When you are writing a book review, the body of the review should answer many of the questions listed in Table 7.1.

The Reviewer's Conclusion

In the end, the reviewer should summarize his or her opinion of the book and which readers are likely to find it useful. In the review of the book *Prognostic and Predictive Factors in Breast Cancer* cited above, the reviewer ends by stating that it "will be a valuable addition to libraries, especially at teach-ing institutions" (Rimm D. Review of Walker RA. Prognostic and predictive factors in breast cancer [New York: Martin Dunitz; 2003]. N Engl J Med. 2004;350:200–201). The pub-lisher may not be overjoyed by this summary, since libraries at teaching institutions are a very small market. For a book to be successful, it must appeal to a larger market, generally of practicing clinicians.

TABLE 7.1 Questions for the book reviewer

Is the book's topic important?
Is the information timely?
Is the content appropriate for the intended audience?
Is the book appropriately organized?
Is the writing clear?
Is the style consistent throughout the book?
Is my favorite topic covered appropriately?
Has the author included appropriate tables and figures?
Are there misspellings and minor errors?
Are there significant errors of fact?
What has been left out?
Is the index adequate to find what I want to find?
Is the book worth the cost?
Does the book fulfill its stated purpose?
How does this book compare to other similar books?
Do you recommend the book and, if so, for which readers?

Contrast this summary with the review by Feldman, which enthusiastically concludes, "*The Atlas of Diagnostic Oncology* is a comprehensive, well-organized, and beautifully illustrated overview of diagnostic oncology. Its multidisciplinary nature will make it a useful educational tool and reference text for practicing physicians and trainees in all fields involving the care of patients with cancer" (Feldman AL. JAMA. 2011;305:306).

What Makes an Excellent Book Review and What Does Not

The excellent book review is informative and brightly written. It offers a personal judgment of the merits of the book, it addresses how the book treats the topic, and it does not rehash the topic itself. But the review must not be excessively amusing. In writing the book review, there is a great temptation for the reviewer to attempt to outshine the author.

With that said, good book reviews often add a little extra. A review of *Dorland's Medical Dictionary* begins by providing some new information. I enjoyed learning the following: "Who uses a medical dictionary? It may surprise some that physicians are probably not the principal users, but rather medical students, other health care professionals, medical transcriptionists, and perhaps even lawyers and journalists" (Fortuine R. JAMA. 2003;290:3225).

I felt compelled to read the review that began, "Have you ever wondered, after a hard week at work, why you decided to become a doctor? If so, you might want to read this book" (McClure I. Review of: Baiev K. The oath: a surgeon under fire [New York: Simon and Schuster; 2003]. BMJ. 2004;328:354).

Sometimes a review walks a fine line between writing vividly and being too clever. In reviewing a book that presents arguments against evolutionary psychology, the reviewer begins, "The contributors to the volume—an eclectic mix of biologists, sociologists, and philosophers—evidently feel about evolutionary psychology the way I feel about squirrels who steal food from the bird feeders in my backyard" (Perlman R. Review of: Rose H, Rose S, eds. Alas, poor Darwin: arguments against evolutionary psychology [New York: Harmony Books; 2000]. The Pharos. 2002;65(3):48–49). Certainly this reviewer is assuming the "rhetorical persona of the book reviewer," described by Salager-Meyer [8].

And sometimes, the reviewer is much too witty for even my taste. The following is the beginning of a review of a book on alternative medicine in America: "Medical doctors and naturopaths work together to manage the publicly-funded King County Natural Medicine Clinic in Seattle. Is this a manifestation of Northwestern coffee intoxication?" (Zaroff L. Review of: Whorton JC. Nature cure: the history of alternative medicine in America [New York: Oxford University Press; 2002]. The Pharos. 2003;66:38).

Yes, I am well aware of the irony that I am reviewing the writing of reviewers. And I am doing so without offering them an opportunity for rebuttal.

Cautions When Writing a Book Review

I have at times been asked to review a book that might be perceived to compete with one of my own books. For example, I have written a book on back-stories of medical history [11]. If I am asked to review a similar book, I will decline. There would be a genuine conflict of interest. This, of course, means that during the publication life of *Medical Writing: A Guide for Clinicians, Educators, and Researchers*, I should also not review any books on medical writing.

The second caution concerns professional relationships. In a critical survey of articles about writing book reviews, Lee et al. point out, "Interestingly, the authors of books under review may be the most avid readers of book reviews. Authors have invested much time and effort into writing their books, and it is not surprising that an author would be curious about how other scholars perceive their books" [7]. I consider the word "curious" here to be a huge understatement. The author will feel the pain of every unfavorable word. Criticizing an author's book in print is like striking someone's child. Even in a balanced review, the negative comments can be taken very personally. If you are asked to review a book written or edited by a colleague who is a personal acquaintance, I suggest that you pass the opportunity to someone else. Declining the review helps assure an unbiased evaluation of the book, and it can prevent the loss of a friend.

As I end my discussion of book reviews, I must mention the issue of *bogus* book reviews online and even the practice of offering bribes for reviews. In 2009, the web site Public Citizen reported a major publisher offering "a copy of the book under review as well as a $25 Amazon gift card" for posting a review to the Amazon or Barnes & Noble web site [12]. The publisher was Elsevier and what happened is confirmed in a comment by the book's editor on its Amazon page: Richard DCS et al., eds. *Clinical Psychology, Assessment, Treatment, and Research*. New York: Academic Press, 2008. I am inclined to believe the claim of the book's lead editor that he and his coeditor were innocent victims of this unfortunate bribery attempt.

Other Medical Publication Models

There are other medical publication opportunities. If you have a special interest, such as poetry or medical history, you might want to consider one of the following. I have listed some journals as examples; I am confident that the models described are found in a variety of publications. If you aspire to write in any of these models, be sure to first identify your target publication, and prepare your submission so that it looks like those that have been published.

Poetry

JAMA publishes a regular column titled "Poetry and Medicine." Some other journals do also. Some recently published JAMA poems have been titled "Lucky," "Superior Canal Dehiscence," and "Neighborhood Playground." The JAMA poem "Autumnal Equinox" begins:

> Today, calm and sunny, dry,
> the sun slips equal to the coming night. . .
> (Halberstadt CS. JAMA. 2016;316:1217)

Rafael Campo of Harvard Medical School asks: "Why should medical students be writing poems?" In fact, why should any of us—clinicians, educators, or researchers—be composing in iambic pentameter? He answers his question with an argument that centers on the thesis that, "Physicians who lack a passion for language or who fail to see beauty will be at a loss to translate these wonders in the most meaningful terms for their lay patients and into the larger society around us" [13]. I think that, of all types of writing, perhaps poetry is the most personally revealing. Even if it were not to make us better diagnosticians or lecturers, a little experience in the art of poetry would probably help us all become better medical writers and maybe even better humans.

As a further incentive, the *Annals of Internal Medicine* offers a prize of $500 for the best poem published in the Journal each year. The winner for 2015 was Lawrence

J. Hergott, MD of the University of Colorado for his poem "Tragedy of Shadows."

About My Practice

Medical Economics, a magazine best known for staff-written articles about practice management and finances, also publishes commentaries about the experiences of their physician readers.

A recent about-my-practice article in *Medical Economics* titled "Making Sense — and Cents" holds that educated patients who understand their illnesses and their management are more adherent and satisfied, helping the practice achieve financial success (Pearson J. Med Econ. Available at: http://medicaleconomics.modernmedicine.com/medical-economics/news/modernmedicine/modern-medicine-feature-articles/making-sense-and-cents).

Another publication that publishes physician-authored practice management articles is *Physicians Practice*, which recently featured an article titled "How I Avoid Burnout" (Norris DJ. Phys Pract. June 16, 2016: Available at: http://www.physicianspractice.com/worklife-balance/how-i-avoid-burnout).

History of Medicine

Some journals publish articles about medical history, a favorite topic of many clinicians. For example, in writing about Civil War medicine, Bollet states, "Supplying armies with fresh vegetables to prevent scurvy was always difficult, even for the tiny, 15,000 man, pre-Civil War United States army. Scurvy was the most common disease reported from frontier posts" (Bollet AJ. The Pharos. 2003;66(4);19–28). And a recent issue of *The Pharos* published an article titled "Lord Byron's Lameness," exploring how the poet's "clubfoot tormented him, both in the degree of physical pain he experienced and in the mental anguish it caused" (Gamble J. The Pharos. Summer 2016; 39).

X-Ray or Photo Quiz

Consultant presents a continuing section, "Photo Quiz." Here authors supply photographs or radiographs accompanied by brief medical histories. The challenge to the clinician is to identify the diagnosis, which is presented later in the journal. A similar feature is found in the NEJM.

Movie Reviews

The Pharos has a regular section titled "Medicine In The Movies." A recent issue reviewed "The Fault in our Stars" and "Me and Earl and the Dying Girl."

A movie review column in a journal tends to be written by the same person each month. However, if you wish to undertake the task, there is no reason that you could not suggest such a column to your favorite specialty journal if none already exists.

Personal Observations and Tales

"A Piece of My Mind" is the title of a feature in JAMA. *Family Medicine* lists these essays under the heading "Narrative Essays." Similar columns appear in many other publications, offering you the opportunity to write about something you feel strongly about. Topics that are fair game include insights from an encounter with a patient, thoughts about the future of medicine, and reflections on how your profession affects you as a person.

A piece titled "Osler in Jail" discusses providing medical care to jail inmates. "Just like on the outside, in jail we ask people about their lives, their jobs, and their family" (Bell JS. JAMA. 2016;315:2523). Another physician describes "A Modern Family," which includes Joe, a schizophrenic man who is no longer institutionalized, and his caregiver, a 60-year-old African American former corrections officer called Miss Elsie. The article chronicles their journey through

Joe's lung cancer, hospice, and eventual death (Colgan R et al. JAMA. 2010;304:2221).

One of the best features of this publication model is that it is egalitarian. Publication is open to all, not just to members of prestigious academic departments. What is submitted is judged solely on its merits—the impact of the message and the clarity of the writing.

Irony and Humor

Some enterprising individuals have conducted tongue-in-cheek research studies, and you may be surprised to learn that some of these articles find their way into print in quite respectable journals. Here are two of my favorites: Two British physicians quantified swearing by surgeons in the operating room. They observed 100 consecutive elective surgical procedures. They found that during an 8-h operating day, there were "16.5 swearing points for the orthopedic surgeons and 10.6, 10, and 3.1 from the general surgeons, gynecologists, and urologists, respectively. In contrast, during 8 hours of ear, nose and throat surgery, little more than one 'bugger' is likely" (Palazzo FF et al. BMJ. 1999;319:1611).

Here is another example of a droll observational study, published and indexed with its abstract available on PubMed. Rockwood and colleagues "conducted a surreptitious, prospective, cohort study to explore how often physicians nod off during scientific meetings and to examine the risk factors for nodding off." Wearing tweed seemed to increase the risk of nodding off; there was less nodding off when speakers were raving or when they dropped the microphone (Rockwood K et al. Can Med Assn J. 2004;171:1443).

Each year in its Christmas issue, the BMJ publishes humorous articles. Examples include "The Darwin Awards: Sex Differences In Idiotic Behavior" (Lemdren BAD et al. BMJ. 2014;349:g7094) and "Case Report of E.T.—The Extraterrestrial" (Scott G et al. BMJ. 2012;345:e8127).

One problem with published satire is that, once ensconced in the literature, "drive-by" researchers may mistakenly take the study seriously. A farcical study on the energy expended by adolescents playing video games has been cited some 400 times. An article titled "Sex, Aggression, and Humor: Response to Unicycling" (Shuster S. BMJ. 2007;335(7633):1320), comparing the responses of men versus women upon sighting a unicyclist, has become evidence supporting a theory proposing that humor has evolved from male aggression and is forever recorded in a book titled *The Male Brain* [14].

Newspaper Column

Some physicians write a column for a local newspaper or send out a monthly newsletter from their practices. In a letter published in *Medical Economics*, one clinician writes: "For the past year, I've used a technique that has generated one or two new-patient visits a week. I write a column called 'A Doctor Speaks from the Heart' for the monthly newsletter of a large retirement community that's located near my practice" (Hoenig LJ. Med Econ. 2004;81(1):13).

Topics that might be discussed in a newspaper column or newsletter include:

- When to call the doctor if a child is sick
- Who should get a flu shot
- First aid for acute injuries
- How to buy medicine at the lowest cost
- Danger signs in common illnesses
- How to prevent falls in the elderly
- Thoughts about herbal remedies

You and I could develop a long list of topics. The key is to keep the contributions short and pertinent. Also, be sure to avoid medical jargon when writing for the public; write headache, not cephalgia. When you undertake to write a column, you are agreeing to produce a written work at regular intervals, and hence the obligation should not be undertaken lightly. However, clinicians who write for the public enjoy the rewards of having readers in their communities remark, "I liked your article in the newspaper this week."

References

1. Apley J. Pleasures of medical writing. Br Med J. 1976;1(6016):999–1001.
2. Jordan EP, Shepard WC. Rx for medical writing. Philadelphia: WB Saunders; 1952. p. 32.
3. Oregon Health Plan. About the Oregon Health Plan. http://www.oregon.gov/oha/healthplan/Pages/about_us.aspx. Accessed 30 Mar 2017.
4. Fontanarosa PB. Editorial matters: guidelines for writing effective editorials. JAMA. 2014;311(21):2179–80.
5. LaVigne P. Letters to the editor. In: Taylor RB, Munning KA, editors. Written communication in family medicine. New York: Springer; 1984. p. 50.
6. Journal of the American Medical Association. Instructions for authors: letters to the editor. http://jamanetwork.com/journals/jama/pages/instructions-for-authors#SecLettertotheEditor. Accessed 30 Mar 2017.
7. Lee AD, Green BN, Johnson CD, Nyquist J. How to write a scholarly book review for publication in a peer-reviewed journal. J Chiropr Educ. 2010;24(1):57–69.
8. Salager-Meyer F. Book reviews in the medical scholarly literature, part II: "This book portrays the worst part of mental terrorism". J Eur Med Writers Assn. 2008;17(3):147–8.
9. Day RA. How to write and publish a scientific paper. 5th ed. Westport, CT: Oryx; 1998. p. 176.
10. Indiana University (Bloomington, Indiana). Writing tutorial services: writing book reviews. http://www.indiana.edu/~wts/pamphlets/book_reviews.shtml. Accessed 30 Mar 2017.
11. Taylor RB. White coat tales: medicine's heroes, heritage, and misadventures. 2nd ed. New York: Springer; 2016.
12. Wolfe SM. Medical publisher offers bribes for writing favorable book reviews: Public Citizen. http://www.citizen.org/Page.aspx?pid=2866. Accessed 30 Mar 2017.
13. Campo R. Why should medical students be writing poems? J Med Humanit. 2006;27(4):253–4.
14. Eveleth R. The ethics of sarcastic science. The Atlantic. 2014;22. http://www.theatlantic.com/technology/archive/2014/12/the-ethics-of-sarcastic-science/383988/. Accessed 30 Mar 2017.

Chapter 8
Writing Book Chapters and Books

*The real point about writing books is that, like mountains, they
are there. Some of us cannot resist the challenge; but it's hardly
rational behavior.*

Alpert T. The A–Z of Medical Writing [1]

In a herculean effort, Sir William Osler wrote the world's first
comprehensive medical reference book, *Principles and
Practice of Medicine*. It was published by Appleton in 1892
and continued in print until the 16th edition, published in
1947. The effort was heroic because Osler wrote every word
himself—no contributed chapters for him—a task that took
3 years. His fiancé refused to marry him until the manuscript
was complete. Following Osler's retirement, later editions of
the book were a collection of contributions by Johns Hopkins
faculty members [2].

Writing and editing medical books and chapters can be a
lot of fun. This activity can also be immensely frustrating, as
you will learn as we go along in this chapter. In the spirit of
full disclosure, over the years, I have edited 18 medical reference books and have authored 11 books for health professionals and five trade books and contributed dozens of book
chapters to the books of various editors. I have my cherished

© Springer International Publishing AG 2018
R.B. Taylor, *Medical Writing*,
https://doi.org/10.1007/978-3-319-70126-4_8

beliefs and pet peeves about putting together medical books. Osler also had some thoughts:

> The most unhappy day of my life was when I sold my brains to the publishers... I must have had neurasthenia or something else, and I beg your pardon for ever having consented to write a book. I have been sorry for students ever since, and trust when *Osler* [his book] goes out of vogue, some one will have ready an easier text.
>
> Sir William Osler (1849–1919), comments
to students about his book [3]

First, I will discuss medical books in general and will offer some definitions. Medical books can be categorized in several ways. One classification is by use: When thinking about medical books by use, we can identify *textbooks*, which are intended to be used by students as part of a course or clerkship; *reference books*, used to look up information; and what I call *enrichment books*, intended to be read for pleasure and personal growth. My textbook *Fundamentals of Family Medicine* (Taylor RB, Ed. New York: Springer; 2003) contains 27 clinical chapters linked by case discussions that all involve members of a large, multigenerational family, plus questions for class discussion. Dambro's *5-Minute Clinical Consult* (published annually by Lippincott Williams & Wilkins in Philadelphia) is one of many broad-based medical reference books; I doubt that anyone other than the editor has ever read it cover to cover. *Stories of Sickness* (Brody H. New Haven, CT: Yale University Press, 1988), an enrichment book written by a philosopher–physician, describes the patient's narration of the experience of sickness as an essential part of the act of healing. Enrichment books can be written for a medical audience, for the so-called lay audience, or both. Books written specifically for the lay audience, such as Jerome Groopman's *How Doctors Think* (New York: Houghton Mifflin; 2007), are called trade books. I will explain more about these book types later in the chapter.

Looking at books another way, there are *edited books* and *authored books*. Edited books contain the works of two or more *contributors* not listed on the cover. With many chapters, often written by several coauthors, large reference books in major medical specialties may have several hundred contributors. If you count the contributors to your own subspecialty's leading reference book, I would be surprised if the total is less than 50, and it is probably over 100 for the largest specialties. Hence, edited books are identified by the name of the editor or, in the case of a book with many editors, by the editor in chief. Edited books may take one of several forms: A true edited reference book has almost certainly been read and actually edited by the persons named on the cover. An anthology or conference proceedings may be compiled without the editor having much ability to edit content or coordinate styles.

A single author or perhaps a small team writes authored books. All names are on the cover as authors. This book is an authored book, written by me, alone. As a broad generality, edited books are more likely to cover a wide spectrum of topics and be larger volumes. Authored books are most likely to be smaller and more focused. As described by LaVigne: "A specialized book, also known as a technical publication, monograph, or scholarly work, is distinguished by the sophisticated level of its content. Since the specialized book is written for an author's colleagues and peers, it does not need to be as comprehensive as a text on the topic, nor as comprehensible as a book written for the general public" [4].

When all the above is considered, your entry into book publishing is most likely to come as an invitation to contribute a chapter to an edited reference book.

Book Chapters

The invitation to write a book chapter is flattering, and, as one who has extended many such invitations, I know that most invitees say "Yes." As a clinician, you are most likely to be invited to write a book chapter if you have a special practice-based interest that you have described in print. This may be considered one of the benefits of writing review articles. Let's say that your special interest is the evaluation of chest pain. You have published several review articles in controlled-circulation medical journals discussing the possible causes of chest pain, the different types of angina pectoris, and the causes of noncardiac chest pain. You have also lectured on the topic. About this time, imagine the plight of a reference book editor whose favorite author on chest pain has decided to retire to a beachfront condominium in Florida. In searching for a replacement, the editor comes across your articles and sends you a letter or an e-mail message. You are on your way to being a book chapter author.

Occasionally an editor needs a chapter on a topic that is rarely covered or an emerging issue on which few have written. In such instances, the volume editor may look for an author who writes on a variety of topics and invite this clinician to take on the "hard to place" topic. In planning the edited reference book *Difficult Diagnosis* (Philadelphia: WB Saunders, 1985), I decided to have a chapter on the evaluation of the patient with hyperhidrosis—excessive sweating. I found no expert who had claimed that topic, and so I asked a generalist colleague if she would be willing to take it on. She agreed and contributed an excellent chapter.

The Invitation to Write a Book Chapter

You feel honored to be selected as a potential author. You are grateful, thrilled, and energized. You want to call today and accept before the editor has a change of heart. But wait. There are some issues to consider.

One of the issues you need not be concerned about is how much you will be paid for your chapter. In almost all instances, the answer is "not very much" or "nothing." Some portion of royalties is sometimes allocated among the contributing authors of a book, but considering the modest sales numbers of even the most popular medical reference books and texts—compared, let's say, to the sales of Harry Potter books—the dollar amounts are tiny. The income, if any, will not compensate for the time involved in writing the chapter. As additional incentives, however, you will (almost certainly) receive a copy of the finished book, an entry on your curriculum vitae, and the editor's endless gratitude.

For the academician, a book chapter invitation presents an important career advancement issue: It is a truism that the greatest academic rewards come from the publication of reports of original research. In the hierarchy of publications that can support a bid for promotion to senior faculty status, book chapters are in the middle of the list, below the research report, meta-analysis, and definitive literature review published in a peer-reviewed journal but above a letter to the editor and book review.

For the clinician, writing a book chapter on your special clinical topic—for example, the treatment of resistant psoriasis or robotic surgery of coronary artery bypass—can help establish your national reputation and thereby stimulate referrals from clinicians who agree with what is in your chapter.

About the Agreement to Write a Chapter

Before accepting the book chapter invitation, there are several questions to ask. These are listed in Table 8.1. I clearly would not accept the invitation to write a chapter unless the

TABLE 8.1 Questions to ask the volume editor when invited to contribute a chapter to an edited book

Who is going to publish the book, and do you have a signed contract?

What other books have you edited and who has published them?

May I review a full table of contents or topic outline, to see what others will cover?

Who will be some of the other authors in the book?

Is there a special format required for the chapter?

What is the space allocation for my chapter (stated in double-spaced manuscript pages)?

What is the deadline for manuscript submission?

May I engage one or more coauthors?

Will I receive payment for my chapter?

Will I receive a copy of the finished book?

editor had a contract with a publisher. I might agree to write contingent upon the editor obtaining a contract, but I would not begin work until publication of the book is assured in writing. Once you are sure that a book contract exists, I consider the two most important questions on the list to be those that concern the page allocation and the chapter deadline. Before beginning to write you must have these items clearly in mind. It is all too easy to write a book chapter that is much too long, and then needs to be cut; this represents wasted effort for both you and the editor.

The deadline is especially important because the editor must receive all manuscripts at about the same time, review them promptly, and get them all in print before the clinical recommendations go out of date. One or two tardy chapters can, and sometimes do, hold up production of a book, ultimately compromising its usefulness (and sales). Or, there is another possibility. Two years ago, my wife and I cruised on the Norwegian Coastal Lines; ours was a working cargo and ferryboat that stopped at more than 40 ports as we sailed down the coast of Norway. Stops at ports of call might be 20 min or 2 h. The captain warned us sternly on the first day, "For those who leave the ship to visit a port, there are no late-arriving passengers. There are only passengers who have been left behind." The editor may decide that your chapter can be "left behind" and go to print without your late-arriving contribution. This happens.

What Is Negotiable?

An agreement to write a book chapter has explicit and implicit commitments from you and the book's editor, aka the compiler. You may be startled to note the casual agreement between you and the compiler, sometimes only a verbal commitment on the telephone. At some later time, the publisher will send you a more formal contract, which has at its core that the copyright to your chapter will be assigned to the publisher.

As discussed in Chap. 4, I advise not being concerned about this copyright assignment. First, it is standard in the trade and is not negotiable. Second, it rarely presents a problem. The only consideration arises when you have an innovative figure, table, mnemonic, or similar entity in your chapter, and you are sure that you will want to use this item in the future. In this case, you may be able to get the publisher to agree that the specific item is included in your chapter for "one-time use." If such agreement is not possible and you still wish to publish the chapter, you should have no problem using your innovative figure or table in later work, but you will need to request permission from the book's publisher for such use. Obtaining permission under such circumstances is usually quite easy.

Table 8.2 lists items that you may or may not be able to negotiate when invited to write a book chapter.

Preparing and Submitting Your Chapter

Writing a book chapter is much like writing a review article, which I described in Chap. 6. They are similar in that you must begin with a limited topic, decide on a concept and

TABLE 8.2 Writing a book chapter: what is negotiable and what is not

---

Possibly negotiable:

   Exact title of the chapter

   Inviting coauthors

   How the topic will be handled

   Headings in the chapter

   Paying for artwork and permissions

   Future use of a specific figure or other item in the chapter without specific permission from the publisher

Probably not negotiable:

   General topic of your chapter

   Deadline for manuscript submission

   Payment for the chapter

   Copyright assignment

   Future use of the chapter as a whole without permission from the publisher

---

structure for what you want to say, do careful research and select references carefully, write a well-organized and authoritative essay, and then summarize while staying within appropriate page limits. But there are differences: The topic is likely to be assigned, the structure and headings may be prescribed, a specific feature such as an algorithm may be required, coordination with other chapter contributors may be needed to avoid overlap, and the deadline may be quite firm to assure timely publication. An example follows.

Earlier in this chapter I mentioned the multiauthor reference book *Difficult Diagnosis*. This book presented the diagnostic approach to a selected group of challenging problems with what I termed "enigmatic clinical presentations." Examples included fever of unknown origin, jaundice, and eosinophilia. Contributors were invited from many specialties. In planning the book, I decided that each chapter should have the same six major headings: Background, including definitions, incidence of the problem, and a laundry list of possible causes; History, to include what I called "high-payoff questions"; Physical Examination, including the significance of key findings; Diagnostic Studies, including laboratory investigations, diagnostic imaging, and other tests; Assessment, to include a diagnostic algorithm; and References, but no more than 25 citations. Therapy was not to be covered unless integral to diagnosis, such as the sometimes helpful response of gout to colchicine. I even wrote a sample chapter, "Acute Headache," and sent a copy to all authors recruited, just to present a model of what I had in mind. The authors selected were seasoned clinicians and distinguished academicians.

Months later, when chapters were submitted, most authors had followed directions. They used my headings, provided tables listing possible causes of dysphagia and hypocalcemia that I still use today, identified high-payoff questions, and constructed useful algorithms. Only a few authors went their own way with different headings and varying concepts for their chapters. When the nonconforming chapters didn't seem to fit, the authors and I negotiated. When the "different drummer" concept seemed to fit the topic as well as my prescribed headings, no change was recommended, although I made a mental note that would influence author selection in a second edition.

In the end, I believe that the contributors and I created a great book. It has innovative features and covers a special group of challenging medical topics. I relate all this because I believe that the success of the book can be attributed to the hard work and skill of authors who, for the most part, followed instructions that called for them to unify headings, limit reference citations, and construct some items—lists of possible causes, high-payoff questions, and algorithms—that readers can find in (almost) every chapter.

Chapter Structure

As noted above, the book editor may be quite specific about concept and headings, or you may be allowed to develop your own approach. The latter is more common, and most book editors do not prescribe structure as precisely as I did with *Difficult Diagnosis*.

I once coauthored a chapter called "Writing a Medical Article" with Joseph E. Scherger, M.D., for a compiled book titled *Written Communication in Family Medicine* [5]. Our topic, as implicit in the title, was on how to write a medical article, and our approach was based on a workshop that we had presented several times. We structured the chapter as a series of ten steps:

1. Conceptualize the subject of the article.
2. Review the literature.
3. Select the appropriate readership and journal.
4. Organize and outline the content of the article.
5. Select a title.
6. Write the first draft.
7. Write the first revision.
8. Submit the manuscript for review by selected colleagues.
9. Write a final draft.
10. Submit the paper for publication.

TABLE 8.3 Classic headings in book chapters on medical diseases

Definition
Epidemiology
Etiology/pathogenesis
Clinical features
Diagnosis, including history, physical examination, and diagnostic tests
Treatment
Prognosis
Prevention

If asked to write a chapter on a clinical topic, such as gastro-esophageal reflux disease or incontinence in the elderly, keep in mind that the classic headings for a clinical chapter in a medical reference book are going to be very similar to those in the *Difficult Diagnosis* book, with treatment and perhaps prevention added. Or you may think of your clinical SOAP note: subjective, objective, assessment, and plan. With a few additions, such as epidemiology and prevention, SOAP is a useful concept for a clinical chapter. If asked to write on a disease topic and given no other instructions, think about the topics in Table 8.3.

Submitting Your Book Chapter

This should be the easy part. Do your best to make it so. If you have carefully followed the editor and publisher's instructions, and have completed your chapter on time, submission should be a breeze. Verify that you have not exceeded your page allocation. Read it through one last time to find the instance in which you have repeated or contradicted yourself. Then, to be sure that you have not forgotten anything, review the checklist in Table 12.2 before sending your chapter to the editor.

Edited Books

In the area where I lived in upstate New York, people had a saying: If you hire six carpenters to do a job, only two will show up; one will have a sore back, and the other one will have to go home to get his tools. There is an analogous saying in medical publishing: If you, as a compiling editor, contract with three authors to contribute chapters and then seek the chapters at deadline time, one will be months behind on commitments that come before your book, one will be on a year-long sabbatical in a remote village overseas, and one will have forgotten about the project entirely.[1]

You as the Initiator of an Edited Book

The initiator of an edited book should have certain characteristics: You should have a fair amount of experience as a book chapter contributor. It would be good to have a name that is well known among potential contributors, but this is not a requirement if you have a very good book idea and a signed contract with a respected medical publisher. You must be a good manager: You will need to keep track of the status of each chapter and its components and to report to your editor from time to time. You must be willing to spend nights and weekends on the project, especially when chapter manuscripts arrive, since they are all going out of date as they sit on your desk. You must be tactful, since you will be dealing with some colossal egos, as a few contributors decide they know better than you how the book should be compiled. And you must be tenacious, since the worst thing you can do in an edited book is let the project die. This death can occur when half the chapters are in hand, and the authors of the other half are behaving like the fictional three authors described above.

Planning an Edited Book

There are major edited books (such as *Harrison's Principles of Internal Medicine*), and there are focused books (such as *Written Communication in Family Medicine*, cited above).

---

[1] If my memory is correct, I read this tale of three authors in the preface to a book published about 25 years ago. I cannot recall the name of the author or book and, to help me avoid accidental plagiarism, I would be grateful if a reader could supply this information for the next edition of *Medical Writing*.

In most areas of medicine, there really is scant room for another major edited book. The issue is not that you could not produce a big book that is better than those available; the truth is that the publisher can rarely afford the financial risk of failure inherent in adding a new expensive product to a crowded market. I find this risk especially pertinent today when physicians first seek information online and not in heavy, printed reference books.

If planning an edited book, think about a focused product. The traditional approach is to marry a group of health problems to an age group, gender, geographic location, or medical specialty. Currently there are books on dermatologic diseases of children, medication use during pregnancy, and geriatric neuropsychiatry. There have been books about gynecologic, behavioral, neurologic, and musculoskeletal problems in primary care.

An early, key decision in planning an edited book on health problems is as follows: Do I want to present my chapters as diagnoses (such as myocardial infarction) or as clinical presentations, that is, symptoms or signs (such as chest pain)? Most medical book editors choose the former. It is handy and traditional. However, patients present to clinicians with complaints, physical abnormalities, and sometimes with unexpected laboratory findings, not diagnoses, which speaks to the utility of symptom-and-sign-oriented books like *Difficult Diagnosis*. As a hint to those seeking contributors, it is much easier to recruit authors to write on diseases than on signs or symptoms. Physicians like to take ownership of a disease, and will write endlessly to hold on to their turf, such as colorectal cancer or psoriasis. On the other hand, few clinicians claim expertise, much less ownership, of clinical presentations such as cyanosis, hemoptysis, or, as mentioned earlier, hyperhidrosis.

At a minimum, you will need to plan the following for your new edited book:

- A compelling need for the book
- A good idea of who will buy the book
- Overall length of the book
- Number and titles of the chapters

- Short description of what should be included in each chapter
- A list of potential authors
- The time and commitment you will need to complete the project

How much time commitment will be needed? Compiling an edited medical book is a 2-year commitment—if all goes well. The good news is that you will not be working constantly for the full 24 months. Editing a book occurs in stages requiring intense effort, alternating with times when the editor has little to do. Here are three major phases when evening and weekend effort will be needed: Phase one is author recruitment. Contacting and reaching agreement with all the book's primary authors will take a lot of effort, as described below. After all authors are recruited, things are quiet while authors write; at least you *hope* they are writing. Phase two comes when all the manuscripts arrive. The manuscript editing time is the busiest of all, because of the need to verify many facts and to negotiate changes with contributors. Phase three is proofreading, which cannot simply be delegated to others. Of course, each contributor should proofread his or her own contribution. In my experience, however, most chapter authors are dismal proofreaders and you, as editor, must take responsibility for all errors by checking every word carefully.

The first step, after planning and committing yourself to your edited book, is getting a contract with a publisher. This is accomplished by submitting a proposal.

The Book Proposal and Contract

What follows regarding book proposals and contracts applies to both edited and authored books.

Finding the Right Editor

Not long after deciding upon the niche-filing edited book you will compile, you must find a publisher. And at that publishing company you must find the "acquisitions editor," the person who can actually offer you a contract (with approval from the publisher, the person who controls the company budget). To locate the right medical publishing firm, look for who produces books in your field. Some publishers bring out a number of radiology and plastic surgery books, those containing many illustrations and requiring specialized production. Some medical publishers prefer primary care books. Another may specialize, to some degree, in psychiatry and psychology books. Check the books on your own bookshelf or in your institution's medical library to see who is publishing in your specialty. Visit individual publisher web sites or Amazon.com.

After you have identified one or two potential publishers for your book, find the acquisitions editor in one of two ways. If you are going to a major medical meeting in your specialty, visit the exhibit booths of the publishers you are targeting. At the booth, you will find salespeople, but also at the meeting may be an acquisitions editor. Ask the salesperson whether the acquisitions editor is at the meeting and, if so, when he or she will return to the booth so that you can discuss your idea. Your best approach may be to call ahead and set up an appointment in advance.

Plan B, if you cannot meet in person, is to use the telephone and network research to track down the acquisitions editor. Let's imagine that you are a radiologist and that you have a great idea for a new book on diagnostic imaging of the brain. Your research has shown that XYZ Publishing Company has a very good list of radiology books. Call the company and ask to speak to the acquisitions editor for medical radiology books. You will probably soon be connected with the office of the person you seek.

Another good way to contact an acquisitions editor is through the publisher's website. For example, acquisitions editors for this book's publisher can be found by visiting http://www.springer.com/gp/medicine/contact-us.

What's Next in Getting a Book Contract?

Tell the acquisitions editor about your proposal, being sure to cover the planning topics listed above. The acquisitions editor may give you some immediate feedback: "We have a book like this in production," "I don't think there is a market for this book," or "Not a bad idea, but here is how I would modify the concept."

In most instances, your idea will be received with some guarded interest, and you will be asked to submit a proposal.

The Book Proposal

Your book proposal is a formal document. By the time it is submitted, you and your acquisitions editor may be on a first-name basis, and you have fully discussed the proposal. You are both enthusiastic. Nevertheless, you should submit a complete, polished proposal, covering all the points listed in Table 8.4. A complete proposal portfolio, with all the pieces, is important because the next task of your acquisitions editor is to present the proposal at the regular meeting of the other editors and the publisher. Here is where your new editor acts as your advocate to get the project approved. At this meeting, his or her most important ammunition is your proposal. In fact, the proposal may be the most important bit of writing you do in regard to your book.

The Contract

The proposal is approved! Hooray! The standard book contract is on its way. Wonderful. But wait. Even though you receive a preprinted contract, it may be useful to know that the publisher has several "standard" contracts that can be used, according to circumstances. Some contract terms may be negotiable, and additions to the contract are possible. A review by your attorney may be helpful, but going over the contract with an experienced book author/editor is likely to

TABLE 8.4 What to include in a book proposal

The cover letter describing the proposed book should include the following topics:

  Book title and any subtitle

  Anticipated length of the manuscript, expressed in single-spaced pages

  Number of tables and figures that will be in the book

  The book's audience, that is, who will buy the book

  The chief competing books, and how the proposed book is different

  Why you are qualified to edit (or write) the book

  Anticipated date of manuscript submission

The proposal should also include:

  A description of the book, including the intent and scope of coverage

  A table of contents

  A sample chapter, to show your style and that you can actually write

  Your curriculum vitae

Optional, but desirable, items to include:

  Expanded outline, showing headings and subheadings

  Annotated table of contents, describing the contents of each chapter

be more helpful (and will cost less). These standard contracts are usually written in plain English, and there are typically not any trick clauses. With that said, there are some key items to review carefully:

- *Royalties:* The standard was once 10% of gross sales at the US retail price and less for foreign sales. About a quarter century ago, however, publishers learned how to cut author/editor royalties without being too obvious. The device was to change the contract to read percent of *net sales,* meaning the amount actually received by the publisher, not the amount charged by the retailer. Since net sales figures are a black box impenetrable to authors, the author/editor who receives 10% of *net sales* may not realize that this is much less than 10% of *gross sales*.

- *Advance against royalties:* Seasoned authors/volume editors should request an advance, as a warranty that the book will actually be published, especially when the book is a major project. Neophyte authors should ask but are often not in a strong bargaining position even though the advance is, in fact, their money, and so it really isn't a cost to the publisher. You are merely getting some of your royalty payment a little early. In the end, if you fail to deliver the book manuscript, you will need to return the advance.
- *Costs related to manuscript preparation:* I always ask that the publisher pay for the cost of preparing figures and the index. Without prior agreement to the contrary, these may be charged to the author and can be an unpleasant surprise on the first royalty statement. If the book contains a lot of art and the publisher cannot agree to pay for all, ask for a grant or an allowance.
- *Author copies:* The contract will state that you get some 6–20 copies of the book. In the case of an edited book, be sure that the contract also states that a copy will be sent directly to each contributor, at no cost to you.
- *Costs related to excessive corrections on proofs:* There is nothing to be negotiated here, but be very aware of this clause. If you start rewriting on page proofs, the cost will quickly exceed your allowance for corrections, and all additional costs will be charged against your royalties.
- *Hold harmless clause:* You assume legal responsibility—that is, you protect the publisher from liability—for any damages caused by the book: libel, slander, and errors that might result in patient injury or death.

There will be some royalty surprises. Some surprises will be bad, some good. Royalties for foreign sales are generally meager; I see no reason why this should be, but it is common. Good surprises will be unexpected, although very modest, payments when your book is translated into Spanish or Japanese. Another nice surprise is the small extra payment showing up on your royalty statement, representing your share of a fee paid by another author who has requested permission to use a table or figure from your book. Increasingly, I receive payment for online versions of my books, and such sales seem likely to outpace print copies.

As with book chapters, copyright to the book will be owned by the publisher. Years from now, if and when the book is out of print, you may request that the publisher return the copyright to you or perhaps prepare a new edition of the book.

Working with Authors

Your contract is signed and in the file. Your outline lists all the chapter titles. Now all you need to do is recruit a lead or primary author for each chapter. I insist that I deal with one lead author. That lead author may invite one or more coauthors, and he or she deals with the coauthors. Coauthors have their names listed on chapters, but usually do not receive copies of the book. The mantra for my edited books is one chapter, one book copy.

Author Recruitment

Selecting the best contributors and communicating clearly with them can prevent hours of aggravation later. If given the choice in authors, I choose reliability over brilliance every time. Enthusiasm for the project is important, and if an invitee begins to haggle over deadline dates and other items, I am likely to break off the negotiation and go on to someone else.

In extending invitations to write, I prefer to speak directly to the potential author on the telephone, especially if this is our first contact. The initial telephone discussion is then followed by a letter with a written agreement (see below). From then on, all interaction will probably be done by e-mail.

Is it difficult to recruit authors to write chapters in books? Not really. It is easiest to solicit contributors to established books—new editions of the ones everyone knows, the ones in their sixth or tenth editions. Recruiting for a new, untested book is a little more difficult. That is why it is so important to have a publication contract before beginning recruitment. My most problematic recruitment was for the books *Difficult Diagnosis* and *Difficult Medical Management* (both published by W.B. Saunders). These were new books, first edition, and they were interdisciplinary. Because of prior publications, my name is fairly well known in my specialty. But radiologists and endocrinologists are very unlikely to know me. However, I had a good concept and a signed contract with Saunders. On my first round of invitations to prospective authors in diverse specialties, my acceptance rate exceeded 60%. Why? Because I invited authors to write on their favorite topics, largely selected by seeing who was writing review articles in controlled-circulation journals, and I believed that these clinicians would want their imprint on their topics in the new book.

Author Agreement

I have each lead author sign my own agreement form. It is probably not a legal document, and later the publisher will also send the more formal author contract that discusses copyright assignment. My agreement is useful when, as sometimes happens, disagreements occur later. It anticipates some of the issues that may arise. My brief agreement form covers six very important topics:

- Chapter topic and title.
- Page allocation.
- Deadline for submission.
- Coauthors are acceptable, but only one complimentary book is allocated per chapter.
- A statement about royalties to chapter authors. I prefer to be realistic: "I hope that you will consider this invitation a great honor, especially because there will be no cash payment for chapters."
- Full contact information, including e-mail address, mailing address, and all telephone numbers, including home number for the prospective author.

After the agreement is signed, I return a copy to the contributor and keep a copy for my files. All my agreements are with lead authors only, not with coauthors.

Author Reminders

Contributors to my edited books receive reminders about their chapters about every 6 weeks. Some are sent by mail, some by e-mail. They may discuss issues such as headings, permissions, manuscript submission, provide a tally of how many chapters have been submitted to date, and so forth. Basically they are all reminders so that my authors do not enter the "forgot about the project entirely" category.

Development Editor

You may be assigned a book development editor, who will help you with issues regarding author communication and manuscript management. Some development editors are very good. The very best will find your errors in grammar, syntax, tense, and even facts. In the end, however, the quality of the book will depend on your efforts and commitment.

Compiling the Book

Months ago you contracted with a number of colleagues to write chapters for your edited book. You have sent periodic reminders. Now the deadline has arrived. Will the book really come together? Will the chapters actually arrive? Will they be as good as you hope?

Fundamentally, there will be two types of problems at manuscript deadline time: One is chapters that arrive and need improvement; and the second problem is those chapters that do not arrive at all.

Editing Chapters That Arrive

Some chapter manuscripts will be better than others. Some will be practically perfect. After all, you have been in frequent contact with all the authors, guiding them during the writing phase. Other chapters will require editing, sometimes a lot of editing. Here we apply the revision principles described in Chap. 3 but with a big difference. Now you are editing someone else's work, not your own. You cannot just make substantive changes; all modifications that might affect meaning must be negotiated with the author. This often means sending the chapter back and forth once or twice before you and the author agree that it is the best that it can be.

Missing Chapters

The authors of missing chapters will offer a variety of excuses. In Table 3.4 I listed some of the many reasons authors fail to complete and submit their manuscripts on time. Of course, as volume editor, you are not really very interested in the excuse, however inventive it may be. You need a chapter manuscript.

When I plan an edited book, I create a set of three "late manuscript" notices. The first begins, "This is a friendly reminder that your chapter was due 2 weeks ago…" The last of the three messages states, "This is the third and final notice that your chapter is late and is in danger of not being in the book. I know you have worked hard on this project, but the book must be submitted and published on time. Therefore, if your chapter manuscript is not on my desk by [you select the date], it will not be in the book. Packages arriving after this date will be returned unopened." By selecting authors carefully, reminding them often, and using late notices when needed, I seldom have problems with missing chapters. But occasionally it happens.

If a chapter actually does not arrive, you must face a choice. One option is to create a chapter on short notice to fill a needed gap in a book. Once while compiling a book on health promotion, I encountered an author who fooled me for weeks after the deadline. "The chapter is almost done." "You will have it next week." Eventually I learned that he had done nothing and was in no hurry to do so. The chapter was about weight control, a topic vital to a health promotion book. To fill the gap, one of the associate editors and I wrote a "weight control" chapter in about 10 days, filled the gap, and submitted an intact book manuscript. The weight control chapter was probably not the best in the book, but reviewers did not single it out for criticism (Taylor RB, Ureda JR, Denham JW. Health promotion: principles and clinical applications. Norwalk, CT: Appleton, Century Crofts; 1982).

Missing chapters force the decision, "Is this chapter expendable?" For the volume editor, the ideal edited books are those such as *Difficult Diagnosis*, which present eclectic topics. Books of this type can be, and often are, published minus several chapters that were originally planned and contracted, but that for some reason did not arrive. In fact, in compiling such books, often with new authors in many specialties, I count on attrition of about 7% of chapters and authors. The more challenging books are those, such as a specialty textbook, that have a sequence of chapters in which not one contribution is expendable. In this case all chapters must be received or created on short notice.

Publication of the Book

You have received all chapters, negotiated editing changes with contributors, added any appendix material, and carefully submitted everything to your development editor or directly to the publisher. Of course, you have kept a copy of everything, just in case.

Here are the steps that follow after the publisher receives the book:

- *Verification:* An editorial assistant will check to see that everything has been received. This person will take a hard look at signed permission forms, and the publisher may refuse to go further if any permission form is missing.
- *Assignment to a production editor:* The project will be passed to a new person, the production editor. This person has the important job of shepherding your manuscript from submission to finished book.
- *Copyediting:* Next the manuscript will have line-by-line attention by a copyeditor who has basically two tasks. One is to fix errors of grammar and syntax without changing meaning. The second is to make decisions about font, page layout, and similar issues.
- *Author review of copyediting:* In many instances, the manuscript will be sent back to you and the contributors to review copyediting changes. At this stage, you will probably see some questions posed by the copyeditor, asking if this fact is true or if you really mean to say that.
- *Marketing questionnaire:* At about this stage, the publisher's marketing department will probably send you a long questionnaire to complete. Questions will concern the key features of the book, the intended audience, the best illustrations, and so forth. Take the time to do a good job on this document, which will be the basis of the marketing program for the book. Be aware that the marketing department staff are generally salespeople, not writers, and are very likely to use the language you submit. Thus you may see your submitted description of the book over and over on Amazon.com and on other sites.
- *Galley proofs:* Galley proofs are your work set in print but not divided into pages. You will review these proofs for errors and return them to the publisher. In some instances, the publisher will skip this step, especially if you have submitted a manuscript with minimal problems and if the copyeditor has asked few questions.
- *Page proofs:* Here is your book set in pages for your final review. At this stage your job is to correct errors. That is all. This is not the time to rewrite to improve phrases or add

new thoughts. Alterations at this stage are costly and may be charged to you.

- *Printing and binding:* This takes a while. During this time, a cover may be created, and you should ask to review the artwork. On several occasions I have picked up errors on covers for my books.
- *Publication:* The book is released. Review copies are sent to major journals by the publisher. Your author copies arrive in the mail. It's celebration time.

After the Book Is Published

Now is the time to take a breather. You have your author's copy of the book in hand. It looks great. You show it to your family and friends, who may actually be impressed. You might even, as I have done for years, frame a copy of the book cover to hang on the wall of your office.

You will wait anxiously for reviews. These take a long time, as might be expected. There is a time lag at each step of mailing the review copies to the journals, assigning the book to a reviewer, and then having the reviewer submit the review, and finally experiencing the interval until publication of the review. You hope for a favorable review, remembering from Chap. 7 that a uniformly positive review lacks credibility.

At this time, create an errata file. As you use the book, you will find small errors, which I hope do not involve drug doses. Keep a file of these spelling glitches and minor factual misstatements, which may be correctable with the next printing.

Also, begin a file on ideas for the second edition of the book, which will come up sooner than you think. Remember that an edited book is a 2-year effort from outline to bookstore. A medical text or reference book has a useful life of about 4 years, as new knowledge makes 5-year-old books seem ancient. Your book has just been published. With a 4-year cycle, this means that you have 2 years to rest (and collect ideas) before you start working on the second edition.

Finally, as volume editor, take good care of your contributors. Send them a letter thanking them for participating. If available, include a copy of the book's reviews. Verify that each lead author receives a copy of the book from the publisher.

Authored Books

Much of what I have presented above about edited books also applies to authored books. The big difference with the authored book, of course, is that an individual or a small team undertakes to write it all.

Sir Winston Churchill, a prolific author who wrote alone, once remarked: "Writing a long and substantial book is like having a friend and companion at your side to whom you can always turn for comfort and amusement and whose society becomes more attractive as a new and widening field of interest is lighted in the mind" [6]. I must say that, although I find revising and proofreading to be chores, I undertake each *writing* session with some relish. I want to find out what I am going to say today. I work alone because I don't want to have to justify each golden phrase to a coauthor who may unreasonably believe that his or her words are even better than mine.

Today not many medical reference books are written entirely by sole authors, as Osler's epic work was. Certainly there are no major, broad-based single-author medical books. On the other hand, there are a number of possibilities for the aspiring book author. Many of these will be enrichment medical books. Here are some diverse examples of single-author enrichment books that have been written over the years:

- Major RH. Disease And Destiny. New York: Appleton-Century; 1936. Major writes of "a dominant role of disease in the destiny of the human race."
- Marti-Ibanez F. A Prelude To Medical History. New York: MD Publications; 1961. The author has compiled his

lectures on medical history given to medical students at the New York Medical College.

- Selzer R. Mortal Lessons: Notes On The Art Of Surgery. New York: Touchstone; 1974. Clinicians and laypersons alike can read about the exact location of the soul and other musings of this articulate surgeon.
- Dirckx JH. The Language Of Medicine. 2nd ed. New York: Praeger; 1983. This physician presents a scholarly treatise on the evolution, structure, and dynamics of the words clinicians use.
- Maynard DW. Bad News, Good News: Conversational Order In Everyday Talk and Clinical Settings. Chicago: University of Chicago Press; 2003. The author discusses information, news, and communication in a variety of settings.
- Meyers MA. Happy Accidents: Serendipity In Modern Medical Breakthroughs. New York: Arcade Publishing; 2007. I hoard curious facts, and hence this is just my sort of book.
- Jauhar S. Intern: A Doctor's Initiation. New York: Farrar, Straus, and Giroux; 2009. This is the story of the author's journey through internship.
- Loop FD. Leadership And Medicine. Pensacola, FL: Fire Starter Publishing; 2009. Written by a surgeon who was once the Cleveland Clinic's chief executive officer, this is a book I wish I had written.
- Mukherjee S. The Emperor of All Maladies: A Biography Of Cancer. New York: Scribner; 2011. The author essentially anthropomorphizes cancer and presents its "biography" over the centuries.
- Colgan R. Advice To The Healer On The Art Of Caring, 2nd ed. New York: Springer; 2013. The advice is presented in two sections: inspirational perspectives from history and practical advice for the modern-day healer.
- Deyo RA. Watch Your Back! How The Back Pain Industry Is Costing Us More And Giving Us Less. New York: Cornell Univ. Press; 2015. Deyo gives us an evidence-based look at how we manage the patient with back pain.

- Kalanithi P. When Breath Becomes Air. New York: Random House; 2016. The book is a memoir of the author's life leading up to his death of lung cancer.
- Taylor RB. Medical Writing: A Guide For Clinicians, Educators, And Researchers. 3rd ed. New York: Springer; 2018. Okay, so I included my own book. It *is* an authored, focused medical book.

What are the commonalities among the books listed above? They are single-author books. They are focused, and generally appeal to clinicians with special interests in medical history, epistemology, language, poetry, or other topics, some outside the medical mainstream.

Notice also that many are not published by the big conglomerate medical publishers. As an example above, I offer Fire Starter Publishing in Pensacola, Florida. Such books are not big moneymakers, and proposals for meritorious projects are often turned down by major publishers with the statement, "This would be a great book, but we cannot project sufficient sales to allow us to publish it." Enrichment books are more likely to be published by university presses, specialty societies, or smaller publishers that can deal with modest print runs. If you love your book and just want to see it in print, then contracting with a small publisher will not be a mistake.

If you decide to undertake an authored medical book, you will follow the same path as described in the section on edited books: Begin by clarifying your concept, and be realistic about potential sales. To be published, you must write on something people will buy. Create a proposal packet, containing all the elements described in Table 8.4. Then find an acquisitions editor, either in person or by telephone. *Do not write the entire book* and then begin to hunt for a publisher. Editors almost always want a role in developing a book's concept and style.

Contracts for authored books differ little from those for edited books. The chief difference would be that there is no provision for copies for contributors; all gratis copies go to you, the author.

The contract will specify a date when the manuscript is due. Be sure to give yourself enough time. Writing a book and doing a good job of it takes time. I suggest allowing yourself 10–12 months from the date of the contract. And that may be optimistic. If you deliver the manuscript early, everyone will be happily surprised.

The big advantage of an authored book is that you are not dealing with egoistic contributors, and you do not need to negotiate changes with others. One disadvantage is that you are on your own, and can go off track, beginning with a good idea and then changing direction or style. While writing your book, I urge that you show consecutive chapters to your trusted colleague reviewer, asking for critical feedback.

In the end, writing a book can be exhilarating. One colleague who wrote a book during a time of major administrative challenges has said, "I wrote the book on evenings and weekends, but at the time it was the only thing keeping me sane." As I write this book, I look forward to envisioning what will come next in each chapter; then I write it. This is the fun of writing, especially book writing, and I hope that all readers experience the pleasure at least once in their lives.

Random Thoughts About Medical Books

Professional Books and Trade Books

Professional/textbooks and trade books live in two different worlds. At a large book publisher's offices, there may be both text and trade divisions, but there seems to be a firewall between them.

Trade books are what general-interest (read: nonmedical) people read. John Grisham and J. K. Rowling write trade books. Dr. Spock's *Baby and Child Care* is a trade book. My first books, in the 1970s, were trade books, until a Harper and Row Publishers trade editor whom I never met did a remarkable thing. I had submitted a manuscript (Yes, I had written the book already, which I would not do today) about a book on symptoms and what diseases they could represent. If an individual had heartburn, might it be gastritis, peptic ulcer disease, or stomach cancer? The trade book editor decided that the book was too technical for a lay audience. Instead of returning the manuscript to me with a form-letter rejection, he sent the book to medical editor Charles Visokay, M.D. Chuck read the manuscript, offered a contract, and Harper and Row Medical Publishers published the book. I have been doing professional medical books ever since that time.

There are tens of thousands of trade books published every year. There are very few authors, like Grisham and Rowling, who make vast sums from their royalties. Most trade authors receive, at best, modest royalties for their efforts. For that matter, neither do medical book authors earn much from their books. For clinicians, the rewards come in professional recognition, career advancement, and perhaps some patient referrals.

I believe that finding a medical publisher is much easier than finding a trade publisher. It seems that everyone in America is writing a thriller, a cookbook, or an autobiography and seeking a publisher. Most trade publishers protect their sanity by considering submissions only through recognized literary agents. Agents, in turn, are besieged by author wannabes and turn away almost all previously unpublished authors.

In medical publishing, there are fewer publishing companies than in the past. The great medical publishing houses are going out of business or consolidating. The merger creating Springer Nature represents only one such example. But there are also fewer prospective medical authors competing for their contracts; aspiring academicians are more likely devoting their energies to research studies, the key to promotion and tenure. And to my knowledge, there are, as yet, no literary agents in medical publishing.

I much prefer the professional medical publishing milieu to the trade publishing process. For one thing, trade publishers are keen on authors promoting their books; think, television appearances.

Do Not Underestimate the Effort

Editing or writing a book is a big effort. Yes, as I mentioned earlier, the intense activity comes in cycles. Nevertheless, preparing any type of book is committing your spare time to the effort. Do not undertake the job lightly. To quote Sir Winston Churchill again: "Writing a book is an adventure. To begin with it is a toy, an amusement; then it becomes a mistress, and then a master and then a tyrant" [6]. If you are planning to commit to a medical book, you must want the project a lot! I have seen clinicians come to hate the books they were working on. A few have given up midway through the project. Giving up on an authored book is bad enough. Abandoning an edited book after colleagues have worked on chapters at your request is devastating—to the authors and to your reputation.

Respect Serendipity and Chance

Howard Conn, editor of *Conn's Current Therapy*, was a Western Pennsylvania small-town general practitioner with an idea: an edited book in which experts told how they treated various diseases. He trudged from one publisher to another until a young editor at Saunders looked past Conn's lack of editorial experience and recognized the merits of the proposal. This editor championed the idea with his senior colleagues. *Conn's Current Therapy*, first published in 1949, sold more than one million copies by the time of Conn's death in 1982 and is still published annually [7].

Here is another story of serendipity: Leon Speroff was lead editor of *Clinical Gynecologic Endocrinology and Infertility* when it was first published in 1973. Speroff was recently interviewed by Marc A. Fritz, who described the book as "the most widely read subspecialty book in the world." In this interview, Speroff tells how he came to be lead editor: "In 1972, Bob Glass approached me in the hallway at Yale. He and Nate Kase were writing a textbook on endocrinology, and Bob asked me to join them, saying that they met every Thursday evening to work on it. During our first meeting, I asked what they had done so far—and the answer was nothing! Being a compulsive organizer, I took the project over, which is how my name got to be listed first on the textbook" [8].

The Market Rules

You and your acquisitions editor must pay close attention to the question, who will buy this book? In today's tight economic times, publishers cannot afford to ignore the market. Long ago, when I was still in private practice, I wrote a short book entitled *Why Doctors Give Children Shots*. The book told the stories of communicable diseases against which we immunize children: smallpox vaccination (I said that this was a long time ago), tetanus, diphtheria, polio, and so forth. I collected some wonderful historic illustrations. It was, in my judgment, a reasonably well-written, vividly illustrated, innovative book. There was only one small problem: Who would buy the book? The kids getting the shots were too young to read a book about medical history, however clearly written. The parents weren't especially interested in the topic, and the book was too consumer oriented for clinicians. I made many unsuccessful efforts to find a publisher. Today the manuscript is in a cardboard box in the attic. I know how to find it, in case anyone wants to publish it.

Book Publishing and Personal Relationships

If you are interested in writing or editing medical books, I urge you to remember what I am about to write. This may be the most useful sentence in the entire chapter: *Medical book publishing is about personal relationships*. As a book editor, you work closely with your contributors. I edited six editions of the large reference book *Family Medicine: Principles and Practice* (New York: Springer Publishers) over 38 years and have just coedited the seventh edition, published in 2017. Many authors contributed chapters over multiple editions.

During the past three decades, I have worked with more than a dozen medical editors employed by five medical publishing houses. Medical editors usually don't fade away; they move from one medical publishing job to another. Relationships continue and are highly valuable when you need access to an editor to evaluate a project.

Nurture your relationships with contributors and with your medical editors. Next to the exhilaration of actually writing, these friendships can be the best part of working on medical books.

About Your Book

Writing or editing a book involves long hours and hard work. As you begin, aim to create the book you would like to read.

References

1. Alpert T. The A–Z of medical writing. London: BMJ Books; 2000. p. 14.
2. Taylor RB. White coat tales: medicine's heroes, heritage, and misadventures. 2nd ed. New York: Springer; 2016. p. 240–1.
3. Osler W. Dr. Osler to students. Oklahoma Med J. 1900;8:53.
4. LaVigne P. Seeking publication. In: Taylor RB, Munning KA, editors. Written communication in family medicine. New York: Springer; 1984. p. 57.
5. Scherger JE, Taylor RB. Writing a medical article. In: Taylor RB, Munning KA, editors. Written communication in family medicine. New York: Springer; 1984. p. 33–42.
6. Churchill W. Quoted in: Humes JC. The wit and wisdom of Winston Churchill. New York: Harper Perennial; 1995.
7. Dusseau JL. An informal history of W. B. Saunders Company: on the occasion of its hundredth anniversary. Philadelphia: W. B. Saunders; 1988.
8. Speroff L, Fritz MA. A way with words: Leon Speroff, MD describes the growth and evolution of reproductive endocrinology. Sex Reprod Menopause. 2008;6(2):6–7.

Chapter 9
How to Write a Research Protocol

He who fails to plan, plans to fail.

Anonymous

No football coach would ever let his team take the field without a "game plan." The research protocol is the game plan for your project, your vision of what you will accomplish when you "take the field" with your research team. The document describes the reasoning behind and the process of the research project that you have in mind [1]. It tells what you hope to accomplish and how you will get it done. It also imposes a discipline, requiring you and your team to anticipate every step of the project before the first subject is recruited. This body of the research protocol more or less follows the IMRAD model, an acronym for the words introduction, methods, results, and discussion. We will return to this model in Chap. 11, which discusses how to write a report of a research study.

For semantic clarity, I want to distinguish between a research proposal and a research protocol. A research proposal, which should be brief, describes a bright idea for a project—with emphasis on the research question you hope to answer. It tells how you might attempt to answer the question, how you will obtain the data you need, a focused literature search, and perhaps the results of a pilot project. The research

© Springer International Publishing AG 2018
R.B. Taylor, *Medical Writing*,
https://doi.org/10.1007/978-3-319-70126-4_9

proposal will help you crystallize your thoughts and will be a useful document when attempting to recruit coinvestigators. A research protocol is the next stage, representing a detailed road map showing how you will successfully complete your project.

Many, perhaps most, research proposals and protocols will be written as an early step in responding to a request for proposal (RFP). Occasionally a brilliant free-range research idea finds needed support (i.e., dollars), but eventually the serious investigator learns that one's research livelihood is dependent on successful responses to RFPs, whether from government agencies such as the National Institutes of Health (NIH) or private foundations. Because of this, it is vital that the person writing a research protocol carefully read the RFP instructions of the prospective funding agency or foundation. Then reread them several times. Failure to follow the instructions to the letter can result in a poison pill, an item at odds with the instructions, which permits the review panel to dismiss consideration of your project and go on to the next. What might be examples? A high-risk item would be a section that describes a generous stipend for teaching medical students or for the services of a paid consultant in instances when these expenditures are specifically prohibited in the RFP. I will return to this issue in the next chapter on writing grant proposals.

I like to think of a research protocol as the framework for the paper that will report the study's findings. To this end, sometimes a good early exercise is to prepare the format for tables that will go in the final report to be submitted for publication. Let us, for example, think about a study looking at the safety of giving live influenza virus vaccine to children with asthma. In the final report, you may have a table describing subjects by age, gender, ethnicity, and other characteristics. You might then have a table of adverse outcomes—asthma attacks, bronchitis, or pneumonia in patients who did and did not receive the vaccine. Then you may have another table showing the incidence of influenza, with and without complications, in both the study group who received the vaccine and

those who did not. In this way, the tables are already concep-
tualized; they await only the data from the study.

The research protocol will almost certainly be submitted
to a "human subjects committee," called an Institutional
Review Board (IRB) at many universities, and perhaps also
to the funding agency (aka grantor), if grant support is
sought. Note that some IRBs have a research protocol tem-
plate that you will be required to follow. You should spend a
lot of time and energy developing the protocol, not only
because it is likely to be a key in securing IRB approval and
grant funding but also because this is the plan you will follow
in the months to come.

The actual research protocol may not be submitted to a
potential funding agency. That document will be a grant proposal, described in the next chapter. For you, the greatest
value of the research protocol will be in clarifying your thinking before you embark on your research journey.

Assembling a Research Team

Two steps precede writing a research protocol: The first is
identifying a researchable question, and the second is assembling your research team. You will note some similarities to
the writing team, described in Chap. 5; a research team differs
from a writing team, however, in that some specialized skills
are needed to plan and carry out the study. Based on the
assumption that you, as the person with the insightful
research question, will be the principal investigator (PI), I
suggest that you consider including one or more of the following team members:

- A clinical epidemiologist. This team member will guide
  planning of the study design, assuring the team uses the
  best method to answer the research question.
- A biostatistician. Although some will differ, I think that
  this individual should be included from the very start. As an
  example, the statistician can determine the sample sizes
  needed and the statistical tests that will be best for the

project. Also, if you wish to make a biostatistician apoplectic, dump a pile of data on his or her desk late in a study and ask if there is a *p*-value somewhere.

- A senior investigator with more experience than you. This person will serve as respected arbitrator when and if differences arise on the team and can be a big help when writing results of the study.
- An aspiring investigator, someone with less experience than you. This individual will bring energy, will learn from the experience, and just may find some way to pay you back some day.
- A project manager. This vital team member will plan and manage budgets, time commitments of various investigators, and all the records that will eventually be submitted to the funding agency.

Elements of a Research Protocol

There is no single, universally accepted format for a research protocol. What is presented in this chapter is expansive. I have listed every topic I can bring to mind, adapted from the World Health Organization Recommended Format for a Research Protocol [2].

Table 9.1 lists the possible elements of a research protocol, although not all research protocols will contain every item on this list. Most research protocols will have fewer topics or will combine some of the items described. For example, separate discussions of safety considerations, follow-up, and quality assurance may not be relevant to your study. On the other hand, you just might list every topic in the order presented here and use "NA" to identify those not pertinent to your study. The order of topics presented can be different in your protocol, but I caution against too much creativity. The format presented here is, more or less, what IRB reviewers and grant funding agencies expect to see. Table 9.1 can serve as a handy way to check your protocol for completion before it leaves your desk. Some comments on the various topics presented are found in the text that follows.

TABLE 9.1 Format for a research protocol: an expanded list of possible elements

---

Project title

Primary investigator (PI) and coinvestigators and their institutions

Project summary: A short overview to orient the reader

Background and rationale: Analogous to the Introduction in a research report

Study goals and objectives: What do you hope to accomplish?

Study design: What type of study is proposed?

Study description and methods: Who will be the subjects and what will you do to them?

Safety considerations: What are the risks to subjects and what will you do about these risks?

Follow-up: What happens after the study is complete?

Data management: How will you deal with the data obtained?

Quality assurance: How will you assure that what is done reflects high standards?

Expected outcomes: What do you think might be found, and why might it matter?

Dissemination of results: Who will be told about your findings?

Duration of the project: How long is each phase of the study expected to take?

Problems that may occur: What are potential difficulties and possible solutions?

Project management: In this project, who is in charge of what?

Ethical considerations: What might be ethical concerns and how will subjects be informed of these issues?

References: What are prior studies that are pertinent to this project?

Budget: What funding will be needed and how will it be used?

Informed consent forms: Forms to be read and signed by research subjects.

Other support: Are there any funding sources that should be disclosed?

Collaborations planned: Will you be working with colleagues outside your designated team?

Links to other projects: Is this proposal the next step in a series of investigations?

Curriculum vitae of investigators

Other research activity of investigators

Clinical trial registration status

Appendix

In presenting some tips about writing a research protocol, I propose that we—you and I—use a hypothetical study, addressing the following question: Are patients who have gastric surgery for weight control at risk of developing serum copper deficiency? This seems a pertinent question, considering the frequency with which such procedures are done today. My choice of a theoretical research project is not a totally random selection. In fact, Prodan et al. did just this sort of study, with results published in 2009 in the *American Journal of Medical Science* [3]. I chose the question of the risk of copper deficiency developing following gastric surgery because it presents a fairly straightforward approach to a potentially important issue, and you will see that our hypothetical study mirrors the Prodan et al. study in various ways.

Project Title

After deciding on a research topic/question/hypothesis, most investigators turn their attention to the project title. This is not a trivial consideration given that, when the final report is eventually published, most readers will scan the titles in the journal table of contents and use this first impression to decide whether or not to read the abstract or even the entire article.

For our study, a reasonable draft title might be: "The Incidence of Low Serum Copper Levels after Gastric Surgery." Or alternatively: "Hypocupremia after Gastric Surgery." The former title tells what I wish to study and is "outcome-neutral." The latter title presumes that the outcome will be lower copper levels in gastric surgery patients and, while this may be the title of the final paper, would be presumptive as a title of a research protocol unless a question mark is added: "Hypocupremia after Gastric Surgery?" To get started I prefer the first title described. For the record, Prodan et al. titled their final, published report "Copper Deficiency After Gastric Surgery: A Reason For Caution."

Acronym-named randomized trials are quite fashionable today. Clinical investigators, whimsical imps that they are, are fond of dreaming up colorful—if sometimes tortured—acronyms, perhaps over a bottle of wine. Here is an example: "The Effect of Hydrocortisone on Development of Shock Among Patients with Severe Sepsis: The HYPRESS Randomized Clinical Trial" (Keh D et al. JAMA. 2016;316:1775).

Stanbrook et al. reviewed acronym-named clinical research trials and what happened to the reports of these studies [4]. They examined 173 consecutive randomized trials reviewed by the Cochrane Heart Group. Of these 173 studies, 59 (34%) had acronymic titles and exhibited the following characteristics:

- Of these 59 studies, 61% were published in just three journals: The *New England Journal of Medicine*, *Circulation*, and *The Lancet*. (Recall that these were heart-disease-related studies).
- Methodologic quality scores were higher than in studies with non-acronymic titles.
- These studies enrolled five times as many patients but had shorter follow-up periods.
- They were no more likely than non-acronymic-titled studies to report positive results.
- They were four times as likely to have pharmaceutical financial support and eight times as likely to have industry-employed authors.

I considered creating an acronym for our modest (and hypothetical) study of serum copper levels in gastric surgery patients. Thus the first title considered, "The Incidence of Low Serum Copper Levels after Gastric Surgery," would yield the acronym ILSCLAGS. Not compelling. The second choice title, "Hypocupremia after Gastric Surgery," results in HAGS. Even worse. I decided against the use of an acronymic title.

When crafting a title, it is helpful to append a descriptor telling the method used, such as randomized controlled trial, case-control, cross-sectional study, or meta-analysis. Our study compares two groups, those who had weight-loss gastric surgery and those who did not. Thus our working title will be "The Incidence of Low Serum Copper Levels after Gastric Surgery: A Case Control Study."

Primary Investigator (PI) and Coinvestigators

Clearly identify the PI and all coinvestigators. Be sure to include—especially for the PI—titles, institutional affiliation, mailing addresses, telephone numbers, fax numbers, and e-mail addresses. Contact information is important, because someone may want to get in touch with you about collaboration in this study or the next or may even want to send you grant support.

Project Summary

Here is where you should explicitly state your research question or hypothesis. Be sure that anyone reading this paragraph has a clear idea of what you hope to learn. A good research question is short, focused, and unequivocal. Most research questions describe something that can be answered with quantitative data, although there are an increasing number of reports of qualitative research, related to topics that defy quantification.

A useful model for stating a research question is the PICO model [5]. Here is how it works and how it might apply to our study of serum copper levels:

P = Population or patients: Patients who had weight-loss gastric surgery
I = Indicator or intervention: Serum copper levels
C = Comparator or control: Patients who did not have gastric surgery
O = Outcome: Differences in serum copper levels

Careful wordsmithing is vital here. Bordage and Dawson describe the research question as the "keystone of the entire enterprise," adding that, "Everything hinges on the quality of the research question, hence its crucial importance" [6].

Many RFPs specify the maximum number of pages permitted, and even if length is not prescribed, keep the Project Summary short—250 words or less and not more than one page in length. Start by using the study title, and follow by briefly telling the rationale and objectives for the project, the research question, the methods and subjects, the duration of the study, and the anticipated outcome. Use language that would make sense to a reader who is not fully familiar with your area of inquiry. This summary page, arguably the most important page of the protocol, must give a crisp and memorable overview, and it must stand on its own, without sending the reader to search items, such as abbreviations, found later in the document.

Background and Rationale

This section, not unlike the Introduction section in a research report (see Chap. 11), tells why the proposed research is pertinent in the context of current knowledge. This section may cover:

- The importance of the topic in the context of current knowledge
- An overview of your approach to the question
- Any results you have already obtained that indicate that the question can be answered by your approach
- How your study will advance medical practice and the health of humankind

Our serum copper level after gastric surgery study is pertinent to medical knowledge because undetected and uncorrected hypocupremia can cause health problems including anemia, neutropenia, optic neuropathy, myopathy, and myelopathy with a spastic gait [3].

You may list current references here or, alternatively, in a separate section (below).

Study Goals and Objectives

The WHO Recommended Format for a Research Proposal describes, "Goals are broad statements of what the proposal hopes to accomplish. They create a setting for the proposal.

Specific objectives are statements of the research question(s). Objectives should be simple (not complex), specific (not vague), and stated in advance (not after the research is done)" [2]. Singh et al. advise that objectives should be specific, measurable, achievable, relevant, and time based, offering the catchy acronym SMART objectives [7]. The objective of our example study might be to determine if patients who have received weight-loss gastric surgery are more likely later to have lower serum copper levels than persons who have not had gastric surgery.

Study Design

Describe your choice of study design—randomized trial, case-control, cohort study, cross-sectional study, or other approach—and why the study design proposed is the best way to answer the research question. For my study of serum copper levels in post-gastric surgery patients, I chose a case control study model. This and various other study design models are described in Appendix D.

Study Description

Here I will begin with a few linguistic tips: First of all, I recommend that you use active voice and future tense. Active voice ("We will draw blood samples" vs. "Blood samples will be drawn") is simply stronger prose. And you should use the future tense because you are describing something to be done, not something being done now or accomplished in the past.

Secondly, describe persons in the study as subjects, not patients. You are not typically in a traditional physician–patient relationship with these individuals.

This section of the protocol often begins by describing the subjects to be in the study and control groups. What will be your sample size? Who will be included and who will be excluded and why (think about the possibility of exclusion bias)? How did you decide on the number of subjects in each group? A too-small sample size may not yield a statistically satisfying answer to your research question, and your study will be criticized as "underpowered."

How will subjects be found? Will you use a newspaper advertisement, search existing hospital records, or use some other method?

Then once you have your subjects, what will you do to them? Describe each step of the study, beginning with enrollment. If subjects are to be randomized, tell the method to be used. Continue to describe what will happen, step by step, all the way through the last follow-up event.

Name the specific statistical tests that will be used to answer your research question(s) or test your hypotheses. In the case of interventional studies, it may be useful here to identify dependent and independent variables. There are a number of statistical tests that can be used, according to the design of your study. In their published study of copper deficiency after gastric surgery, Prodan et al. used independent t tests and Fisher exact tests for comparison of continuous and categorical variables, respectively [3]. In my opinion, the diversity and complexity of the statistical tests that might be used just serve to emphasize the importance of a research team member with statistical expertise. And here is a sobering thought that will be pertinent when you write the final report of your study: According to Bordage, the most common reason manuscripts are rejected by peer-reviewed scientific journals is incomplete or inappropriate statistics [8].

Safety Considerations

This section is about risks to the subjects, especially pertinent when patients will take drugs or undergo procedures. Tell the risks, including possible drug side effects, allergic reactions, or procedural complications. Then describe what you will do to reduce risk and what will happen if adverse events occur.

Rid et al. have proposed a framework for assessing the risks associated with a research project [9]. They call this method the systematic evaluation of research risks (SERR) and base the method on four steps:

1. Identifying potential harms associated with the project
2. Categorizing the magnitude of the potential harms described
3. Quantifying or estimating the likelihood of each potential harm occurring
4. Comparing the likelihood of each potential intervention-related harm with what might occur with a comparable activity

For my study involving determining serum copper levels in study and control group subjects, I believe that the chief risks are those associated with obtaining blood samples. In the study cohort, the surgery is completed before the study begins.

Follow-Up

Here you should tell what, if anything, will happen to subjects after the research study is completed. In my study, patients found to have significant hypocupremia will be referred to their personal physicians for further evaluation and management.

Data Management

As things move along, you will accumulate data—information about subjects, consent forms, laboratory reports, tables of results, and so forth. How will these data be coded and entered into computer files? How will you assure that data are both accurate and complete? Especially when your study involves human subjects, you should tell how you will maintain security of these data. Identify who will do these tasks, ideally the project manager on your team.

Quality Assurance

You should tell how you will pay attention to the fundamentals of good clinical practice, especially important when human subjects are involved. How will you determine best practice in the conduct of the study? Will there be an independent oversight committee?

Expected Outcomes

The ideal clinical study will have an impact on some segment of the population. In the case of my small study on the risks of copper deficiency following gastric surgery, the results will either be helpful in alerting physicians to a potential adverse outcome of an increasingly common procedure or serve to be cautionary to patients considering gastric surgery for weight control or for other reasons.

Duration of the Project

Here is where you should present a timeline, which may help you identify possible bottlenecks, such as the possibility that you may not find as many qualifying subjects as anticipated. The timeline also may be useful later when writing a grant application. Table 9.2 presents a sample timetable that would be appropriate for my gastric surgery/serum copper level study. Figure 9.1 presents the same information in tabular form.

Dissemination of Results

Who will be told of your findings? Are you targeting a specific journal or a clinical specialty as the eventual reader of your study report? Do you plan to present to a specific specialty group or at a future scientific meeting? Will study participants be informed of the outcome of the study? Under this

TABLE 9.2 Sample timeline for a not very complicated 18-month project

Research Question:
Are patients who have gastric surgery at risk of developing serum copper deficiency?
Year one:
Months 1–3
Identify potential subjects who have had a history of partial gastric resection
Identify potential control population with no history of partial gastric resection
Assure that controls match study subjects relative to age, gender, and concurrent illnesses
Months 4–6
Recruit study and control subjects
Months 7–9
Collect serum samples from study and control subjects
Months 10–12
Analyze data and determine conclusions
Year two:
Months 13–15
Plan report of study
Months 16–17
Present report at national meeting
Month 18
Submit final report for publication

heading, the WHO research protocol advises discussing "who will take the lead in publication and who will be acknowledged in publications, etc." [2].

In the case of our hypothetical study of the possible occurrence of low serum copper levels following gastric surgery, I think that the information would be especially pertinent to certain groups of physicians: surgeons, notably bariatric surgeons, and also generalists, including general internists and family physicians, who will see these postoperative patients in their continuity practices. Whether to aim for publication in a surgery or a generalist specialty journal will be a decision for the research team to ponder.

Project Activity	Months 1-3	Months 4-6	Months 7-9	Months 10-12	Months 13-15	Months 16-18
Identify study subjects	X					
Identify control subjects	X					
Assure matching study/control subjects	X					
Recruit study and control subjects		X				
Collect serum samples from study and control subjects			X			
Analyze data; determine conclusions				X		
Plan report of study					X	
Report study at national meeting						X
Submit final report for publication						X

FIG. 9.1 Sample timeline presented as a figure. Research question: *Are patients who have gastric surgery at risk of developing serum copper deficiency?*

Problems That May Occur

Research trials are not exempt from Murphy's law: If something can go wrong, it will. Use your imagination to think of possible problems and what you would do to remedy them. Here is an example: In our hypothetical study, a potential problem might be discovering that my surgery subjects turn out to have a much higher incidence of a concurrent disease, such as inflammatory bowel disease, than my control subjects. What would I do about this?

Project Management

In this section, tell the specific role and duties of each research team member, including the all-important project manager. Reaching consensus on these issues can prove vital to success, and misunderstandings about the assignment of responsibilities can spell trouble. For these reasons alone, this section of the protocol should be the subject of informed agreement by all on the team.

Ethical Considerations

Ethical issues are a chief concern of the IRB. The IRB's scope of interest includes hospital chart reviews, questionnaire studies, and anything that involves human bodies, tissues or fluids, or information. They will ponder any discomfort or even pain associated with a study intervention. For example, in my study, there will be blood samples drawn. Does the potential outcome of the study justify the admittedly small discomfort that will be experienced by subjects?

In any study involving drugs, there is the risk of adverse reactions. Are there any hazards to subjects that might not be readily apparent, such as the long-term risk involved in studies involving radiographic imaging? Does the potential benefit of the study justify such risks?

Will participants be paid to participate in the study? If so, is the amount being offered "correct," that is, enough to compensate for their time without being such a large sum that persons step forward as volunteers who really should not do so?

Do subjects have the right to withdraw from the study without physical risk and without the threat of being punished—that is, of having subsequent care withdrawn?

All of these issues, and perhaps more, should be discussed in a carefully worded informed consent document, which is appended to the research protocol.

References

This will be a list of published reports that serve as background to your proposal.

For my hypothetical study, I would certainly list the 2009 Prodan et al. report and others.

Budget

In this section, describe the funding that will be needed to complete your project, including justification of how every dollar will be spent. If there is an RFP involved, you need to read the RFP carefully to see what expenditures are allowed and what are not. Can you, for example, budget for administrative assistance, student research workers, or travel to present findings at a scientific meeting? Although the budget section of your research protocol may be of only passing interest to the IRB, it will be a key part of your eventual grant proposal, described in the following chapter.

Be sure your budget figures are realistic and accurate. An underpowered budget—not nearly enough money to do the job—is as bad as an underpowered study. Budget preparation is not time for guesswork.

Other Support

Here is where you should reveal any funding—such as a pharmaceutical company grant—that might not otherwise be apparent in your protocol.

Collaborations Planned

Is your project being done in concert with investigators outside your research team, perhaps even in other institutions? If so, you will eventually need letters of agreement from these individuals.

Links to Other Projects

Is the proposed project somehow related to some other research project? Because academicians tend to develop "career topics," such links are not uncommon [10]. Statements here may document compelling evidence of your leadership in this topic. Or they may raise suspicion that this is a "chain letter" project (see Chap. 12).

Curriculum Vitae of Investigators

Append the curriculum vitae of each member of the research team. Follow any RFP instructions as to format and number of pages desired.

Other Research Activity of Investigators

The principal investigator and coinvestigators should briefly describe their current research projects, the amount of time devoted to each, how long each project will last, and the sources of funding.

Clinical Trial Registration

International Committee of Medical Journal Editors (ICMJE) member journals now require, as a consideration for publication, registration of the study in a public trials registry before the enrollment of the first subject [11]. This rule was implemented to counter the practice of selective reporting of trials—if the drug had desired result, the results were published, but if the drug tested seemed no better than placebo, the study data languished in someone's desk drawer. Furthermore, the US Food and Drug Administration requires clinical trial registration 21 days after the first subject is enrolled. I recommend that your research protocol mention the status of your clinical trial registration. Full information is available at http://clinicaltrials.gov.

And in the future, we may see mandated data sharing to provide other researchers with access to your data. The ICMJE "proposes to require that authors include a plan for data sharing as a component of clinical trial registration" [12].

Appendix

This section should contain a copy of the informed consent form. You may also list here the literature reviewed, if not presented above, as well as other items that do not logically fit in the outline above.

What Makes a Good Research Protocol

Fundamentally, a good research protocol provides enough detail that could allow another investigator to do the study and arrive at comparable conclusions.

The best research protocols have some characteristics in common:

- Early overview, described above as the "Project Summary": Begin with a brief but crystal-clear synopsis of the project that helps orient the reader to what is coming later.
- Logical progression of ideas: Use the outline described here to lead the reader, point by point, to a clear understanding of what you plan to do and how you will do it.
- Carefully constructed headings: The research protocol is really an essay. Use headings to announce how ideas are grouped.
- Clear prose: Remember that the person reading your protocol, such as a member of your Institutional Review Board, may not be familiar with your field at all.
- Completeness: Anticipate the questions a reader might have, and try to provide answers.

Common Problems in Research Protocols

This section describes mistakes we make in research planning and protocol writing (or perhaps in writing, in general). Some of the common ones are:

- Inadequate literature review, conducting a quick survey when a systematic review is needed. Don't propose to do what has already been done.
- Vague research question: Often this means the question is too broad or unanswerable and needs to be focused.
- Flawed research design: Do not select a study type that will not answer the question. Much time and effort will be wasted. Most research failures can be traced to the early planning stages.
- A project too ambitious for your research skills or for the institutional resources available to your team.
- Too many objectives and research questions: I think a study can answer up to three related research questions. More than that suggests a lack of focus. I once encountered data from a study that had listed 57 research questions. Although the investigators succeeded in collecting some data, when ultimately preparing a paper, they struggled to find just a few questions whose answers had statistical significance. ("Isn't there a meaningful p-value anywhere is the mess?") They never succeeded in writing a publishable paper.
- Inadequate number of subjects to answer the question: Do not count on the IRB to alert you to this problem, which poses no risk to subjects, even though it wastes the time of willing volunteers.
- Inappropriate plan for statistical analysis: The statistician is planning to use the wrong tests to look at the data.
- Poorly written consent form: Your IRB will send the consent form back for rewriting if it is not comprehensive and legally sound.
- A budget inadequate for the project or even too high.
- Failure to reach consensus on all aspects of the protocol. The discipline of preparing—and struggling to group agreement about—a research plan will prove invaluable if there are later disagreements within the research team.
- Underestimating the time needed to complete all the steps—including peer review and institutional review—needed to get the grant out the door on time.

Cover Letter to the Institutional Review Board

Securing approval from your Institutional Review Board can be a speed bump that delays submission of your grant proposal. Keep in mind that the IRB is interdisciplinary; members at the table may include biologists, anatomists, physicians in diverse specialties, and, in some cases, community representatives. I urge that your research protocol be accompanied by an easy-to-understand cover letter [13]. With the recognition that some of what I list below repeats what is in your protocol, here are some suggested topics for this somewhat brief letter:

- Title of the project.
- Why is your department undertaking this project?
- Is what you propose invading another department's turf? If so, have you discussed this with them?
- How many subjects are involved, and what is the time frame for the proposed research?
- Is there a scientific spin-off for your department and the university?

Final Steps

After the research protocol is written (and rewritten a few times), what then? As with all writing products, I recommend that you next have it reviewed by your "critical reader" colleague, described in Chap. 3. This person will help you identify problems with organization, syntax, and grammar that may detract from the merits of your idea. If the critical reader colleague is not research savvy, especially in your area of investigation, I suggest that you next have the document reviewed by an experienced investigator. (Following my own advice, I have had the manuscript for this chapter reviewed by our department's most skilled researchers.)

Then your research protocol is ready for consideration—and, we hope, prompt approval—by the Human Subjects Committee/IRB. With that approval in hand, you are ready to work on your Application for Grant Funding.

References

1. O'Brien K, Wright J. How to write a protocol. J Orthod. 2002;29(1):58–61.
2. World Health Organization Recommended Format for a Research Protocol. http://www.who.int/rpc/research_ethics/format_rp/en/. Accessed 25 Apr 2017.
3. Prodan CI, Bottomley SS, Vincent SS, et al. Copper deficiency after gastric surgery: a reason for caution. Am J Med Sci. 2009;37(4):256–8.
4. Stanbrook MB, Austin PC, Redelmeier DA. Acronym-named randomized trials in medicine—the ART in medicine. N Engl J Med. 2006;355(1):101–2.
5. Glasziou P, Del Mar C, Salisbury J. Evidence-based medicine workbook. London: BMJ Books; 2003. p. 40.
6. Bordage G, Dawson B. Experimental study design and grant writing in eight steps and 28 questions. Med Educ. 2003;37(4):376–85.
7. Singh S, Suganthi P, Ahmed J, Chadha VK. Formulation of health research protocol—a step-by-step description. NTI Bull. 2005;41(1&2):5–10.
8. Bordage G. Reasons reviewers reject and accept manuscripts: the strengths and weaknesses in medical education reports. Acad Med. 2001;76(9):889–96.
9. Rid A, Emanuel EJ, Wendler D. Evaluating the risks of clinical research. JAMA. 2010;304(13):1472–9.
10. Taylor RB. Academic medicine: a guide for clinicians. New York: Springer; 2006. p. 136.
11. DeAngelis CD, Drazen JM, Frizelle FA, et al. Clinical trial registration: a statement from the International Committee of Medical Journal Editors. JAMA. 2004;292(11):1363–4.
12. Taichman DB, Backus J, Baethge C, et al. Sharing clinical trial data: a proposal from the International Committee of Medical Journal Editors. PLoS Med. 2016;13(1):e1001950.
13. Guidelines for cover letter accompanying a clinical research protocol. VU University Medical Center Amsterdam. https://www.vumc.com/branch/cca/research/CWO/9640719/. Accessed 25 Apr 2017.

Chapter 10
How to Write a Grant Proposal

The relatively young woman stood up from her computer and replied while sipping her coffee: "It is hard work and it requires a lot of dedication. I know it's going to be many hours before I finish this grant and I know the chances of getting funded aren't in my favor. But, it's a labor of love because I'm discovering a cure for cancer."

From an article by American physician and educator Chip Souba [1].

The engine of America's clinical investigation enterprise is fueled by grants. In fact, so is some of medical education, by virtue of government and foundation grant funding for educational programs. One of the big surprises I encountered upon leaving rural practice and entering academic medicine in 1978 was the discovery that there was no pool of money to fund my salary. In short, I was expected to bring in almost all my support. There were other funding sources, such as private philanthropy and endowments, but for most of us in the United States, funding the salary that supports our teaching efforts meant seeing patients or writing successful grant proposals. Things have not changed over the past four-plus decades. An academic appointment is not a meal ticket; it is a hunting license.

Fortunately, there has historically been a lot of money available: The US National Institutes of Health (NIH) commits more than $30 billion annually to medical research,

© Springer International Publishing AG 2018
R.B. Taylor, *Medical Writing*,
https://doi.org/10.1007/978-3-319-70126-4_10

largely awarded through approximately 50,000 competitive grants to more than 300,000 investigators in some 2500 institutions in the United States and around the world [2]. In addition, tons of private money, donated to nonprofit organizations as tax-deductible gifts, are available as grant funding. While all this funding could easily cover your salary and mine for many years, getting access to the money requires knowledge, effort, and perseverance.

Seeking funding via grants in the United States uses a "tournament" model that involves competition, recruitment of star players, and both winners and losers [3]. In regard to recruitment, would you believe that if your academic department has a nationally recognized, highly productive grant-getter, other institutions are constantly wooing this person? These "rainmakers" are the champions in the grantsmanship competition. As to winners and losers, failing to acquire grant funding can be a major problem for a faculty member, one that could lead to job loss, not only for the investigator but for everyone on his or her research team.

The purpose of writing a grant proposal/application is to get an award—money that will support your project over a few years. At this point it may be instructive to be clear about the words we use. You and I write *grant proposals*; in doing so we hope to get *grant awards*. Thus, saying that I am hard at work "writing a grant" is semantically incorrect, even though this is the common parlance we use today.

There are actually two types of awards. We most commonly think of the *grant* award, often funding basic science or clinical research. Classically, the applicant generates the research idea, and the grant recipient has some flexibility in using the money to complete the project. On the other hand, the *contract* award, often used for applied research, is an agreement to do something the funding agency—such as a state agency or pharmaceutical firm—wants done. A state agency, for example, may award a contract to survey generalist physicians regarding their ability and willingness to provide mental health services in the face of reduced availability of psychiatric referrals for Medicaid patients. In the case of a contract, expect greater control by the funding agency and strict accountability for the money spent.

In some ways, a grant application will resemble a research protocol, described in the previous chapter, but there are important differences. Fundamentally, the research protocol is a document created for you and your team, even though it may be shared with the Institutional Review Board and perhaps others. To reprise the sports metaphor, it is your "game plan," a series of steps to which you all agree. In contrast, the grant application is written for an outside audience—specifically for the panel of experts who will review your request for funding. As I have written grant proposals, I have occasionally reflected that the dozens of pages being written will actually be read completely by only a handful of people—perhaps only two—who will then describe the proposal, as they understand it, to the review committee. I'll return to this below.

Where the Money Is: Government and Private Grant Funding Sources

To begin at ground level, there are two major funding sources: government and private. Government sources may be federal, state, or local. Private grant and contract funding sources include foundations, corporations, or professional associations.

Government Funding Sources

State and local grant funding agencies are often politically grounded, and funding may be awarded as contracts that advance favored agendas such as care of the homeless, rather than based on the likelihood of providing new knowledge. If you or your department has a contact in the state, county, or city government, you may have a chance of receiving state/local funding for a project. An example of such a project might be a needed statewide survey of the impact of high professional liability rates on procedure-oriented specialists in regard to their willingness to accept indigent patients for care. Or county leaders might need a survey of physicians as they assess the need for more or fewer hospital beds in the future. If offered such a contract, you must consider your need for salary support as well as the direction this might take your personal research agenda.

There are a number of granting agencies in the federal government, offering opportunities of various types. For example, there are primary care training grants available through the Bureau of Health Professions (BHP) of the Health Resources and Services Administration (HRSA). For the academic clinician and researcher, the important funding source is the National Institutes of Health (NIH), whose mission is "to seek fundamental knowledge about the nature and behavior of living systems and the application of that knowledge to enhance health, lengthen life, and reduce the burdens of illness and disability" [4]. I urge you to learn about NIH grants and funding early in your career. A good beginning web site is the NIH Guide to Grants and Contracts, available at http://grants.nih.gov/funding/index.htm.

Because the NIH is the source of so many funding opportunities, its policies and attitudes are especially important to the academic clinician who aspires to do serious clinical research. According to Kotchen et al., "A perception exists among clinical investigators that the NIH peer review process may discriminate against clinical research." With that as a background, these authors studied outcomes of grant applications submitted to the NIH by MDs vs. non-MDs and those involving human subjects vs. those that did not. They conclude: "Although physicians compete favorably in the peer review process, review outcomes are modestly less favorable for grant applications for clinical research than for laboratory research" [5].

Here is another interesting statistic: The number of research trials underwritten by the NIH is declining. From 2006 to 2014 the number of NIH-funded trials decreased by

TABLE 10.1 Selected funding databases and web sites

Agency for Healthcare Research and Quality (AHRQ) Grants On-Line Database (GOLD): http://www.ahrq.gov/cpi/about/otherwebsites/gold.ahrq.gov/index.html
Research Portfolio Online Reporting Tools (RePORT). Provides access to reports, data, and analyses of NIH research studies. https://report.nih.gov/
Federal Register: http://www.gpoaccess.gov/fr/index.html
The Foundation Center: A source for "fundraisers and grantmakers solving social problems through philanthropy. http://foundationcenter.org/
Grants.gov: A portal to search for federal grants in diverse areas. http://www.grants.gov
Health Resources and Services Administration (HRSA): Offers health-related grants in various areas. https://www.hrsa.gov/index.html
National Institutes of Health, Office of Extramural Research home page. Describing grants and funding through the NIH. http://grants.nih.gov/grants/oer.htm

24%. And during that same time, the NIH budget fell by 14%, adjusted for inflation [6].

Table 10.1 lists selected grant and contract databases. The sites here may include both government and private funding opportunities.

Nongovernmental Grant Sources

Foundations, societies, corporations, and associations can be a rich source of funding support and are a good place for the new faculty member to get started. There are independent, sometimes regional, foundations, such as the Northwest Health Foundation or the Paul G. Allen Foundation for Medical Research, serving the Pacific Northwest area of the United States. There are health-company-related foundations, such as the Aetna Foundation or the Robert Wood Johnson Foundation, and charitable family foundations, such as the Ford Family Foundation. Almost any major organ or disease you can name has a foundation; examples include the American Heart Foundation, the American Lung Association, the National Stroke Association, the American Cancer Society, the American Diabetes Association, the Alzheimer's Association, and several foundations focused on autism. Funding for research projects may also be available from your specialty society, which may have its own foundation, such as the American Academy of Family Physicians Foundation. In addition, there are many grants available from business and industry; some of these are available to clinicians and academicians, and others are for projects outside the realm of medicine and science.

If you are a faculty member considering sending a grant proposal to a private or corporate foundation in your state, I urge that you contact your academic medical center (AMC) grant office. That office is charged to coordinate grant requests submitted to various agencies, especially those that are "local." Their reasoning is as follows: The institution looks foolish if a local foundation receives several proposals from your institution, with one investigator unaware of the other's submission. Even worse, your heartwarming grant award of $10,000 today may be blamed for a later rejection of a million-dollar proposal if the grantor chooses to make only one award to a single institution.

Another type of private funding is related to research conducted by pharmaceutical companies or corporations making medical or surgical equipment. One of the big surprises of young faculty members may be the amount of corporate-sponsored research conducted in AMCs. Such research might be part of a larger collaborative study with you as a listed coinvestigator. It is much more likely, however, that your role will be to submit research data, based on a company-generated protocol that is being used in a number of institutions. You may have no control over what goes into the final paper and, in fact, are unlikely to see your name in print when the results are published in the medical literature. Of course, without being listed as a coauthor on a published report, the effort is valueless when you become a candidate for promotion. "Then why do this research?" you ask. The answer is money, and the monetary rewards for providing pharmaceutical research services are quite high. Many medical school departments and divisions depend heavily on this income to support the salaries of faculty and staff.

Early Steps in Writing Grant Applications

Here I will present some generalities that apply to various types of funding proposals. A noteworthy exception to what follows is pharmaceutical company contract research, in which you simply agree to abide by the terms of their contract offer—or decline to participate.

The Request for Proposal

Grant awards often begin with a request for proposal (RFP), an invitation by a granting agency—government or private—to submit an application. There will be a description of the type of projects that will be considered, specific instructions, a cap on the amount that may be requested, and a submission deadline. In some instances, there will be a funding priority—an item that, if included in the grant proposal and approved, adds points to the final funding score, moving the application higher in the funding queue. As a hypothetical example, the American Diabetes Association might seek proposals that study the impact of homelessness on the management of diabetes mellitus, with a maximum award of $100,000 over 3 years, a deadline for submission about 4 months in the future, and a funding priority for proposals that target Native American homeless subjects.

Study the RFP carefully before taking the fateful step of beginning to outline a grant proposal. Be very sure that your idea for a project fits exactly with what the funding agency is seeking; in the hypothetical study above, writing a proposal examining the impact on homeless Native American subjects of having an *alcoholic* family member in the household will probably be a waste of effort.

Reviewing What Has Worked in the Past

In a world as competitive as grant-getting, it seems strange that successful grant applications to government agencies are available for your review. Revealing such information would be unheard of in industry. In some cases, when there are repeated cycles for similar initiatives, past award-winning applications can serve as helpful models for your grant. Even if you do not read every word of every grant, a quick review can tell you who are writing the grants (the principal investigators) and what is contained in the summaries. To view information on successful NIH grants, access the Research Portfolio Online Reporting Tools (RePORT) at: http://report.nih.gov/index.aspx.

In fact, if you are especially keen on seeing the entire text of a specific grant, you can do so under the Freedom of Information Act (FOIA). You will need to contact the NIH Freedom of Information Office Coordinator for the Institute in question; begin by accessing http://www.nih.gov/icd/od/foia/coord.htm. Expect to pay a fee for processing and handling.

Foundations and other private sources will generally supply you with a list of projects they have funded recently, but beyond this, you may need to talk to the authors of the grant applications.

The Program Officer

Most federal and private grant funding agencies will have a designated program officer (sometimes called a project officer) for each grant solicitation. This person is a very valuable contact. I advise early contact by telephone. A face-to-face meeting would be even better but is often not possible because of geographical distance. Be ready to give a brief description of your project. Then ask open-ended questions:

- How well do you think my ideas match the intent of the proposal?
- What might be the problems with my idea?
- What else would you suggest be included?
- Is there something you would do differently? Do you see a fault in my thinking?
- What other suggestions would you have?
- What else should I know?

The program officer is likely to know a great deal about the project and the agency. It is his or her job to help you present the best proposal possible. Contact the program officer early and often as you work on your proposal.

Do not call the program officer with foolish questions that are readily answered in the RFP or on the grantor's web site. Also, don't call to ask questions such as, "What types of proposals are likely to be funded this year?" Or "Should I send a copy of my curriculum vitae with the proposal?" Be sure your questions are thoughtful and carefully constructed.

Just one word of caution: The role of the program officer is to be helpful and supportive. However, this person is not a decision-maker when the time to review your proposal comes.

Encouragement by your program officer does not predict or connote approval.

The Letter of Intent

Many foundations request a letter of intent briefly describing your project. Some federal and state funding sources are adopting this concept, and you may see the terms "proposal concept paper" or "white paper." This concise overview of your idea allows both the funding source and you to decide early if more effort is warranted. If a letter of intent is requested, think your project through carefully, pay attention to the length of letter requested (one page, two pages, or some other length), and be sure to answer all questions included in the instructions.

If you are provided no prescribed format for a letter of intent or proposal concept paper, use the following as topics for the paragraphs in your letter:

- Project summary: This is a two- or three-sentence overview of your idea and why the project is appropriate for the agency you are contacting.
- Significance of the project: Tell the problem you intend to address.
- Approach to the problem: Tell how you will address the problem and how your approach is different from other past efforts.
- Request for funds: Describe why you will need money to complete the project, with a brief overview of how funds will be used.
- A sentence thanking the potential grantor for considering your proposal, followed by your signature and full contact information.

I like letters of intent, because they can provide a preview of potential success or failure, without the full effort of preparing a long grant proposal. With that said, however, I would not submit a letter of intent without having had a conversation with the program officer.

Planning the Budget

Some say that this is the second task, right after deciding on the concept for your proposal. The budget is often prepared by working with a project manager. The effort is certainly important because asking for too much may sink your proposal; requesting and getting a too-small grant award can cause you to be underfunded. Whatever you put in your budget, be sure to justify every item in your application. If you ask for travel funds, tell why specific travel is needed to make your project a success. If you request money for photocopying or postage, describe what you plan to copy and mail. Also, you must master the somewhat arcane terms used in grant budgets, including direct and indirect costs, the latter now called (at the NIH) "facilities and administrative costs," and TBA, which stands for "to be added," and may refer to faculty, staff, or equipment—all dependent on successful funding.

A Title for Your Project

In the end, your proposal will be presented to a review committee that will judge its merits. I am an advocate of making the topic and the outline of the project easy for the reviewers to remember. Sometimes the key is a catchy acronym, as discussed in Chap. 9. A few years ago, our department submitted a federal training grant to support a 3-year program to teach our residents about advocacy (for their patients), cultural competence, and ethical issues in medicine. It became the ACE program; the acronym made little sense in an academic setting, but the three-letter word represented a memory device to help the review committee recall the three main components of the project. The project was, in fact, approved and funded.

Another training grant proposal consisting of what was, frankly, a jumble of unrelated projects was approved and funded in part, I believe, because we linked them together with the memorable title, "The New Physician's Black Bag for the 21st Century." Today I can't recall what we stuffed in the "black bag," but I do remember the title of the project.

The Grant Proposal

A good idea for a project is important, as is early contact with the program officer, but success ultimately depends on a professionally prepared grant proposal. In many instances, and especially with nongovernmental funding agencies, your grant proposal can be crafted to address the mission and goals of a grant funder, emphasizing how you will address their published objectives. Table 10.2 tells basic components of a grant proposal, written assuming that you are the princi-

TABLE 10.2 Basic outline of a grant proposal

Executive summary (abstract): briefly describe the proposal
Overview of institution: describe your institution and project team
Problem/background: the problem and rationale for what you plan, typically based on a literature review and/or preliminary studies
Project objectives: your hypothesis or the aim of the project
Project method: what do you plan to do?
Subjects, methods, and analysis
OR
The proposed educational program or other activity
Timeline: show what you plan to do and when
Budget and budget justification
Other funding
Plans for future funding
Appendix/supplementary items:
Support letters
Affiliation agreements
Biographical summaries of investigators
References
Other items

pal investigator (PI) and grant proposal author. Some of these items are similar to headings in the research protocol, but others are not, because grant proposals may describe projects, such as proposed training programs, rather than research.

Executive Summary

Also sometimes called the abstract, this short but vitally important component of the grant is intended to provide early orientation for the reader. In the case of NIH grant applications, the abstract may be used in deciding which study section should review the document. In some proposals, the summary may be as short as three sentences, and brevity is better than excessive length. Because it is short, it must engage the reader's attention early and whet the appetite for more. Here is an example of a three-sentence executive summary, based on the hypothetical gastric surgery/copper deficiency study I used for a model in Chap. 9. This summary tells my research question, how I will approach the question, and how the answer to the question might affect clinical practice.

> We propose to determine if patients who have received weight loss gastric surgery have lower serum copper levels than individuals who have not had gastric surgery. We will do so by means of blood samples obtained from cohorts of patients who have and have not had gastric surgery in the past. The outcome of this study can help determine if post-gastric surgery patients might be at risk for hypocupremia, which would have implications for long-term post-operative management.

In the case of foundations that may have lay donors who take an interest in what is funded, you may consider submitting two types of summaries: The first is the scientific abstract, intelligible to scientists with training and experience in the area of the proposal. The second is the layman's abstract, written in terms intelligible to the general reader.

I suggest that you write the executive summary early, and then return to it from time to time, making sure that it is as good as it can be.

Overview of Institution

This section, generally only a few paragraphs long, should describe your organization in a way that suggests that it has the wherewithal—experience, trustworthiness, resources—to support your project and to manage funds properly. Describe important institutional accomplishments. Important evidence of all of this is a past record of research success, especially with big-budget projects. If you are part of a very large institution, be sure to identify your role, perhaps including an organizational chart.

This section should be included even if you and your team have a past track record with the funding agency. Remember that funding agency personnel can change and institutional memory is short.

Problem/Background

In this section, you will explain the problem and why it is important, based on a selective literature review or sometimes, in the case of a major research endeavor, a systematic review (see section "Biographical Summaries of Investigators"). In the case of copper deficiency following gastric surgery, I would point out that hypocupremia in adults can cause neurologic manifestations including progressive sensory ataxia and weakness in the extremities, as well as anemia and neutropenia [7–9].

If you have done preliminary work or pilot studies, describe them here, especially if this work has resulted in publications.

If you are citing just a few references, they may be listed here, at the end of this section. If the list of citations is longer, and/or citations also occur elsewhere in your document, they should all be listed below under a separate heading "References" in the Appendix. In most cases you need cite only very pertinent studies that are integral to your proposal. Do not append a long list of references intended chiefly to impress reviewers.

Project Objectives/Research Question

Here, in the case of a request for research support, you tell your specific aims and hypotheses. This section is described by Inouye and Feillin as "the most important section of the grant" [10].

Not all requests are for hypothesis-based research support, and, if this is the case, the project objective should be stated clearly. Here are some examples:

- We propose to develop, teach, and evaluate a course for second-year medical students presenting the recognition, management, and prevention of domestic violence.
- We propose to plan, conduct, and evaluate a 1-year leadership fellowship for primary care physicians who have completed residency training and at least 3 years of practice.

Following the initial statement of the project's objectives, you should spend a paragraph or two presenting the elements involved, including primary and secondary hypotheses, if any. Your writing here may seem to repeat what was said in the Executive Summary. This reiteration is acceptable, even desirable, because you want the reader to have your aim clearly in mind while he or she is reading the rest of the document.

Project Methods

How you will achieve your objectives is going to be vital to success, both in attaining grant funding and in carrying out your project. Writing this section is easier if you have previously prepared a comprehensive research protocol. Topics to be included in proposals related to clinical research include study design, availability of subjects, inclusion and exclusion criteria, the intervention strategy, safety considerations, data collection methods, how data will be analyzed, and the outcomes to be measured. I recommend using subheadings when writing this section, to be sure that each topic is fully described.

Inouye and Feillin emphasize the importance of the Project Methods section: "The most common general issue (in grants reviewed) is that the methods were underdeveloped" [10]. They recommend that grant application writers devote at least half of their total page allowance to the Methods section.

Timeline

Include a timetable for completion, such as the one developed when writing your research protocol (see Table 9.2 or Fig. 9.1). Be careful that your timeline is consistent with the grant funding available.

Budget and Budget Justification

If there is a major difference between the research protocol and the grant proposal, it is here. Because the chief objective of writing a grant application is to convince someone to give you money to support your project, you need to submit a carefully crafted budget complete with prose that explains every planned expenditure, practically down to the last paper clip.

What might you ask for in your budget? The answer to this question depends on the rules of the funding agency and, often, the stipulations in the RFP. Follow guidelines carefully, so that you do not compromise your credibility and perhaps even your application's approval, by requesting forbidden funding. Examples of items that may be subject to funding prohibitions are equipment such as computers and administrative expenses such as secretarial support. Here is a list of items that you should consider when crafting your budget:

- Personnel, including salary support for the PI, coinvestigators, and research associates
- Independent contractor expenses
- Consultant costs
- Supplies, including paper, envelopes, and printer ink
- Clinical items, such as needles, syringes, and laboratory supplies
- Equipment, including hardware, software, and sometimes even furniture
- Fees paid to subjects
- Space or equipment rental
- Travel expenses to project sites
- Conference expenses to present results of the project
- Miscellaneous costs such as advertising, copying, printing, insurance, and postage
- Facilities and administrative costs

Bordage and Dawson recommend presenting the budget in three sections: (1) funds needed for year 1; (2) funds requested for the remaining period of support; and (3) the budget justification [11]. The budget justification is the section that tells the need for each item in the budget and when the money will be spent. Although some agencies ask only for global budgets, most require detailed justification of every item requested in the budget. For major expenses, include how you determined the anticipated costs, perhaps even appending estimates from vendors.

Other Funding

This can be a good thing. Agencies, especially private foundations, favor projects that have been able to attract support from various sources. Such support can add credibility to your proposal.

Plans for Future Funding

Funding agencies generally like to look to new projects and don't favor funding the same endeavors over and over. For this reason, if your project is to continue beyond the period of initial grant funding, you should state how this will occur. A clinical trial, such as my post-gastric surgery/copper deficiency study, may be projected to be complete on the very day grant funding ceases. On the other hand, in the case of training grants, which typically fund 3-year programs, the recipient is often asked to describe how the educational program will continue after grant funding runs out. Our medical school department currently has several programs that we now self-fund years after grant support ended.

Appendix/Supplementary Items

This is the "attic" of a grant proposal—where you put stuff that may be needed, sometime. Inouye and Fiellin caution never to put anything in the Appendix that you actually want the reviewer to read. "The grant should stand alone, and appendices should only provide supporting materials. The reviewers may not receive or read the appendices" [10]. With that admonition, I submit that there are some items that have to go somewhere, and this is usually it. These may include support letters, affiliation agreements, consent forms, and more.

Support Letters

Support letters are often requested by agencies. For example, in a medical school, you may need a support letter from your dean or from the chair of a department whose cooperation will be vital to the project's success. If such a letter is needed, ask for it early; your letter writer has things that are higher on his or her personal to-do list. I have found that I get the promptest response when my request for a support letter includes a draft of what I want in the letter.

Affiliation Agreement

Some of these are already in the institution's files. If a new document is needed, follow the advice given just above under "Support Letters."

Consent Form

If there is a consent form that participants will sign, include a copy in the Appendix.

Biographical Summaries of Investigators

When biosketches are requested, there is often a prescribed format—often as regards what to include and a limit on pages. Follow instructions.

References

If your proposal calls for a long list of reference citations, put it here.

Other Items

Here you may append requested items such as a list of your board of directors, a copy of your Internal Revenue Tax Exempt Letter, or a current financial statement.

What Makes a Good Grant Proposal

Fundamentally, the grant proposal applicant most likely to be funded is the one who seems to be thoughtful, capable, and professional. The grant application document should reflect these attributes. The following are a few principles that apply to grant proposals of all types:

- Tell your idea early in the proposal. Do not make the reader wade through three pages of "rationale" and "obstacles to be overcome" before finding the project overview on page 4.
- Use the language in the RFP. If the RFP states that the foundation seeks grant proposals to "determine ways to improve the nutritional status of homeless women in large cities," you should use exactly that language to describe your project. You will also need to determine what is meant by "nutritional status," "homeless," "large cities," and even "women." Are 13-year-old homeless females "women"?
- Craft your project description carefully, and then use the same words in the same manner over and over. This assures that, after reading the document, the reviewer will recall the keywords. Thus, in the ACE program described above, I used the words *advocacy*, *cultural competence*, and *ethical issues in medicine* repeatedly, in exactly the same way each time.

- Make the document visually interesting. The reviewer will probably receive a number of grants to read, and you want to capture his or her attention. Try to avoid using very long paragraphs. Use tables to present data, when possible. If you see a section of prose extending to several pages, consider inserting headings to break up the long string of paragraphs. Notice on this page that I have used bullet points to avoid large blocks of prose.

- The document should use the font and margin size recommended in the RFP. If none is recommended, use size 12 font. Margins should be 1 in. or more on sides, top, and bottom. Don't try to gain a few more words by crowding your pages. This can annoy your reader, and you do not want an angry reviewer.

- Document assertions with data and sources. Cite the literature if appropriate, but don't let your grant proposal become a literature review with 90 citations.

- Peer review is an important part of grant proposal writing. Just when you think you are done and everything is perfect, submit the grant to one or more experienced and trusted grant-getting veteran colleagues, asking for criticism. Where are the errors? Can you detect cognitive dissonance? Is something important missing? Do not rush this volunteer peer reviewer, who is likely to be as busy as you. Allow up to 2 weeks for the peer review, just one more reason to start early and stay on schedule.

- Start early and finish early. Try to finish the proposal well ahead of the deadline. I hate last-minute, frantic rushes. Your institutional research services office—which must read and approve your project before it can be submitted—probably dislikes last-minute problems even more than I do. Grant deadlines for various agencies come in cycles, and all grants must be vetted by your institutional office of research services (or some office with a similar title). Hence, if you have a grant headed for the NIH, it is likely that there are a number of other grants from other departments at your institution that have the same deadline. For this reason, it is best to be at the head of the line by completing your grant proposal early. A late submission will not get the attention from the offices of research services that it deserves, a problem that becomes even worse if there is an issue with your proposal.

A Little About the Grant Review Process

Your grant proposal has been approved by your department chair and the institutional research services office. The prospective grantor has received it. You are in the tournament. Next it goes to a review panel, termed a "study section" at the NIH. In a typical grant review panel, all reviewers will have access to your grant. Some may read it completely; others will scan it. At the table, one of the reviewers will be selected to present it to the group. What are the implications of this method?

First, be sure that your proposal is appropriately titled in a way that accurately describes the project and that the reader can recall a day later.

Next, what most review panel members will read is the executive summary. The reviewer who presents your proposal to the review panel is likely to begin his or her presentation here, perhaps reading it word by word, to others around the table. Be sure to tell the readers your concept, the keywords, and the approach you will use throughout the proposal.

In various grant application review settings, there will be a "score," based on either the total or the average of scores submitted by the reviewers present. The scores of all proposals will become a continuum when it comes to deciding funding. What you will eventually hear is that your proposal is:

- Approved without modification to the project or budget. Congratulations!
- Approved, with modification to the project and/or budget. This is usually also considered good news.
- Approved, but not funded. Your grant received a good score, but the agency ran out of money as they funded proposals with even higher scores. Here is where funding preferences may sometimes be the key to success or failure.
- Rejected. This means that your proposal's score fell below the level needed for approval and funding.

If your proposal was rejected or approved but not funded, you should request a copy of the reviewers' written comments, which can guide your decision as to whether or not to resubmit the grant in the next submission cycle. If you do decide to resubmit, the reviewers' comments will be valuable as you modify the proposal.

As you read the reviewers' comments, you might find a remarkable diversity of opinion among members of the panel. You might even conclude that one or two members of the review panel did not understand the proposal, if they read it at all. Recognize that review panel members are selected based on expertise in some key area which may be very different from your specialty, or perhaps to reflect some diversity in constituencies, and there may be considerable differences in their individual knowledge of your project topic.

As you consider modifying and resubmitting the proposal in the next cycle, ask the program officer for any suggestions that might be helpful. Does the program officer think you might have a reasonable chance of acceptance if you resubmit? Are there any special parts of the grant proposal that the program officer thinks especially merit change? Perhaps there is a problem that was not covered in the reviewers' comments.

To learn more about the NIH review process, go to What Happens to Your Grant Application at https://public.csr.nih.gov/aboutcsr/NewsAndPublications/Publications/Documents/yourapplicationflyer.pdf.

Thoughts About Getting Grants

Grantsmanship

Being a well-funded grant writer is one of academia's most valued skills. It can be especially useful because many research grants can be moved from one institution to another; they follow the principal investigator, who may actually move an entire research team. In the academic world, this is powerful.

You can learn to be a skilled grantsperson by pyramiding your experience. Begin by joining a research team of people more experienced than you, and being willing to do the "grunt" work of organizing boilerplate, getting letters of support, and writing budget justifications. Do whatever is needed to be a good team member, learn the process, and be a true coinvestigator on the project. Your next step is to plan your own project, organize your own research or project team, and write a grant in which you are the principal investigator. All tournament champion, "all-star," grant-getters started with small projects and later expanded their horizons as they gained experience.

It is also helpful to volunteer to serve on your AMC's Institutional Review Board, which can be an eye-opening introduction to the many types of grant proposals considered and the issues that arise around the table.

After you, as PI, have submitted a grant or two and have befriended a program officer, ask the program officer how you can become a member of a grant review panel for the granting agency. Serving on a national review panel is a highly valuable experience because you get to see the grants that others have written and learn why some succeed and some are rejected. In addition, during the review process, you will spend time with leaders in your field from across the country.

In the end, the top grant-getters share certain characteristics. In addition to good writing skills, they have the administrative ability needed to lead a team, the integrity to do the best work possible, the salesmanship to convince grantors that they are best suited for the job, the imperturbability to endure rejection, and the persistence to revise and resubmit over and over until successful.

If and When Your Grant Is Rejected

Yes, you will have a proposal rejected, probably more than one, during your career. For example, the Research Project R01 grant, the classic NIH grant, is an award made to support a discrete, specified, circumscribed project to be performed by the named investigator(s) in an area representing the investigator's specific interest and competencies, based on the mission of the NIH. The 2015 R01 success rate for all investigators was 14% [12]. Grant-getting seems to be the inverse of Pareto's 80:20 "rule," which holds that 80% of your efforts will succeed and 20% will fail. (If you are not familiar with Pareto's rule, check it out through Google.) In the instance of grant application submissions, more than 80% of our efforts may be unsuccessful. What should you do when you receive the notice of rejection of your grant proposal, which will often be in the form of an aggravating form letter?

Let me begin with what you do not do. You do not blame your grant program officer; this person has tried to help you, had no vote in the review committee's decision, and stands ready to help you in the future. Do not risk losing a friend.

Do not act while angry. Do not call the agency and accuse the review committee of being a clan of Neanderthals who would not recognize the merits of the wheel. Do not impugn their motives or their honesty.

What should you do? First, consult with your coinvestigators and plan your telephone inquiry to the agency. Write out a script with your questions. Begin by biting your tongue and thanking the agency for their thoughtful review. Then inquire, "What could I do that would improve the proposal?" "What can you can suggest to help us in the future?"

You want to find out what sort of rejection was received. Was it an "oh, so close" no? Or was it a "this-was-really-awful-proposal" no? Did you almost make the cut, and fall short by just a few points? Or did the review committee truly loathe your application and wish never to see it again?

I mentioned earlier that one of the attributes of the successful grant-getter is persistence. After your anger and disappointment subside and after getting all the information you can from the rejection letter agency, you and your team should have a strategy meeting. If your proposal was not truly terrible, but just not good enough, and if you still think it might match with the mission of your targeted funding source, then dust it off, make revisions based on feedback received, and resubmit at a later time. Many grant proposals, especially NIH grant applications, succeed only on the second or third submission.

If you still think you have a great, and fundable, idea but conclude that resubmission to the initial target agency is not going to succeed, then your initial application can probably be revised to meet the requirements of another agency. And the reworked and improved application may well be funded.

Common Errors in Grant Proposal Writing

Beginning grant proposal writers make some classic errors; experienced academicians also sometimes make missteps [13]:

- Ignoring the instructions. When agencies have a surplus of grant applications, the first cut may be those who did not follow instructions precisely. Here is an example that is extreme but true. In 2003, a drug and alcohol treatment center in Oregon had two grants rejected by a federal agency because of the width of page margins. The center had submitted funding requests totaling $703,000 but "missed out because the application margins were two-tenths of an inch too small" [14].
- Failure to define and document the problem you intend to solve. Here a needs assessment is often helpful [15].
- Failing to recognize signals in the request for proposal. If the RFP seems somehow peculiar, as though one needs to have very special attributes in order to carry out the project, it is just possible that it is "wired." This means that a specific institution already has an inside track, may even have had a hand in writing the RFP, and your proposal will fight an uphill battle.
- Not listening carefully to the program officer. You have just described your idea to the program officer, who replies, "What you are describing is not exactly what we usually fund." Of course, you can ignore this comment, spend weeks preparing a grant application, and receive sympathetic reviewer comments ("I wish we could have approved this well-written proposal, but …") along with your rejection notice.

- Carelessness. Do not submit a grant with grammatical or typographical errors. Avoid excessive use of abbreviations or abbreviations that send the reader scrambling back 20 pages earlier to figure out meaning. Do not submit a grant with misstatements or outdated information. Avoid topic-specific jargon. Such errors can only harm your chances of success.
- Failure to adequately justify your budget requests.
- Injecting guaranteed failure into the proposal. One example is targeting the wrong population. I once sat in a review panel for HRSA training grants. These specific grants involved training medical students and residents. One of the most comprehensive and articulate grants we considered during the 2-day meeting involved a longitudinal educational program in an integrated continuum from college to residency. But the grant funding was intended only for medical students and residents, not college students. We turned to the program officer, who stated that this grant could not qualify for funding. Fatal error. Next grant.
- Submitting to the wrong agency. Some grantors fund research; some fund education and training. Do not waste your time by mixing these up. If you intend to combine research and training in a grant, discuss this early with the program officer.
- Overestimating your capability. Grantors always consider if the PI has the experience and resources to get the job done. Begin with modest achievable projects with reasonable budgets. Then, after a few successes, think about more ambitious projects with larger budgets. Eventually you may qualify to write the grant for the Big Project, but this must be earned by a track record of earlier successes. A step-by-step, patient approach offers the best chance of being a winner in the tournament of grants.

Where to Learn More About Getting Grants

There is much more to learn about getting grants. Table 10.3 has some suggestions for further study.

TABLE 10.3 Information sources about grant seeking

Articles and books

Bauer DG. The "how to" grants manual: successful grant seeking techniques for obtaining public and private grants. 8th ed. Lanham, MD: Rowman and Littlefield; 2015

Browning B. Perfect phrases for writing grant proposals. New York: McGraw Hill; 2007

O'Neal-McElrath T. Winning grants: step by step. 4th ed. San Francisco: Jossey-Bass; 2013

Coley SM, Scheinbert CA. Proposal writing: efficient grantsmanship, 4th ed. Thousand Oaks, CA: Sage; 2013

Keinholz M, Berg JM. How the NIH can help you get funded: an insider's guide. New York: Oxford University Press; 2013

Kotchen TA, Lindquist T, Malik K, Ehrenfeld E. NIH peer review of grant applications for clinical research. JAMA. 2004;291:836–43

Reef-Lehrer L. Grant application writer's handbook. 4th ed. Boston: Jones & Bartlett; 2005

Web sites

Developing and writing grant proposals. Catalog of Federal Domestic Assistance. U.S. General Services Administration: http://www.cfda.gov/public/writing.pdf

National Institutes of Health Office, grants and funding: https://grants.nih.gov/grants/oer.htm

National Institutes of Health Office of Extramural Research, types of grant funding: http://grants.nih.gov/grants/funding/funding_program.htm

Selected organizations

Agency for Healthcare Research and Quality (AHRQ)
5600 Fisher Lane
Rockville, MD 20857
http://www.ahrq.gov

National Institutes of Health (NIH)
9000 Rockville Pike
Bethesda, Maryland 20892
http://www.nih.gov

National Science Foundation
4201 Wilson Boulevard,
Arlington, Virginia 22230
http://www.nsf/gov

References

1. Souba C. Perspective: the language of leadership. Acad Med. 2010;85(10):1609–18.
2. National Institutes of Health. Overview. https://www.nih.gov/about-nih/what-we-do/budget. Accessed 28 Apr 2017.
3. Freeman R, Weinstein E, Marincola E, Rosenbaum J, Solomon E. Competition and careers in bioscience. Science. 2001;294:2293–4.
4. National Institutes of Health. Mission and goals. https://www.nih.gov/about-nih/what-we-do/mission-goals. Accessed 28 Apr 2017.
5. Kotchen TA, Lindquist T, Ehrenfeld E. NIH peer review of grant applications for clinical research. JAMA. 2004;291:836–43.
6. Ehrhardt S, Appel LJ, Meinert CL. Trends in National Institutes of Health funding for clinical trials registered in ClinicialTrials.gov (Research letter). JAMA. 2015;314(23):2556–7.
7. Kumar P, Hamza N, Madhok B, et al. Copper deficiency after gastric bypass for morbid obesity: a systematic review. Obes Surg. 2016;26(6):1335–42.
8. Papamargaritis D, Aasheim ET, Sampson B, le Roux CW. Copper, selenium, and zinc levels after bariatric surgery in patients recommend to take multivitamin-mineral supplementation. J Trace Elem Med Biol. 2015;31:167–72.
9. Robinson SD, Cooper B, Ledahy TV. Copper deficiency (hypocupremia) and pancytopenia late after gastric bypass surgery. Proc (Bayl Univ Med Cent). 2013;26(4):382–6.
10. Inouye SK, Feillin DA. An evidence-based guide to writing grant proposals for clinical research. Ann Intern Med. 2005;142(4):274–82.
11. Bordage G, Dawson B. Experimental study design and grant writing in eight steps and 28 questions. Med Educ. 2003;37(4):376–85.
12. National Institutes of Health Research Project Success Rates by Type and Activity for 2015. https://report.nih.gov/success_rates/Success_ByActivity.cfm. Accessed 28 Apr 2017.
13. Liu JC, Pynnonen MA, St John E, Couch ME, Schmalbach CE. Grant-writing pearls and pitfalls: maximizing funding opportunities. Otolaryngol Head Neck Surg. 2016;154(2):226–32.
14. Center loses grant by slimmest of margins. Oregonian. p. D2. Accessed 3 Dec 2003.
15. Harris M. Ten mistakes to avoid when writing a grant proposal. GTC Grant Training Center. 29 Aug 2014. http://granttrainingcenter.com/blog/ten-mistakes-to-avoid-when-writing-a-grant-proposal/. Accessed 28 Apr 2017.

Chapter 11
How to Write a Report of a Research Study

In questions of science, the authority of a thousand is not worth the humble reasoning of a single individual.

Italian physicist and philosopher Galileo Galilei (1564–1642*)*.

Galileo, a leader in the Scientific Revolution that followed the hyper-religiosity and doctrinaire thinking of the Middle Ages, was a champion of reasoning. Ideally, of course, reasoning is based on observed facts — data — and medicine science's best format for data presentation and analysis today is the report of a clinical study.

In the *Journal of the American Medical Association* (JAMA) is a report of a study intended "to investigate the associations between major classes of psychotropic medications and violent reoffending." The researchers followed 22,275 released prisoners over a mean follow-up period of 4.6 years. They found that the rates of violent reoffending were lower when subjects were receiving psychotropic drugs compared with periods when they were not dispensed these medications (Chang Z et al. JAMA. 2016;316:1798).

A study reported by Lauch et al. described the use of cabbage leaf wraps as therapy for treatment of symptomatic osteoarthritis (OA) of the knee in 81 patients, finding "cabbage leaf wraps are more effective for knee OA than usual

© Springer International Publishing AG 2018   289
R.B. Taylor, *Medical Writing*,
https://doi.org/10.1007/978-3-319-70126-4_11

care, but not compared with diclofenac gel" (Lauche R et al. Clin J Pain. 2016;32:961).

In *Epidemiology* is the report of a study that examined the risk of fatal myocardial infarction in persons exposed to aircraft noise (Huss A et al. Epidemiology. 2010;21:829). Following analysis of 4.6 million individuals over 5 years, the authors concluded that there is, indeed, a dose-related association between aircraft noise and death from myocardial infarction, independent of possible confounding factors such as particulate matter air pollution and socioeconomic status of the municipality.

According to a report published in *Pediatrics*, the use of probiotics, specifically *Lactobacillus reuteri*, can reduce daily crying episodes in colicky babies, a conclusion based on a randomized, double-blind, placebo-controlled trial involving 50 infants (Savino F et al. Pediatrics. 2011;126;e526).

A research report in the *New England Journal of Medicine* (NEJM) titled "Effect of Short-Term vs. Long-Term Blood Storage on Mortality after Transfusion" found "no significant difference in the rate of death among those who underwent transfusion with the freshest available blood and those who underwent transfusion according to the standard practice of transfusing the oldest available blood" (Heddle NM. NEJM. 2016;375:1937).

Preparing the report of original research is arguably the most challenging undertaking in medical writing. It is not necessarily that writing the report is so complicated, because the model is prescribed. In a sense, you need only to fill in the blanks. The challenging part is that one needs to have completed a research study and have the resulting data available. What follows assumes that you have completed that task and are composing your research report for publication.

Because there is a prescribed model, writing the report of original research has one advantage over other types of medical writing. You will not need to dream up a concept and structure for the article. In previous chapters I discussed diverse ways to approach the review article, editorial, book chapter, and other models of medical publication. For the report of original research, there is only one model, called IMRAD. This acronym stands for the major parts of a research report: introduction, methods, results, and discussion. The IMRAD format is what editors are accustomed to reviewing. It is what clinicians and scientists are used to reading. Deviating from this format risks summary rejection. I describe the IMRAD format below.

The rigid format for the report of original research highlights the fact that research reports are intended to be recorded in the scientific literature and subsequently cited by others; they are not really written to be read, as most of us think of reading. They are intended to be repositories of scientific data rather than literary gems. They just happen to be written in prose. Day has summarized this viewpoint very well: "Some of my old-fashioned colleagues think that scientific papers should be literature, that the style and flair of an author should be clearly evident, and that variations in style encourage the interest of the reader. I disagree. I think scientists should indeed be interested in reading literature, and perhaps even in writing literature, but the communication of research results is a more prosaic procedure" [1].

With that said, I still plead with authors, even those composing research papers, to construct paragraphs thoughtfully, avoid long and convoluted sentences, select words carefully, avoid the use of jargon, and express their ideas as clearly as possible.

Thinking About the Research Report

For the clinical investigator, getting research results published can be the difference between professional success and failure in the academic medicine arena. It can determine whether or not one gets the big grant or receives tenure. Entire academic careers have been built on a single groundbreaking research study, carefully reported in a prestigious journal. Whether you are a patient care physician or a research-track academic faculty member, whether you have done a bench project in the laboratory or a randomized clinical trial, remember that your research is not completed until the results are reported in print.

The five papers I cited above all had research questions that provoked my interest and perhaps yours. The paper describing less violent reoffending in released prisoners when taking psychotropic drugs seems to provide some data supporting an assumption we have long held. I had never heard of cabbage leaf wraps for treatment of knee OA, but this safe and inexpensive remedy may appeal to some patients who favor alternative medicine. Although I had never thought much about the issue before I read the title, I wanted to know if aircraft noise might be associated with death from myocardial infarction. I was intrigued by the well-designed study of the use of probiotics in colicky babies. The finding that "old" bank blood is just as good as the freshest blood helps to support standard blood bank practice. Because these and other research reports have implications for daily practice and public health, I briefly summarized the study outcomes, even though this is a book about writing and not clinical science.

I mention the above—about my interest in the research questions that prompted the studies—because you may be tempted to stretch the definition of research too far. As a surgeon, you may consider reporting the findings of your last 200 cases of lumbar laminectomy or laparoscopic cholecystectomy. If you are an internist, you may believe that your colleagues are keenly interested in how you treated 100 consecutive patients with congestive heart failure. Such studies do not set out to answer a clinical question and generally do not have anything important to say. They may qualify as quality improvement efforts, but are not likely to result in a publishable research paper.

A research report describes your research, whether it involves humans, rats, or a meta-analysis of previously published studies. In general, you generate a research question and then collect data to answer the question. "Data mining," sifting through tons of data to find something, *anything* that has statistical significance, is not good research, and a paper describing such a method will be deemed inferior by an informed reviewer.

Then there are "parachute trials." These studies get their name from asking the fanciful research question: Are parachutes effective in preventing major trauma related to gravitational challenge? (Smith GCS et al. BMJ. 2003;327:1459). For example, would we really need to report a study showing that antibiotic therapy of meningitis is more effective than watchful waiting? Consider the study of "Genetic Evidence for Causal Relationships Between Maternal Obesity-Related Traits and Birth Weight," showing basically that overweight mothers had overweight babies (Tyrrel J et al. JAMA. 2016;315:1129). Or perhaps even the previously cited report that released prisoners taking their psychotropic medication exhibited less violent behavior. Yes, data mining and parachute trial reports are published, but the best hypothesis-based studies have the best chance of acceptance in the leading journals.

When planning a research report, be aware that competition for publication space in leading refereed journals is intense, and research papers are typically rewritten several times before final acceptance. Ultimately, your clinical research paper will be judged by its impact on your specialty and on the greater body of medical knowledge, as evidenced by its citation in other research articles, review papers, and textbooks.

Just before launching into a discussion of how to write a report of hypothesis-based research based on the quantitative scientific model, I want to acknowledge another branch of research that also is reported in the literature—qualitative research. This type of research, which medical science has borrowed from our colleagues in sociology and anthropology, does not generate piles of data. Instead, we find terms such as focus groups, studying stories, and mixed methods research [2]. The IMRAD model, describe below, does not readily lend itself to reports of qualitative research, which tend to use more innovative styles, prompted by the nature of the results being reported. Here, we will examine how to report the results of traditional quantitative research.

The Expanded IMRAD Model

The IMRAD model of research reports has evolved over generations of scientific publications. It has at its core four elements:

- Introduction: Why is the topic important, what prior research has been done, and what question did you set out to answer?
- Methods: Who were your subjects and what did you do to them? How did you analyze the data?
- Results: What did you find out?
- Discussion: What do your findings mean? What are the cautions regarding interpretation?

These four items are the foundation of IMRAD. Research papers, however, have more than just the four main components, and I am going to present an expanded IMRAD model. Keep in mind the four key elements as we explore the IMRAD model and more, beginning with selection of the title for the report.

Those reporting on scientific research should also consult the EQUATOR (Enhancing the QUAlity and Transparency Of health Research) network, an international collaboration that aims to promote accurate and reliable reporting of health research studies. The web site provides reporting guidelines for the various types of health research studies: randomized trials, observational studies, systematic reviews, and so forth. The EQUATOR network site is available at http://www.equator-network.org.

Title

The title is the "label" for the paper. The title must tell, more or less, what was studied. An early question the writer must answer is this: Should I reveal my conclusion in the title?

One of the studies cited at the beginning of the chapter is titled "Association Between Prescription of Major

Psychotropic Medications and Violent Reoffending After Prison Release." If I read only the title and have no other background knowledge, I might misunderstand the authors' meaning and presume that prescription psychotropic medications lead to violent reoffending after prison release. In fact, the study showed just the opposite. Therefore, I believe that a better title would be "Prescription of Major Psychotropic Medications Reduces Violent Reoffending After Prison Release." Might the title of the cited article called "Aircraft Noise, Air Pollution, And Mortality From Myocardial Infarction" be improved by stating that, yes, there does seem to be an association between aircraft noise and myocardial infarction?

A title telling your conclusion is called a declarative title. For example, the "fat mothers/fat babies" study cited above might have been titled "Genetic Evidence Found for Causal Relationships Between Maternal Obesity-Related Traits and Birth Weight." Note the insertion of a verb in the title. Whimster writes: "I believe that readers need a verb in the title, such as a newspaper headline usually has, and that to be meaningful it should convey the message, as in: 'Rickettsial Endocarditis Is Not A Rare Complication Of Congenital Heart Disease In Dental Practice: A Report Of Five Cases'" [3]. Some journals encourage such titles, while others discourage or even prohibit them. A study by Wager et al. found "no evidence that the use of a declarative title affected readers' perceptions about study conclusions" [4].

Sometimes we authors dream up witty titles. Consider the following title: "It's B-A-A-A-A-A-A-Ck Again, Or How To Live With The New APA Manual: Reprise For Edition 6" (Baggs JG et al. Res Nurs Health. 2009;32:477). Generally, editors counsel against using clever phrases in titles and rightfully so.

Note how often colons show up in article titles. They allow progression from the general to the specific, all in an integrated title phrase. An example is the title "A July Spike in Fatal Medication Errors: A Possible Effect of New Medical Residents." The authors discuss the general problem and then the approach used in the research. The reader has a better idea of the article's contents than if only the first phrase was listed.

Today it is fashionable to title a research study with an acronymic name and to carry this over into the title of the research report. An example is "Effect of Laparoscopic-Assisted Resection vs Open Resection on Pathological Outcomes in Rectal Cancer: The ALaCaRT Trial" (Stevenson ARL et al. JAMA 2015;314:1356). The ALaCaRT acronym is derived from the Australian Laparoscopic Cancer of the Rectum Trial. Consider also "Anticholinergic vs. Long-Acting Beta-agonist in Combination With Inhaled Steroids in Black Adults with Asthma: the BELT Randomized Clinical Trial" (Wechsler ME et al. JAMA 2015;314:1720). The BELT acronym comes from "The Blacks and Exacerbations on LABA vs Tritropium (BELT) Study," which I submit seems to be a bacronym, a word (BELT) turned into an acronym by creating a phrase to match the letters.

An article's title can influence the citation rates. Jacques et al. studied citation rates of articles published in three prestigious journals. They found: "The number of citations was positively correlated with the length of the title, the presence of a colon in the title and the presence of an acronym. Factors that predicted poor citation included reference to a specific country in the title" [5].

On a technical basis, the instructions for authors may prescribe a word or character limit for the title. Also, I believe that titles should not contain acronyms or abbreviations, no matter how widespread the author and editor consider their use.

Authors

The chief issues in an authorship of a research report are generally twofold: (1) Who is an author? (2) How shall the authors be listed?

As discussed in Chap. 5, everyone who contributed substantially to a research project and preparation of the report should be listed as author. Furthermore, each author should have participated sufficiently in the work to take public responsibility for appropriate portions of the content [6, 7].

What about adding author names of those who have contributed very little? Strasburger describes the problem: "Fiction is written by one individual; medical articles may be written by committee. There is no such thing as 'author inflation' in fiction, simply because there is no need for it. Medical writers must publish or perish, academically. Fiction writers must publish or perish, existentially" [8]. Despite the need to avoid perishing, it is inappropriate to have your name listed if you have not met the criteria listed in the previous paragraph. You must not become an perpetrator of author inflation.

No department chair or research director should insist on being named as an author unless he or she has made a significant contribution to the study and to writing the paper. Authorship listing by administrative fiat is academic malpractice. Adding the name of a prestigious senior faculty member as the final entry on a long author list might help get the paper a better review, but including the well-known name implies that person's active participation in the project. Gratuitous addition of an author name—honorary authorship—is ethically inappropriate.

The order in which authors are listed on a research report should be decided very early in the process, generally during one of the first meetings of the research group planning the study. Changes in the rank order can be made later if contributions of individuals to the project do not turn out to be what was originally planned.

The first author should logically be the one who has done most of the work on the study being reported. Generally this is the person who led the research team and who has created the early drafts of the paper. From then on, authors should be listed according to how much they contributed to the study and the report. As one whose last name begins with a letter toward the end of the alphabet, I have never considered alphabetical listings of names to be fair to the Taylors, Washingtons, and Zells of the world. And Alpert, citing his mentor, reminds us, "The fastest way to make an enemy is to fail listing someone as an author who thought they should have been included" (Alpert JS. Am J Med. 2015;128:551).

A quirk of citation listing holds that when the paper is used as a reference in other studies, if your paper has seven or more authors, only the first three are named and the rest will join the et al. army of obscurity. Johnson has given us a humorous poem titled "Buried in the Et Al" (Johnson DH. The Pharos, Summer 2016:35) that include the memorable lines:

> I made a contribution,
> But got no attribution.
> … buried in the "et al."

Abstract

The Abstract is an author-generated synopsis of the paper. Many advise that the final version of the abstract should be the last item written, since only then will you know exactly what is in the paper that you are summarizing. When writing an abstract, select each word as if your paper's being read depended on it and jettison verbal clutter ruthlessly.

In general I have always taught that the abstract should mirror the IMRAD structure of the paper. That is, the paper's introduction, methods, results, and discussion (conclusions) should each be presented in a sentence or two, and many good abstracts have exactly four short paragraphs. According to the International Committee of Medical Journal Editors (ICMJE) recommendations, "The abstract should provide the context or background for the study and should state the study's purpose, basic procedures (selection of study participants, settings, measurements, analytical methods), main findings (giving specific effect sizes and their statistical and clinical significance, if possible), and principal conclusions" [6].

Many abstracts set the stage by starting with an unassailable general statement. Here is an example: The abstract for a report titled "A Prospective Study of Sudden Cardiac Death among Children and Young Adults" begins with the sentence, "Sudden cardiac death among children and young adults is a devastating event" (Bagnall RD et al. NEJM. 2016;374:2441).

The current trend is for journals to require structured abstracts [9]. This means that information in the abstract is presented according to specific headings that differ a little with each journal. All structured abstracts will include the four key components of the IMRAD model, although synonyms for these headings may be used, including some variations such as "Context" and "Main Outcome Measures." Some journals prefer abstracts with full sentences; others encourage the use of phrases. Here, from the *Archives of Surgery*, is what we find in a well-written structured abstract for a paper titled "Risk Factors for Lymphedema in a Prospective Breast Cancer Survivorship Study" (Kwan ML et al. Arch Surg. 2010;145:1055):

Objective: To determine the incidence of breast cancer-related lymphedema (BCRL) during the early survivorship period as well as demographic, lifestyle, and clinical factors associated with BCRL development.

Design: The Pathways Study, a prospective cohort study of breast cancer survivors with a mean follow-up time of 20.9 months.

Setting: Kaiser Permanente Northern California medical care program.

Participants: We studied 997 women diagnosed from January 9, 2006 through October 15, 2007, with primary invasive breast cancer and who were at least 21 years of age at diagnosis, had no history of any cancer, and spoke English, Spanish, Cantonese, or Mandarin.

Main outcome measure: Clinical indication for BCRL as determined from outpatient or hospitalization diagnostic codes, outpatient procedural codes, and durable medical equipment orders.

Note that so far, only one section — *Participants* — contains a complete sentence. Later in the abstract, under *Results* and *Conclusions*, paragraphs become longer and the style changes from phrases to complete sentences.

The instructions for authors for the *Journal of the American Medical Association* state, "Reports of original data should include an abstract of no more than 350 words using the headings listed." These headings are: Importance, Objective, Design, Setting, Participants, Intervention(s) or Exposure(s), Main Outcome(s) and Measure(s), Results, Conclusions and Relevance, and Trial Registration. The JAMA Instructions for Authors goes on to tell what should be presented in each section of the abstract [10].

The tight word limitation and the many topics to be covered serve to get the important data into tightly written abstracts but at the expense of some very complicated, number-laden, and almost incomprehensible sentences in the Results section. For brevity, most journals allow incomplete sentences in the abstract.

On a technical basis, descriptions of work that has been done (*Methods* and *Results*) should be written in the past tense. An explanation of what you think (*Discussion*) is written in present tense, often with a phrase such as "We conclude.…" In the spirit of intellectual honesty, the abstract must never contain a conclusion that is not supported by what is in the body of the paper.

Be sure to end the Conclusions and Relevance section of the abstract by telling the results of your research. Curiously, some authors seem to want to keep their conclusions a secret. Consider the following from a trial of fecal microbiota transplantation (FMT) to treat relapsing *C. difficile* infection: "This preliminary study among patients with relapsing *C. difficile* infection provides data on adverse events and rates of resolution of diarrhea following administration of FMT using frozen encapsulated inoculum from unrelated donors" (Youngster I et al. JAMA. 2014;312:1772). Wonderful. But what were your conclusions?

Clinical Trial Registration

For all clinical trials, the name of the trial registry, registration number, and URL of the registry must be included. A list of acceptable trial registries can be found at http://www. icmje.org.

Keywords

In some instances you will be asked to identify Keywords. Keywords can be what keep your report from being lost in the information jungle. They are part of the retrievability process that can contribute to the number of times your paper will be cited. In the instructions for authors, many journals request that you submit a short list of keywords or phrases. These will be used to cross-index the article; they may or may not published with the abstract. Terms from the Medical Subject Headings (MeSH) list from the US Library of Medicine should be used if possible. For more information on MeSH, see https://www.nlm.nih.gov/mesh/ and Chap. 1 of this book.

Introduction

Finally we arrive at the "I" in IMRAD. The introduction should identify the problem you set out to solve. In a sense, it describes the context of the study. In general terms, the introduction should cover three areas:

- *Problem statement*: What is the general nature of the problem that merits valuable journal space and the reader's attention?
- *Background and work to date*: What are the most pertinent, timely published studies that relate to the problem?
- *The research question*: What is the specific, focused question(s) that you set out to answer? If you have a formally stated hypothesis, here is where it should be presented.

The Problem

The Introduction classically opens with a broad statement that puts the problem in context. The introduction to a paper on aspirin and colorectal cancer begins, "Colorectal cancer is

the second most common cancer in developed countries..."
(Rothwell PM et al. The Lancet. 2010;376(9754):1741).

Good introductions are often written as a three-level
"inverted pyramid." The broadest statement comes first.
Here is an example: Primary care clinicians encounter many
patients with headaches. Next comes a more narrow statement: The clinician treating a headache patient is always
aware that, in a few individuals, the cephalgia might be the
tip-off to a life-threatening disease. This might be followed by
an even more specific statement setting out the purpose of
the study: This study examines patient records to identify
symptoms and signs that might identify persons most at risk
for life-threatening causes of head pain who should be
referred for diagnostic imaging.

Background

Describe the key work that has been done on the topic to
date. Do not present an exhaustive literature review dating
back to the Renaissance. Be very selective and include only
articles that have a direct bearing on your research question.

Research Question

State clearly the question you are trying to answer. One
focused question is usually better than many. The question
may be stated as a query or perhaps as a hypothesis but often
is phrased as a statement of intent: In the study of aircraft
noise and fatal heart attacks, the research question is stated:
"We examined residential exposure to aircraft noise and
mortality from myocardial infarction, taking air pollution
into account."

To inform the reader as to what your study is all about, it
is vital that you articulate the research question clearly in the
introduction. I wish that writers of research reports would all
do so and would frame their research questions as direct queries or even as hypotheses. For example, the authors of the
paper on blood storage and mortality, cited earlier in the

chapter, state clearly, "Our goal was to determine whether the in-hospital rate of death among patients requiring transfusion was lower among those who received blood after short-term storage than among those who received blood after long-term storage" (Heddle NM et al. NEJM. 2016;375:1937).

However, many authors are less explicit, and I have learned to be content with somewhat vaguely stated research questions such as: "The purpose of this study was to investigate both early and late dumping syndromes after gastrectomy for gastric cancer in 2 high-volume centers in Japan" (Mine S et al. J Am Coll Surg. 2010;211:628). At this point in the paper, I am still not aware what question the authors set out to answer.

Technical Issues in Writing the Introduction

When writing your introduction, use the present tense to describe the general nature of the problem and the background work. Then the research question, if presented as a statement, is usually in past tense, as in the examples above.

The ICMJE recommendations advise, "Do not include data or conclusions from the work being reported" [6]. Not everyone agrees with this stance. Both Day [1] and Whimster [3] advocate stating the conclusions early in the article, and not keeping the reader in suspense, as you would with a whodunit mystery novel. The best spot for the important implication for translation of your findings to clinical practice may be in the introduction. In this area where controversy exists, use your best judgment, based on the data you are presenting.

Methods

The Methods section, sometimes called Participants and Methods or perhaps Methods and Materials, should describe a logical experimental approach. Because this section presents a number of topics, subheadings are often used. The Methods section of the article mentioned above about aircraft noise and fatal MI has five headings: Study Population, Outcomes, Exposure to Aircraft Noise, Exposure to Air Pollution, and Statistical Analysis. In the article about blood storage and mortality after transfusion, the Methods section has six subheadings: Study Design, Patient Population, Randomization and Intervention, Outcomes, Data Collection, and Statistical Analysis.

Fundamentally, this section needs to describe the subjects, what you did to them, and what statistical methods you used. After writing the first draft of the Methods section, ask yourself whether what you are presenting allows *reproducibility*. That is, could a trained investigator in your field replicate your study, given the information you have provided?

Methods should not include numerical data, which should be presented in the Results section.

Subjects

Describe the subjects studied, including age, gender, and other important characteristics that may be pertinent to the study. The ICMJE Recommendations state that when authors use such variables as race or ethnicity, they "should define how they measured these variables and justify their relevance" [6].

Tell also whether any potential subjects were excluded and why they were excluded, if there is a meaningful reason. For example, in a study of the use of probiotics to reduce infant colic, subjects with chronic illness or gastrointestinal disorders were excluded (Savino F et al. Pediatrics. 2011;126:e526).

Methods

Here you describe what was actually done to the subjects. Also, if appropriate, describe any data collection tools, such as survey instruments. If apparatus was used, identify the item and manufacturer. Be sure to identify all drugs by generic name; adding the trade name is optional but is useful for the practicing clinician. Be sure to include medication doses and routes of administration.

Statistics

Describe the statistical methods used, "with enough detail to enable a knowledgeable reader with access to the original data to verify the reported results" [6]. This generally means identifying specific tests used. In the study of aircraft noise and fatal MI, the description of the statistics used begins, "We analyzed the association between aircraft noise and cardio-vascular mortality using Cox proportional hazard models, with age as the underlying timescale."

In an effort to make this book more useful for those involved in research studies, I have added a lexicon explaining commonly encountered methodological and statistical terms. (See Appendix D.) In the meantime, here are some thoughts, several taken directly from the ICMJE recommendations [6], about the use of statistics in presenting reports of clinical research studies:

- Avoid relying solely on statistical hypotheses testing such as P values, which fail to convey important information about effect size [6].
- When data allow, present quantifiable findings with appropriate indicators of measurement error or uncertainty (such as confidence intervals) [6].
- When describing the statistics you employed in analyzing data, specify the statistical software package(s) and versions used [6].
- Don't hesitate to seek help with statistics. It is easy to get lost in the unfamiliar forest of statistical analysis. A study by Strasak et al. found, "Five of 31 papers for the New England Journal of Medicine (NEJM) (16.1%) contained usage of wrong or suboptimal statistical tests, either because of incompatibility of test with examined data, inappropriate use of parametric methods, or use of an inappropriate statistical test for the scientific hypothesis under investigation" [11].
- Finally, you should never allow a pharmaceutical company or other research sponsor to do the statistical analysis of your data [12].

TABLE 11.1 Sources of statistical information for medical writers

Bland M. An introduction to medical statistics. 4th ed. New York: Oxford University Press; 2015
Everitt BS. Medical statistics from A to Z: a guide for clinicians and medical students. 2nd ed. London: Cambridge University Press; 2007
Good PI, Hardin JW. Common errors in statistics (and how to avoid them). 4th ed. Hoboken, NJ: Wiley; 2012
Hastie T, Tibshirani R, Friedman J. The elements of statistical learning: data mining, inference, and prediction. 2nd ed. New York: Springer; 2013
Kirkwood B, Sterne J. Essential medical statistics. 3rd ed. Hoboken, NJ: Wiley-Blackwell; (for release in 2020)
Lang TA, Secic M. How to report statistics in medicine: Annotated guidelines for authors, editors, and reviewers (medical writing and communication). 2nd ed. Philadelphia: American College of Physicians; 2006
Peacock JL, Peacock PJ. Oxford handbook of medical statistics. New York: Oxford University Press, 2011
Scott I, Mazhindu D. Statistics for healthcare professionals: an introduction. 2nd ed. Thousand Oaks, CA: Sage; 2014

Table 11.1 lists some publications that may be helpful for the statistically challenged.

Results

What did you discover at the end of your research trial? Describe your findings in a logical sequence and do so fully, yet succinctly. To support my plea for readability in research reports, I like the image created by Alexandrov: "Make data presentation so clear and simple that a tired person riding late on an airplane can take your manuscript and get the message at first reading" [13]. (As a physician, I find this a slight challenge, given that with the imperfect pressurization of aircraft cabins, there is a measureable decrement in blood oxygen saturation and hence in cerebral oxygenation, at 35,000-feet elevation.)

I have sometimes said, only partly in jest, that the ideal Results section has a single sentence, "The results are presented in Table 1," followed by a single, carefully constructed table. In reality, presenting research results is never this simple, but the use of tables and figures can help organize numbers in ways that cannot be accomplished in words. Also, the Results section should begin with some explanatory prose before sending the reader to the first table. Keep in mind that figures are expensive to produce and tables are a leading source of error. On balance, however, most Results sections benefit from one or more tables or figures. The article on blood storage and mortality after transfusion, described earlier, has three figures and two tables.

Tables and figures for all types of publication models are discussed in detail in Chap. 4. Here I will only emphasize the importance of creating a legend for each that explains the table so that it can be reasonably understood without referring to the accompanying text. That is, a lecturer can readily incorporate your table with its legend into a PowerPoint presentation (with credit to you, of course) with minimal explanatory prose.

Tables and figures should not duplicate data presented in the text. Select only one location to present the numbers.

Discussion

In Chap. 1, I stated that each article must face the "So what?" question. The Discussion section should answer that question by stating the relationships among facts discovered, relating them to prior studies (the ones you mentioned earlier in the introduction), and postulating what it may all mean—the conclusions. Discuss the results, but do not restate what has already been said under Results. A good way to begin this section is with the phrase: "Our study showed…" [13].

The Discussion section is where you might describe your opinion of the novelty of your findings or how they may affirm or contradict previous research or experience in the field. For example, in the study of psychotropic medication and violence after release from prison described above, the authors write: "There has been uncertainty about whether treatment for released prisoners with mental disorders should focus on crimogenic rather than mental health-related factors. The current observational study supports the potential role of treating psychiatric disorders, including by psychotropic medication" (Chang Z. JAMA. 2016;316:1798).

The Holy Grail in all of this is *generalizability*: Can what you discovered in your study be extended to the population at large? Or does what you have found apply only to your group of subjects, a weakness of the small sample or the single-institution study? In an ideal world, your findings have implications for similar patients elsewhere, the obvious advantage of the large trial involving thousands of subjects in various sites, such as the aircraft noise vs. fatal myocardial infarction study mentioned at the beginning of the chapter.

State any weaknesses of the study design, or these will surely be described enthusiastically by reviewers or in letters to the editor. The Discussion section is also where you should tell about any factors that may have biased collection of the data, such as unexpected events, attrition of subjects, or mid-study changes in methods, such as terminating one of the study groups. The aircraft noise study, for instance, describes the possibility of bias in the coding of deaths. Here is also where you describe any disagreement among coauthors regarding the interpretation of results.

In the last paragraph (where the grazing reader may go right after reading the abstract), present a summary of your conclusions and what your team thinks they mean. State the implications for others in your field and perhaps how the findings of your study might translate to patient care in the office or hospital. Write this paragraph very carefully. It represents the outcome of months of effort.

References

Your references are where you have obtained background information; the list indicates your awareness of prior work in the area of your research. A focused list of citations is more valuable to your reader — and to you, as author — than a very large collection of papers including some that are only slightly related to the topic of your article.

References serve other purposes. Readers often use them as part of their own research on topics. For these individuals, your list is already a little out of date by the time it is published, but it can be a useful starting point at times. Your reference list also represents a sort of "merit badge" for the authors, indicating that you valued their papers enough to cite them as credible sources.

When using a reference citation to support a statement, be sure that you are conveying the actual meaning of the author. I have seen too many references used to support statements when the paper cited says something entirely different. Today, the ready availability of PubMed and other sites makes it easy to match author assertions and the actual words of authors.

The technical considerations of presenting references are similar for all publication models and are presented in Chap. 4, along with the most familiar models (Table 4.2). Here I will list just a few additional suggestions and comments:

- The ideal reference citation is the original research source.
- Avoid citing the "gray literature," such as working papers, white papers, and conference abstracts.
- If in doubt in listing the name of a journal, write it out, because, for example, "Psych" could mean psychiatry or psychology. PubMed provides a guide to standard abbreviation of journal titles.
- By custom, a journal with a single word title, such as *Nature* or *Science*, is written in full and is not abbreviated.
- A paper accepted for publication, but not yet published, can be cited as "in press" or "forthcoming." If the paper is published before your article goes to press, the citation can be updated in page proofs to provide the details of publication.
- Try to avoid using web sites as references in a scientific report; these sites contain a lot of specious data and outright fiction.

- If you must cite a web site: Because the site of electronic citations can change or disappear altogether, the author citing a web site should print out a copy of the online material, in case it is requested later.
- Never cite a source you have not read and copied for your electronic or paper files.

Acknowledgments

Some papers have a final section listing those who assisted with the work. This includes everyone who helped with research project or manuscript preparation, but did not meet the criteria for authorship, such as a person who provided purely technical support or assistance with the report or a department chair who provided encouragement (and perhaps some research time), but was not part of the research team. For example, at the end of his article "How to Write a Research Paper," Alexandrov states: "The author is not a native English speaker. I am indebted to John Norris, MD, FRCP, for—among many things during fellowship training—his patience with my 'a's' and 'the's' and the first lessons in study design, analysis, and presentation" [13]. If financial or material support has not been disclosed elsewhere, it should be included here.

There is one important caveat: Be sure that all the people you thank are pleased to be acknowledged and that they actually agree with the substance of the paper. Being mentioned allows readers to infer that those acknowledged support the data and conclusions, whether this is true or not. For this reason, you must have written permission from all persons listed in the acknowledgments. Some journals have specific online forms for this purpose; others will accept a signed note on a letterhead.

Avoiding Common Problems in Reports of Clinical Studies

What are the common mistakes seen in reports of clinical studies? Despite the many hours of labor that go into scientific manuscripts, there are a few errors that occur even with the most experienced medical researchers and writers. Maybe some creep in as unhappy compromises during group word-smithing. Others may be the result of midnight editing, when not all the mental light bulbs are on. Whatever the reason, we make mistakes in following the recipe for writing research reports. To help you avoid these missteps, I offer the following to act as a checklist to use when you think your manuscript is done.

- Be sure to prepare a Title Page listing the article title, the names and affiliations of all authors, sources of support such as grants, the number of tables and figures, a word count, and anything else requested in your target journal's instructions for authors.
- Remember that the title page should specify the "corresponding author"—the author who will represent the research team in conversations with the editor—along with this individual's full contact information.
- Check once again to assure that your title accurately describes your study and that it just might prompt the casual reader to learn more.
- Ask yourself: Have I stated the problem clearly?
- Perform a last-minute review of the literature to assure that you have not overlooked a recent key report.
- Review the Results section of your research report to be sure that it does not contain background information (which should be in the Introduction).
- Ask yourself: Have I tried to put too much in my tables and figures?
- Also check to be sure that you have not repeated the same data in tables, figures, and text.
- Verify that interpretation of what you found is in the Discussion section and not in Results.
- Remember that the Discussion section is not the place to introduce new information.
- Eliminate overused words, overly clever phrases, and clichés. The word "impact" comes to mind here.
- Be sure your conclusions are consistent with the data, even if you are disappointed with the outcome.

- Consider ruthless removal of anything that causes you to think, "I just want to get this fact in print."
- Reconsider acknowledgments: Remember that leaving someone out can lead to hard feelings.
- Assure that you have clearly identified any potential conflict of interest.
- Have a last meeting of the research/writing team to assure that everyone knows exactly what is being submitted and that all agree, once again, on the initial target journal.

Thoughts About Research and Research Reports

Quality Writing and Research Design

Medical composition is a laudable skill, one that we should all work to improve. Wager, in an article telling "What Medical Writing Means to Me," observes that medical writing "inhabits a strange boundary zone between science and art" [14]. When it comes to writing a report of a clinical research study, however, the art of medical writing skill must take a back seat to research design. Have you ever read a research report and wondered whether the skillful prose—perhaps composed chiefly by an editorial assistant—masks questionable methods or unjustified conclusions? As Dirckx has written, employing no less than four metaphors, that one should guard "against the temptation to cover his lack of information with a rhetorical snow job, to palm off muddy thinking under a veneer of smooth writing" [15]. Medical writing, especially in the case of research reports, is chiefly about medical science, and here art cannot trump science.

Stating What You Really Think

Reports of research studies are often written by committee; the members seek consensus on what will appear in print. Perhaps this is why the final version of the paper does not always include the heartfelt opinions of some researchers on the team and often does not reflect the diversity of author opinions. Richard Horton, editor of *The Lancet*, surveyed contributors to ten research articles published in *The Lancet*. Thirty-six of 54 contributors to the ten articles responded to questions in a qualitative analysis. The research question in the study was: "To determine whether the views expressed in a research paper are accurate representations of contributors' opinions about the research being reported" [16]. The study found unreported concerns about study weaknesses and disagreements among authors about findings and their significance. The study concludes that one remedy for the problem of suppressed opinions may be structured Discussion sections in research papers, as we now see in Abstracts.

Research Mentors

Research is best undertaken in teams, and members of the team bring different skills, one of which may just be mentoring. Research mentors can be especially important team members, who provide nurturing and guidance to the less experienced. They help keep young researchers on track, which can yield surprisingly good outcomes. Hoff writes: "When I finished medical school, I did not intend to do research as part of my life in surgery. That all changed when I met a mentor who inspired me during my training days. I had some protected time, assembled space and equipment, developed a hypothesis, and went to it. I'll never forget my first experiment and publication. Frankly, it was my best" [17].

Getting Your Research Report in Print

General Douglas MacArthur once said, "There is no substitute for victory." In academic medicine, there is no substitute for publication. You can have a brilliant idea, perform groundbreaking research, and write the results with great proficiency, but if the paper is not published—so that it can be cited, criticized, or praised—then the effort has been largely wasted. The advancement of science depends on sharing knowledge in print. Chapter 12 discusses how to achieve publication, for your research report or other publication models.

References

1. Day RA. How to write and publish a scientific paper. Westport, CT: Oryx; 1998. p. 34.
2. Cohen DJ, Crabtree BF. Evaluative criteria for qualitative research in health care: controversies and recommendations. Ann Fam Med. 2008;6(4):331–9.
3. Whimster WF. Biomedical research: how to plan, publish, and present it. New York: Springer; 1997. p. 101, 105.
4. Wager E, Altman DG, Simera I, Toma TP. Do declarative titles affect readers' perceptions of research findings? Research integrity. Peer Rev. 2016;1:11.
5. Jacques TS, Sebire NJ. The impact of article titles on citation hits: an analysis of general and specialist medical journals. JRSM Short Rep. 2010;1:2.
6. International Committee of Medical Journal Editors. Recommendations for the conduct, reporting, editing, and publication of scholarly work in medical journals. http://www.icmje.org/recommendations/.
7. Meyer H, Varpio L, Gruppen L, Gurjit S. The ethics and etiquette of research collaboration. Acad Med. 2016;91(12):e13.
8. Strasburger VC. Righting medical writing. JAMA. 1985;254(13):1789–90.
9. Nakayama T, Hirai N, Yamazaki S, Naito M. Adoption of structured abstracts by general medical journals and format for a structured abstract. J Med Libr Assoc. 2005;93(2):237–42.
10. Journal of the American Medical Association. Instructions for authors. http://jamanetwork.com/journals/jama/pages/instructions-for-authors#SecAbstractsforReportsofOriginalData.
11. Strasak AM, Zaman Q, Marinel G, Pfeiffer KP, Ulmer H. The use of statistics in medical research: a comparison of The New England Journal of Medicine and Nature Medicine. Am Stat. 2007;61(1):47–55.
12. Gotta AW. Review of Taylor RB. The clinician's guide to medical writing. Ed. 1. New York: Springer-Verlag, 2005. JAMA. 2005;293(9):1142.

13. Alexandrov AV. How to write a research paper. Cerebrovasc Dis. 2004;18(2):135–8.
14. Wager E. What medical writing means to me. Mens Sana Monogr. 2007;5(1):169–78.
15. Dirckx J. Dx+Rx: a physician's guide to medical writing. Boston: G.K. Hall; 1977. p. 99.
16. Horton R. The hidden research paper. JAMA. 2002;287:2775–8.
17. Hoff JT. Research by academic surgeons. Am J Surg. 2003;85(1):13–5.

Chapter 12
Getting Your Writing Published

There is no form of lead poisoning which more rapidly and thoroughly pervades the blood and bones and marrow than that which reaches the young author through mental contact with type-metal.... So the man or woman who has tasted type is sure to return to his old indulgence sooner or later.

American physician and author Oliver Wendell Holmes, Sr. (1809–1894) [1]

Today, more than a century and a half after Holmes penned the words quoted above, we no longer use lead type. Submitting manuscripts, checking revisions, and proofreading today are all online, with even the fate of printed pages containing actual ink becoming a question for the future. And thus, while we may not develop classical "lead poisoning" today, some of us will "suffer the indulgence" to write described by Holmes and long to see our words published, whether on paper or on the web.

This chapter is the longest in the book, if for no other reason than getting your work published often turns out to be the most challenging phase of the medical writing process. You are entering the world of editors and publishers, a place where you will encounter rules and perils unlike those found in the clinical practice, the classroom, or the laboratory. Yet another reason for this chapter's length is that this is the area of most change since the last edition, and some of these changes are not good.

© Springer International Publishing AG 2018
R.B. Taylor, *Medical Writing*,
https://doi.org/10.1007/978-3-319-70126-4_12

Let us reprise on the path to publication: You had a great idea for a review article, case report, editorial, or letter to the editor. Maybe you completed a research project. You developed the concept—how you would handle the idea. You have written the paper, revised it at least three times (see Chap. 3), and had it critiqued by your harshest reviewer colleague before preparing the final draft. In short, you have been able to write it up. These are all important steps; the next is getting your work in print. Notice that I say, "Next next step," not "final step," because, as I will explain at the end of the chapter, there are things to consider even after publication. What follows are hints as to how to get your work published. The advice is general and applies to all the publication models discussed in the book, not only to research reports.

Fundamentally, publication follows an invitation by an editor that is accepted by the author after having submitted a manuscript for consideration. Of course, along the way there will be peer review, editing changes, and sometimes a major revision or two. But, following negotiated changes, author and editor must both say, "Yes."

In fact, you and the journal editor have compatible goals. You, as the author, want your work in print as soon as possible. The editor needs high-quality articles for publication, in most cases each month. You and the editor need one another. As King writes, "Authors and publishers thus live in symbiosis. The unpublished manuscript accomplishes nothing for its author, and a journal without manuscripts speedily dies" [2].

Planning Your Article Submission

Submitting Your Article to the Right Journal

Choosing the journal for first submission is an important step that should begin as you conceptualize the paper, as discussed in Chap. 1. Here are some tips on selecting your "target journal."

Pay attention to how often the journal publishes papers similar to yours. What topics are generally presented in the journal?

If you have a paper on a general medical topic, such as irritable bowel syndrome, depression, or chest pain, your range of journal possibilities is wide. If your paper describes a urologic surgical procedure or a method of teaching psychologic assessment of the geriatric patient, your choices are more limited.

Sometimes you will sense an unmet need. If your research shows that the *Annals of Internal Medicine* has published no articles on dermatologic topics over the past few years, that finding can mean one of two things: Either the journal editor considers skin disease articles outside the scope of the journal, or the editor has received no useful submissions in this area and would welcome your paper on current approach to the patient with hives.

There is an interesting web site that may prove useful: http://jane.biosemantics.org/. Here you can type in the title or abstract of your article, and the site will generate a ranked list of possible journals for publication. Just as a test, I made up a title: "The Use of Vanilla Extract Reduces the Frequency and Severity of Migraine Headaches." This web site suggested, quite logically, that the best journal for my paper would be *Headache*. Also high on the suggested list were *Neurology* and *The Clinical Journal of Pain*. Down on the list was *The Journal of Headache and Pain*, clearly tagged as open access. Not bad. Try this web site with your next paper.

In selecting your target journal, consider the following factors:

The Variety of Article Formats

Some journals accept almost no articles that are not research reports. Others limit themselves to review articles. Some publish case reports; other journals never do so. In some journals you will find invited editorials—that is, written by persons who are not the editor of the journal. In other journals, only the editor writes the editorials. Here are two ways to check on the variety of article formats published: (1) Scan several recent issues of the journal, which is also helpful in determining the scope of topics, the usual writing style, and what authors are publishing in the journal; and (2) review the instructions for authors, which will probably describe the types of articles published, with some guidelines for the preparation of each. Fortunately, both the table of contents for recent issues and instructions for authors for almost all journals are available online, with no need to make a trip to the library.

The Journal's Impact Factor

For the author submitting a research report, the impact factor becomes a two-edged sword. On one hand, the impact factor of the journal in which your article is published is the key to having your findings widely cited [3]. On the other hand, and this is why I bring up the impact factor again, a journal's high impact factor reduces your chances of acceptance. The most prestigious journals receive huge numbers of submissions. The greatest number of submissions is likely to go the major broad-based journals with high impact factors and acceptance rates often below 10%.

Aiming High: The Controversy

Some investigators submit their papers first to one of the most prestigious journals. Of course, there is only a slim chance of acceptance, but the authors generally recognize this fact. What they seek is a critical review of the paper by experts. In recommending rejection, the peer reviewers will identify the weaknesses of the paper. This allows the author to fix the problems before submitting the paper to what was always the true target journal.

One disadvantage to such a practice is that it delays publication. The turnaround time in peer review and editorial decision-making can be measured in months. For a paper that has very timely data, this delay may actually work against publication.

The larger question is the ethical issue of seeking what is really a free consultation regarding your paper, when you know that your chances of acceptance approach is zero. Yet one goal of volunteer peer reviewers must be to help investigators and authors prepare the best papers possible.

Working with Journal Editors

Working with editors means recognizing and respecting what they want from you. Norton, an assistant editor of the *Journal of the American Academy of Dermatology*, writes, "I would be proud if every article published in the Journal were novel, interesting and important—in other words, if every article were both readable and worth reading. (I'd also like it if every article were eloquent, funny, and short). The editors would love to receive manuscripts that are perfect when first submitted, but these papers rarely exist. The peer-review system is intended to select the most worthwhile papers and nudge them along toward that elusive perfection" [4].

"Read the instructions, Grandpa." This was my then 5-year-old granddaughter's directive when mixing ingredients to make pancakes, starting a board game, or trying to operate a new electronic gadget. My granddaughter was on the right track. Journal editors earnestly wish that more authors would actually read—and follow—the instructions for authors. Failure to do so results in extra work for both the editor and author. It can cause delays, as the manuscript is returned for the missing pieces. Sometimes failure to follow directions can result in summary rejection (see below), simply because the manuscript was egregiously nonconforming.

If you read author instructions carefully, you may learn some very useful facts. One of these has to do with getting an early opinion from the editorial staff. For example, the *New England Journal of Medicine* (NEJM) offers a presubmission inquiries/fast track: "Send your summary via our Rapid Review request form. You should hear back from us within 36 hours. Rapid Review allows a manuscript to be reviewed by the Journal, and a decision on publication will be reached within two to three weeks. A Rapid Review does not in any way guarantee acceptance of the manuscript nor does it promise rapid release if the paper is accepted. Each of these decisions will be made separately" [5].

Good Manuscripts and Bad: What Editors Think

Here is what one editor thinks about good and bad articles:

> Wonderful articles are alike in so many ways. They have a concise introduction that proposes a testable hypothesis, a methods section with a good study design, a results section in which the statistical analysis addresses clinical relevance as well as statistical significance, and a discussion in which points are made succinctly and are based on evidence, not conjecture. In wonderful articles, the prose is clear, fluent, and direct. On the other hand, unhappy articles are often uniquely bad, each with its particular combination of distinctive flaws [4].

In an insightful, but humorous editorial in *JAMA*, Grouse identifies a "rogues' gallery of medical manuscripts" [6]. The following sections describe a few of the perpetrators.

The Clone

The clone is born as a researcher attempts to publish two or more papers based on data in a single study. The act of submitting clone articles is sometimes called fractionated publication, salami science, or duplicate publication. Von Elm et al. reviewed 56 systematic literature reviews that included 1131 main articles. They report, "Sixty articles were published twice, 13 three times, 3 four times, and 2 five times" [7].

Academic institutions must bear some responsibility for this behavior, as promotion and tenure committees carefully count the number of publications listed on a candidate's curriculum vitae (CV). Journals contribute to the problem with a reluctance to publish long research reports. Nevertheless, the clone wastes valuable journal space by repeating background material, methods, and often-similar conclusions in several papers.

The Chain Letter

The chain letter is a variation on the clone. In a chain letter, a research group lets each member be the first author by submitting an ongoing series of papers that present just a little more data from an ongoing study plus a great deal of previously published results. Each version of the chain letter varies a little in the list of authors and in the title of the article.

The Attention Grabber

In this manuscript, the authors may have conducted perfectly good research, but they postulate sometimes-outrageous conclusions that go beyond their data. In many cases, the discussion suggests some breakthrough in the diagnosis or treatment of disease that is sure to be reported in the media. An egregious variation on this behavior is when the authors release their findings to the media just as their scientific article goes to press.

The Shell Game

A shell game occurs when an author submits the identical paper to more than one journal at a time. Playing the shell game is risky and some say unethical. The player "wins" when one journal accepts the paper, and it is rejected by all the others. The player loses when two or more journals accept the article, and all but one must be told (or learn) of the ruse. The shell game wastes reviewers' and editors' time. It can make for duplicate publication if the author doesn't withdraw the paper from all but one publication. Journal editors hate shell game players.

The Ambush

In his paper, the author launches a missile aimed at a colleague in the field. The Background or Discussion section of the paper contains a cleverly crafted criticism of the colleague's work, perhaps including an attack on the individual.

The Zombie

This describes a manuscript that never dies. When a journal rejects an article in no uncertain terms, it means that the editor does not want to see the manuscript again. The author's job is to make any needed changes, and then submit the article elsewhere. Do not let your manuscript become a zombie by resubmitting it to the editor who rejected it without that editor's invitation to do so.

Technical Requirements for Publication

By now you have selected the best journal for first submission, contacted the editor or decided why you should not do so, and made sure your manuscript will not be considered one of the "rogues' gallery" described above. It is time to take care of the last technical details of manuscript submission.

Submission Letter

A submission letter should accompany every manuscript, from research report to letter to the editor. Also sometimes called the "cover letter," the submission letter provides information about your paper and about you as the author(s). The letter should be addressed to the journal editor, by name. Identify the title of the paper just before the salutation in the letter. Table 12.1 describes the contents of a comprehensive submission letter.

TABLE 12.1 Contents of cover letter accompanying an article manuscript submitted to a medical journal

Letter item	What to include
Introductory paragraph	Identify the accompanying manuscript and indicate that you are submitting it to be considered for publication. In some instances, you should identify the type of paper you are submitting, e.g., report of original research, brief report, case report, or other format
Word count	Cite the number of words in the manuscript. Your word processing program will give you the needed number

(continued)

TABLE 12.1 (continued)

Letter item	What to include
Specific author contributions	Many journals ask that you describe each author's specific contribution to the research and writing. For example, did an author recruit the subjects, collect data, provide statistical analysis, or edit the manuscript?
Contact author	Identify the one author who will respond to correspondence and who can answer questions about the study. Provide full contact information
Copyright relinquishment	Many journals insist that the cover letter relinquish copyright if the article is published. See the journal's instructions to authors to determine if this is needed in the letter and, if so, to note the exact wording to be used
Conflict of interest disclosure	Describe any industry sponsorship of the study, contractual agreements with industry, consulting or speaking agreements, or even stock ownership if there might be a perceived conflict of interest
Author approval	State that the manuscript has been read and approved by all the authors and that the requirements for authorship have been met by each
Duplicate submission or publication	State that the contents of the paper have not been published previously and that the manuscript has not been submitted elsewhere. State if an abstract has been presented at a scientific meeting
Special requests	Try to avoid special requests. However, in the case of cutting-edge scientific research, there may be a valid reason for requesting that a certain individual not be used as a peer reviewer
Thank you	Thank the editor for considering your manuscript for publication
Author approval	All authors must approve the submission letter

Not all journals require a separate submission letter. The *New England Journal of Medicine*, for example, states: "You do not need to send a separate cover letter file with your online submission. Instead, we offer a text box in which you can type your information, or you can cut and paste from a previously written letter. This box can also be left blank, if you wish" [5].

Title Page

The title page gives important data about the paper and the authors. The title page should include the following items, which are consistent with both the recommendations of the International Committee of Medical Journal Editors (ICMJE) [8] and the instructions for submission to the *New England Journal of Medicine* [5]:

- The article's title
- Each author's name, academic degree(s), and institutional affiliation
- The name of the department(s) and institution(s) where the work was done
- Disclaimers, if any are appropriate
- The corresponding author's name and full contact information
- The name and address of the person to whom reprint requests should be addressed or a statement that no reprints will be available
- Sources of support, such as grants
- A running head (a short version of the title) that will appear on each manuscript page

Literature Review Update

Just before submitting the manuscript, repeat your literature review. Important papers may have touched on your topic since you did your original literature search. Be sure that there has been no "breakthrough" study that should be acknowledged in your article. Assure yourself also that no one has recently published a paper just like yours. Having someone beat you to publication on a topic should not discourage you from submitting, but you should know that the playing field has changed.

What to Submit and in What Order

When you finally have collected all the pieces, it is time to assemble your submission folder. Unless specifically instructed otherwise, assemble your materials as follows:

- Submission letter
- Title page
- Abstract
- Keywords
- Body of the text
- Acknowledgments
- References
- Tables with legends, each on a separate page
- Figures with legends, each on a separate page

Check the instructions to authors carefully if you are submitting artwork that is not appropriate for online submission. When you are all ready to submit, review the checklist in Table 12.2 to help ensure that you are not forgetting anything.

Electronic Submission of Manuscripts

Today almost all journals require electronic submission of manuscripts, whether as an e-mail attachment, on a compact disk, or by uploading to the journal's web site. This saves time and money for the journal and facilitates the peer-review process; no paper, no delay in the mail. Different journals have different requirements. For example, the NEJM states: "All text, references, figure legends, and tables should be in

TABLE 12.2 Manuscript checklist for journal article or book chapter submission

Use 12-point font unless the instructions specify otherwise
Leave the right margin of the manuscript unjustified (i.e., ragged)
Identify all abbreviations when first used in the text
Use nonproprietary names of drugs
Check all references for accuracy and completeness
Confirm that all references are cited in the text
Be sure you have disclosed any possible conflict of interest
For all borrowed materials, send a consent form signed by the copyright holder
Include informed consent to use images that may identify human subjects
Keep a copy of everything, which will be used later to check proofs

one double-spaced electronic document (preferably a Word Doc). You may either insert figures in the text file or upload your figures separately. We prefer the former, but this may not work well for complicated graphics, which should be sent separately" [5].

As one who has made the transition from carefully mailing manuscripts to submitting electronically, I can attest that the online way is not necessarily easier than the old method. To check my belief, I spoke with my colleague Rick Deyo, MD, MPH, who has published scores of highly regarded papers in top journals. Loosely quoted, here is what Rick told me: "I allow 2–3 hours for an electronic submission. This is even for journals with which I am familiar. Some want all parts of the manuscript bundled; some want them submitted separately. I may have to look up coauthors' addresses and e-mail addresses. Or they will request an extra document. There is always something. It takes time."

The "always something" can be unique to the journal. For instance, the *British Medical Journal* asks authors of research reports to complete a "What this paper adds" box, providing a thumbnail sketch of what the article contributes to the literature, which assists readers who are seeking a quick overview [9].

Here is a special caution when uploading to a journal site. Never attempt to compose online. You are likely to be timed out and lose what you created—very frustrating. Instead, compose everything on your computer so that you can copy and paste to appropriate locations on the journal's site.

Other than the above, submitting online is a lot like mail-in submission used to be. You still need all the manuscript "pieces," and the checklist above is still pertinent. What's different is that there is no envelope, no postage, and no lost packages, and, once the system is mastered, things move much faster. And reviewers no longer receive manuscripts with smudges and coffee stains.

Some Mistakes Made in Submitting Manuscripts

The discussion above will help you avoid most technical manuscript submission errors. Here are some additional ways authors go wrong.

Relying on Your Spell-Checker

Your Microsoft Word spelling and grammar utility is excellent, but it will not detect all errors. For example, type in the following:

> Eye no hat correct spellings is important, and sew eye was care full to us the spell checker.

My Microsoft spell-checker accepted this sentence as correct.

> Also, proofread to be sure words are left out, especially if the omission can change meaning.

Whoops, again! In reading, did you notice the omission of the word "no" from the example sentence, an omission that my spell-checker also approved?

Touting Your Paper

Do not use your submission letter to tell the editor that yours is a *very important* paper. Editors look at many articles and can recognize those that are important, especially with the advice of peer reviewers. Your paper is not a used car to be "sold," claiming to report the greatest advance since Wilhelm Conrad Roentgen took a snapshot of his wife's hand in 1895.

Seeking Perfection

Earlier in this chapter, I quoted Norton about the quest for "elusive perfection." In fact, your paper will never be perfect, either in content or manuscript preparation. Do not undertake multiple, but trivial, revisions. At some time you must say, as all writers and artists must eventually do, that this is as good as I can reasonably make it and I am going to declare it done.

Journal editors want pertinent, timely, and well-written articles and will make allowance for small deviations from minor technical requirements so long as they do not interfere with reading, reviewing, or editing the manuscript. That is not to say that the editor may not require corrections before the manuscript is published. The point is that you should do your very best when writing a paper. However, do not fret about whether the terminal page numbers in references should be written in full or truncated. Such minor variations will not cause rejection, and perseveration over trivia can only interfere with your writing success.

The Review Process

Your manuscript has been received by the journal and has been sent for review. Your article was not summarily rejected and sent back immediately by the editor as being "not appropriate for consideration by the journal." That would have meant that the editor believed the work to be outside the journal's field or that it is libelous, blasphemous, hopelessly incomprehensible, or totally irrational. This sort of summary dismissal is called a "desk rejection." You have passed the first hurdle [10]. Things are now in the hands of the peer reviewers.

In 1665 Henry Oldenbert, the founding editor of the *Philosophical Transactions of the Royal Society* in London, devised the peer-review system used today. Here is what you need to know.

Peer Review

The Role and Duties of the Peer Reviewer

The journal editor selects peer reviewers who will read and comment on your paper. Many are senior academicians and investigators. All are volunteers, and they do a lot of work for no pay. Peer reviewers, sometimes called referees, can be a very big help to you, even if your paper is ultimately rejected.

If you wish to be a peer reviewer, send a letter and your curriculum vitae to the journal editor, and volunteer to serve. State the areas in which you have some expertise and are willing to review papers. The editor will reply and perhaps add you to the review team. Editors want their peer reviewers to have certain traits. Peer reviewers should be knowledgeable in the topic under consideration, intellectually honest, and time-sensitive. The author and editor cannot wait 6 months for a paper to be reviewed. In reviewing reports of clinical studies, a peer reviewer should know research methodology and basic statistical analysis. In the end, the peer reviewer helps to improve the paper, making it clearer, more informative, and often shorter—even if the paper is ultimately rejected by the journal. (Remember that the paper will then be revised and submitted to the next journal on the author's list.) These are exactly the traits you hope for in the reviewer who evaluates your paper.

The duties of a peer reviewer can be summarized as follows:

- Accept a paper to review only if the job can be completed within the time specified in the editor's request.
- Agree to referee papers only in your, the reviewer's, areas of expertise.

- Maintain confidentiality about the paper.
- Disclose any possible conflict of interest, and decline a review if there is any potential difficulty.
- Write a thoughtful review that is honest and free of bias.
- Aim to make the paper the best it can be, balancing criticism with suggestions for improvement.
- Avoid excessively harsh comments, especially those that could be interpreted as a personal attack on the author(s). The opportunity to comment anonymously on unpublished papers can bring to the surface heretofore-submerged sadistic traits, which must be recognized and stifled.
- Submit the review promptly. The authors of the paper are anxiously awaiting a verdict.

The peer reviewer never contacts the author directly. In most cases, but not all, the name of the author is not present on the paper being reviewed. Remember that the author's name goes only on the title page, which is generally not sent to the peer reviewers. There are exceptions. The last paper I reviewed contained the names of the authors, and there had been no effort to "blind" the review. Even when the names of authors and institutions are absent in blinded reviews, the peer reviewer who is working actively in the field can often deduce the source of the paper based on the topic, methods, and even writing style.

I think of the roles of a peer reviewer and a practicing clinician as somewhat similar. Both are expected to exhibit ethical behavior and to be committed to providing high-quality service. Both the reviewer and clinician should be knowledgeable, capable, and thorough in what they do. Both need to examine details while keeping a broad perspective. Both must be reliable and trustworthy and believe that they serve a worthy purpose. And, if careless, both can cause a lot of harm.

The Role and Duties of the Editor

The editor makes the final decision about acceptance or rejection of an article. Of course, an editor's decision is based strongly on the recommendations of the peer reviewers.

Although it is significant that most papers are sent out to three reviewers, not two or four, the final decision is not a "vote." Editors are paid to make judgments, and they make the final call.

Editors, like peer reviewers, must be honest, ethical, unbiased, responsible, and detail-oriented. They must also be literate, knowledgeable, and compulsive as to deadlines. After all, most journals must be published every month, some more often.

The editor serves as the buffer between the author and the peer reviewers. As such the editor must be able to deal with authors who are disappointed or angry. In other cases, the problem is tardy or sloppy authors. A good editor can handle all these problems with tact and grace.

What Actually Happens

Here is a quick summary of what occurs when you submit an article to a medical journal. You will establish an identity on the journal's manuscript tracking system, following which you will send your manuscript online. Your article will be assigned with an identification number, and you may be asked for some additional data, such as release forms or identification of an "archival author," who will be responsible for maintaining records of the study.

Next, the editor or assistant editor looks over the article quickly to see whether it merits peer review. As discussed above, articles with topics outside the journal's scope or those that are carelessly prepared will be immediately returned to the author. Those that survive the initial screening are sent to referees for peer review, a process that has changed little in decades. The editor's choice of reviewers is probably more intuitive than scientific, something along the lines of: "I think so-and-so would be a good person to look at this report."

After (what we hope is) a careful reading, each referee prepares an evaluation. Most evaluations have two parts: one part is for the editor's eyes only, and one part is sent to you, the author. The part sent to you can be quite valuable—or not—as discussed below.

When all reviews are received, the editor makes a decision and lets you know the outcome of the process. If you have not heard about a decision in a reasonable time, let's say 6–8 weeks from the time of submission, it is a good idea to contact the journal. For example, your paper may be in a pending file while the assistant awaits receipt of a third review, due from a referee who has left for a 4-month trek in Nepal. Some journals offer a way to keep track of the process. For example, the *New England Journal of Medicine* allows authors to track the status of manuscripts through the author dashboard of their ScholarOne Manuscripts system [11].

Possible Responses from the Journal Editor

The journal editor's decision will come as a letter that indicates one the following: rejection, revision, or acceptance.

Rejection Letter

The rejection letter is the one you really don't want to receive. The editor will probably avoid the word "reject" and instead will euphemistically state that it "does not meet the Journal's needs." (Note that editors always refer to their publication as "the Journal," with a capital "J.") The editor is not only saying that, after careful review, your paper will not be published in their Journal. This response also connotes that it cannot be improved to make it consistent with their standards. The editor simply does not want to see your paper again.

Unless you have had the bad luck to compete with an article in press that is very similar to yours, the rejection will be attributed chiefly to the evaluations of the referees. These comments will usually be sent to you, and you should read them very carefully. The decision to reject will almost certainly be based on one or more of the reasons listed in Table 12.3.

TABLE 12.3 Classic causes of article rejection

Topic considered unimportant or outside the area of interest of the journal's readers
Outdated or inaccurate information
Inadequate literature review
Faulty scientific method or statistical analysis
Conclusions that are inconsistent with the data
Clumsy structure to the article
Poor writing
Suspected bias, plagiarism, duplicate publication, inappropriate criticism of colleagues and their work, or other ethical concerns

Your first reaction will probably be denial. Could this editor really have rejected my paper? Could there be a mistake? Maybe this rejection notice was meant for someone else. Then you read the reviewer comments and become annoyed, actually furious. How could they miss the point of my paper? Did the referees read the paper at all?

Next you settle down and consider appealing the decision. Should you request reconsideration? Actually, this sometimes works, but not often. Your appeal must be rational and civilized. Describing the referees as troglodytes will not advance your cause. A reasonable appeal letter should politely refute the reviewers' criticisms point by point, citing evidence. Show how your paper will be especially important to the journal's readers and how this point may have been overlooked. Indicate any recent publications that validate your findings and conclusions. Type your brief, let it sit for a day or two to cool off, and then revise to expunge any hint of anger. Then send the appeal, and prepare to be rejected again. According to an editor at the *British Medical Journal*, some 20% of appeals are successful (Smith R. The inside view of writing for medical journals. Available at: http://www.pitt.edu/~super7/14011-15001/14851.ppt).

Then sadness sets in. Maybe I am not cut out to be a medical writer. Perhaps I should spend my spare time working in the yard or traveling to Europe. How could I have ever had the hubris to think that I could get my work in print?

By this time have you recognized your progress through the classical stages of bereavement—denial, anger, bargaining, depression, and acceptance—described by Elisabeth Kübler-Ross [12].

The final step is to accept the judgment of journal number one. At this point, you should use this opportunity to improve the paper. Seek the nuggets of truth in the reviewers' remarks. Yes, I know that at least one of the reviewers seems to have totally misunderstood the paper, and maybe there is a message there. Make the appropriate revisions, and update the literature search and references, especially if a few months have passed. Then submit the paper to another journal. Do this soon to help prevent becoming discouraged. As a hint, subsequent submissions are sometimes more successful when sent to more specialized journals, especially those with lower rejection rates than the *Journal of the American Medical Association* or the *New England Journal of Medicine*, both of which reject more than 90% of submissions.

When preparing the second submission, read the journal's instructions, and make sure your manuscript complies with its technical requirements, which are sure to differ from those of the previous journal. Basically, the second submission should have no indication that this is not the first time the paper has left your desk. There is, of course, the chance that one of the reviewers for the second journal may be the very same person who was a referee for the first publication, an occurrence most likely in limited scientific fields.

Even the best writers suffer rebuff at times. Bryson describes the comments of a journal editor upon receiving an advance copy of Charles Darwin's *On the Origin of Species* in 1859. He counseled Darwin that the book, although meritorious, would never appeal to a wide audience. The editor, in a helpful mood, undoubtedly noting the many pages about birds in the book, suggested that Darwin write a book about pigeons. "'Everyone is interested in pigeons,' he observed helpfully" [13]. I recommend that you save all rejection letters. Put them in a folder in the back of your file. Medical writers all receive many such letters, and the file may eventually overflow. Years from now you will read them and chuckle.

As I leave the grim topic of rejection letters, allow me to indulge my sense of humor by describing what I consider some amusing examples.

- "Dear Contributor. We are returning your dumb story. Note that we have not included our return address. We have moved to a new office, and we don't want you to know where we are" (Source: Peanuts cartoon in *The Oregonian*, March 5, 2004).
- "Your work was good and original. Unfortunately the good bits were not original and the original bits were not good." Richard S. Smith, former editor of BMJ tells that this was a rejection letter actually used at the BMJ during his tenure [14].
- "I am returning this otherwise good typing paper to you because someone has printed gibberish all over it and put your name at the top" (Source: Writing quotes. Available at: http://www.quotegarden.com/writing.html).
- And my favorite, a letter sent to a writer by a Chinese publication: "We have read your manuscript with boundless delight. If we were to publish your paper it would be impossible for us to publish any work of a lower standard. And as it is unthinkable that, in the next 1,000 years, we shall see its equal, we are, to our regret, compelled to return your divine composition and beg you a thousand times to overlook our short sight and timidity" [15].

Revision Letter

This is a much better letter to receive than the rejection letter. Be aware that the revision letter, sometimes called the modification letter, can be misleading. It can begin with the cunning phrase, "I regret to inform you that your paper does not meet the Journal's requirements in its present form." Oh, sadness and gloom! But read on. The next sentence may be, "However, if you make revisions as suggested by the peer reviewers, we will be pleased to reconsider your submission." Hooray! This is actually a conditional acceptance letter. If you agree with the suggestions offered by the referees, you should make the recommended changes and thank the reviewers in your resubmission letter. Your resubmission cover letter should also indicate where changes were made and how they relate to the comments of the referees and editor.

In a descriptive analysis of manuscripts submitted to and eventually published by the *Annals of Internal Medicine*, Purcell et al. identified five leading types of problems prompting manuscript changes during peer review and revision. These were "too much information, too little information, inaccurate information, misplaced information, and structural problems." They further state, "Changes most often occurred because information was missing or extraneous" [16].

In modifying your paper, focus your effort on the suggested changes. Consider the language offered by your reviewers, which should be used in any letter responding to reviewer comments. Does some of this language also belong in your paper? Do not add new data or conclusions, which can only give the editor and referees something new to criticize. Make surgical repairs and resubmit before the editor has a change of mind.

One dilemma you may face is the revision letter that invites you to cut your paper to 500 words for a brief report or even shorten and resubmit as a letter to the editor (see Chap. 7). This calls for some soul-searching, discussion with coauthors, and perhaps consultation with a trusted senior advisor. On one hand, such an invitation suggests virtually certain publication in a journal high on your list. On the other hand, you have to give up on full presentation of your data and conclusions. I can only recommend that your writing team struggle to a unanimous decision.

Acceptance Letter

Someday you might receive the following letter:

Dear Contributor:
The three referees and I have all read your paper.
We agree that your hypothesis is inspired, your methods are flawless, your results are brilliantly stated, and the conclusions are

logical and important. We have no suggestions to make and wish
to publish the paper as submitted.
Yours truly,
The Editor

But I don't think that letter will ever come. Through the first
two editions of this book, I have offered the following: If you
submit a research report to a major referred clinical journal
and it is accepted upon first submission without a single revision, let me know and I will take you to dinner the next time
you are in Portland, Oregon. So far, no one has taken me up
on the offer. I now live in Virginia Beach, Virginia, and the
offer for a free dinner in my hometown following uncritical
first-submission acceptance of your pristine paper by a
respected publication still stands.

Most acceptance letters follow one or more revisions. This
is probably a good idea, because the revisions, based on
reviewer comments, usually result in better papers in print.
After all, the real goal of peer review is the make the report
the best it can be.

Whose Papers Are Published and Why?

In the next few paragraphs, I shared some of the dark secrets
of medical publication, especially in regard to research
reports. Tell no one what you read next!

Some Concerns About Peer Review

Peer review may not be the pristine process we imagine.
Conflicts of interest are rampant, especially in focused
research communities. There are only so many investigators
who are experts on, as a whimsical example, the new vaccine
against male pattern baldness. Few people would have the
expertise to review papers in this area, and all may be at different stages along the same path to a very lucrative discovery.
Is it possible that the reviewer might make use of the information in the paper being reviewed? Such use would be

unethical, but I suspect that it might happen. Or might a reviewer unfairly criticize a paper that seems a few months ahead of his own submission of parallel findings?

Few studies have examined the peer-review process, but I found one that is quite revealing. The research question had to do with positive-outcome bias by reviewers. Emerson et al. fabricated two versions of a well-designed randomized controlled trial, differing only in the principal end point—positive outcome vs. no difference. The papers were submitted to 238 reviewers for two prestigious orthopedic journals; 210 reviews were returned. The investigators report: "Reviewers were more likely to recommend the positive version of the test manuscript for publication than the no-difference version (97.3% vs. 80.0%, $P < 0.001$)" [17].

Okike et al. studied single-blind review (author identities revealed to reviewers) vs. double-blind review (author identities concealed from peer reviewers). They found "Reviewers were more likely to recommend acceptance when the prestigious authors' names and institutions were visible (single-blind review) than when they were redacted (double-blind review)…" [18].

Smith considers peer review to be slow, expensive, and wasteful [14]. Yet today we have nothing better to offer, and medical writers need to cope with its inefficiencies and caprice.

Your Native Language Matters

When we consider the worldwide scientific community, it becomes apparent that more than half of all published research reports are written by authors whose first language is something other than English. If you speak English as your native language, you have an advantage over others around the world. A study by Coates et al. found, "The acceptance rate of non-mother English tongue authors is generally a lot lower than that for native English tongue authors" [19]. A survey of Korean authors submitting papers in English-language journals revealed that the respondents perceived the "linguistic elements of journal papers" to be the most problematic area [20].

The fundamental issue seems to concern language problems in manuscripts, rather than discrimination against international contributors. Imagine yourself as someone struggling to master a language in which we drive our cars on parkways and park in driveways. Our patients describe feet that smell, noses that run, and heartburn that doesn't relate to any type of cardiac disease. In this book, I am guilty of using idiomatic metaphors such as "game plan," "sweepstakes," and "shell game." Consider yourself, as one who speaks English daily and other languages infrequently or not at all, being required to submit your scientific paper in the Russian or Japanese language. My manuscript would surely be full of grammatical errors. This helps explain the study findings by Coates et al. that, in submissions to the journal *Cardiovascular Research*, "The US/UK acceptance rate of 30.4% was higher than for all other countries. The lowest acceptance rate of 9% (Italian) also had the highest error rate" [19]. Simply stated, the authors conclude that with articles of equal scientific merit, a poorly written, grammatically challenged article is more likely to be rejected.

About Author Affiliations

An eye-opening article all medical writers should read was published in 1982 in *Behavioral and Brain Sciences*. Authors Peters and Ceci wondered about the adequacy and fairness of peer-review practices. Here is what they did: The authors selected 12 articles by researchers in highly respected United States psychology departments like Yale and Harvard. Each of these articles had been published in a different, prestigious American psychology journal with high rejection rates (80%) and non-blinded peer reviewers. The authors substituted fictitious author names and institutions (something like the Mountain View Center for Human Potential) for what had been listed on the original papers. The manuscripts, with only author names and institutions changed, were then retyped and formally resubmitted to the same journals that had peer reviewed and published them 18–32 months earlier.

What happened to the 12 papers? Thirty-eight editors and reviewers evaluated the altered articles; only three detected the ruse. Nine of the 12 articles were earnestly reviewed, resulting in an editorial decision. In the end, eight of the nine were rejected. Sixteen of 18 referees had recommended against publication. In many cases, the referees described "serious methodological flaws."

Peters and Ceci ponder the possibility "that systematic bias was operating to produce the discrepant reviews. The most obvious candidates as sources of bias in this case would be the authors' status and institutional affiliation" [21].

In getting published, who you are, where you work, what language you speak daily, and who reviews your paper may profoundly influence whether your paper is accepted or rejected.

Competition for Journal Space, Industry-Sponsored Studies, and Editorial Conflict of Interest

Here is another little-recognized truth about medical publication. You and your writing team seeking publication are up against a formidable opponent—the industry-sponsored study. Seventy percent of studies published in the five leading medical journals are funded by industry [14].

We begin with the fact that publication space is precious, especially in the top-rated journals (read those with the high impact factors). Then consider the money, research know-how, and writing skills available to pharmaceutical firms—those companies that have a vested interest in clinicians prescribing their products. Is it any wonder that industry-sponsored studies achieve better journal "placement" than nonindustry-sponsored studies? Here is an example: In a Cochrane Database Systematic Review of 274 published influenza vaccine studies, Jefferson et al. "found industry funded studies were published in more prestigious journals and cited more than other studies independently from methodological quality and size." In this review there was also a difference in positive outcomes that, as noted above, helps assure publication: "Studies funded from public sources were significantly less likely to report conclusions favorable to the vaccines" [22].

Then there is the issue of multiple publications [23]. In a study of published trials of selective serotonin reuptake inhibitors submitted to support a bid for marketing approval in Sweden, Melander et al. found that "21 studies contributed to at least two publications each, and three studies contributed to five publications" [24]. All of these clones and chain letters increase the number of papers competing with your paper and mine for publication. Duplicate publication can also confound review articles and meta-analyses.

All the above is bad enough, but there is one additional concern—editorial conflict of interest. Here I am going to quote Smith, whom I remind the reader is former editor of the BMJ:

> This is a very important point: there are journals which are making millions of dollars out of reprints of these articles. *The Lancet* makes more money out of selling reprints of drug company sponsored trials than it does from subscriptions or straight advertising. Take the VIGOR study, which was published in the *New England Journal of Medicine*—all the information was released—the manufacturer bought a million dollars' of reprints, by no means uncommon, and of course the profit margin is huge. If you sell a million dollars' worth of reprints the profit is about $700,000 dollars, maybe $800,000, and that goes straight through to your bottom line, so more and more editors and publishers are under tremendous financial pressure. Think of the conflicts of interest for an editor. You know which trials will make that kind of money. If you publish it, you have $800,000 profit; if you don't publish it, you might have to find that $800,000 in some other way, which is of course extremely difficult. I think it is a very, very stark conflict of interest, more stark than many researchers experience [14].

And it is a handicap for the researcher seeking publication of a report that will not inspire a pharmaceutical company to purchase thousands of reprints. This economic reality represents an example of publication bias.

Peer-Review Fraud

We have recently seen instances of peer-review fraud, what Haug calls "hacking the scientific publication process" [26]. According to Haug, "In August 2015 the publisher Springer retracted 64 articles from 10 different subscription journals 'after editorial checks spotted fake e-mail addresses, and subsequent internal investigations uncovered fabricated peer-review reports,' according to a statement on their website." About 15% of article retractions are attributed to this scam.

Here is how peer-review fraud occurs. An author writes a paper and submits it to a journal, along with a list of suggested reviewers, complete with e-mail addresses. But the names of the suggested reviewers are bogus, and messages to the e-mail addresses given go directly to the nefarious author, who submits a series of favorable reviews for his own paper [26].

After Your Article Is Accepted

Finally, the acceptance letter arrives. No more worrying, and no more revisions. Your article is on its way into print. There are now three items to consider: proofreading, preventing errors, and what to do after publication.

Proofreading

Upon acceptance of your article, a copy editor will buff it for publication, tidying up errors of grammar and syntax. The copy editor is your friend. With a degree in English literature or some similar liberal arts credentials, the copy editor is there to help you and the editor publish the finest article possible. There may be minor alterations to improve clarity and eliminate ambiguity, and you may find very long sentences divided into two, and even some subheadings added in long expanses of text. The changes made will reflect standing orders from the editor about style and should not affect meaning.

Although you may or may not see the "marked-up" manuscript, you will definitely receive proofs to review. Occasionally you will be sent *galley proofs*—your manuscript set in print but not yet formatted to the journal page. Some journals always send galley proofs, while others send galleys only when they anticipate that the author will want to make some more changes. Prior to publication, you will definitely receive *page proofs*, with your article formatted to the journal page, perhaps even with the page numbers in place.

Read every word in the proofs carefully. Begin by checking the page proofs against the manuscript. Has anything been omitted or jumbled? This happens. Try reading out loud, which helps you assume the role of the reader. Use your computer search function to find the errors you know you often make—for example, *its* instead of *it's*—and overused pet words such as access or paradigm. Some authors prefer to print out the proofs and work from paper, rather than staring at a computer screen. If there are numbers and totals in the paper, get out your calculator to recheck math.

Beware of the printer's devil, today sometimes called the computer devil, which can change words like *for* to *of* and *antenatal* to *antinatal*. Do all the reference citations appear in the text, and do the numbers match the reference list? Pay special attention to tables and figures, where the printer's devil likes to lurk. In 2016, the *Annals of Family Medicine* published corrections to a previously published article with 17 specific errors in the tables and figures (Corrections in: Knottnerus BJ et al. 2016;14:399).

In the proofs, there may be queries to "Au." You must answer these questions precisely. Do not waffle, give both sides to an answer, or respond with a long explanatory paragraph. The editor is asking you for a decision about an issue in your paper. Make the decision and incorporate it in the text in an efficient, workmanlike manner.

Keep in mind that proofreading is intended to correct errors. You may be tempted to add new material during proofreading. A new study was published since your paper was submitted, or a new drug has been introduced. If you propose to add to the paper, I advise that you call the editorial office and discuss what you have in mind. Some editors will approve adding sentence or two or perhaps a reference. In the case of books, I can attest that too many changes can result in a charge against royalties.

If adding a reference, ask about numbering. In some journals, the author need not renumber all 90 references when adding one more in proofs. Instead, go to the appropriate location in the text, and, in the reference list, add the new number with an "a." Thus, if the new reference follows reference 45, the new addition will be reference 45a as a text citation and also in the reference list. This convenience saves time and cost and avoids many subsequent numbering errors.

There are proofreader's marks used as shorthand to identify corrections and changes in proofs in those instances when you receive a marked-up paper manuscript or galley proofs. These are found in Appendix B.

Return the manuscript promptly; the journal probably has already reserved space in an upcoming edition. If your work is a book chapter, there is probably a date scheduled with the printer for the entire book. Keep a copy of the corrected proofs. You spent valuable time and mental energy on the changes. Assume that the version you are returning to the journal will get lost in the ether of hyperspace.

Good writing is hard. Good proofreading may seem even harder because it is not creative. Proofreading can be mind-numbingly dull, and this is a danger, because it is very easy to have errors escape into print.

About Errors

Whenever I have published a book and have the first copy in my hand, I can unfailingly open the book to the exact page with a misspelled word. It may be the only error in a 1200-page book, but it seems to jump out at me.

Sometimes mistakes in print are called *errata*, as though the Latin word makes them seem less serious. Errors find their way into print in many ways. Some begin with the author and some with copyediting, and some seem to appear for mysterious reasons. It really doesn't matter how they occur, it is the author's job to discover and crush errors. If you think errors won't occur, examine Fig. 12.1a, b carefully. They are from a published article about medical publications. Do you see the error? Hint: The lines in Fig. 12.1b are correctly labeled. Now look at the two *arrows* pointing to the single line and the other "*arrow-less*" line in Fig. 12.1a.

One hundred years ago, *The Lancet* apologized for using the words "a sour correspondent," insisting that it should have been "as our correspondent" (JAMA 100 Years Ago. JAMA. 2001;286:140). The University of New South Wales has advertised for a mathematics research assistant who would work in a "3/4 research and 1/3 teaching position." The September 24, 2014 issue of JAMA has an article titled "Effect of Enhanced Information, Values Clarification, and Removal of Financial Barriers on Use of Prenatal Genetic Testing: A Randomized Clinical Trial." But in the table of contents on the journal cover, the study is identified by "Effect of Enhanced Information, Effect of Enhanced Information, Values Clarification, ... (Kuppermann M et al. JAMA. 2014;312:1208). This duplication of a phrase in the table of contents is not the fault of the authors but must have embarrassed someone in the journal office.

Today some major medical journals seem to have a monthly column correcting errors in recently published papers. Most errata are of minor significance, other than the damage to the self-esteem of the authors. Much more egregious, even dangerous, are errors involving drug doses. I received a copy of the 16th edition of the *Handbook of Antimicrobial Therapy* published by the Medical Letter on Drugs and Therapeutics. The handbook came with an attached warning label:

> On page 130 the pediatric dosage of doxycycline (combined with quinine sulfate) for treatment of chloroquine-resistant *P. falciparum* malaria should be 2 mg/kg/d × 7 d.

In fact, on page 130 of the handbook, the dose is listed as 30 mg/kg/d × 7 d. This is much more worrisome than incorrect fractions in a job advertisement.

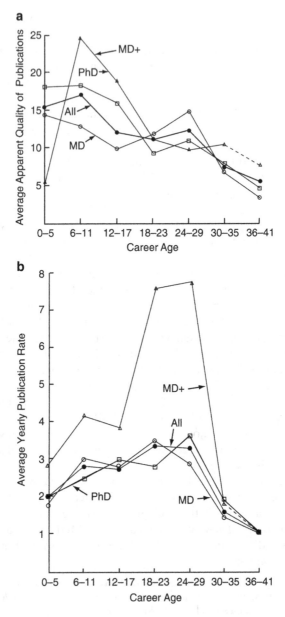

Fɪɢ. 12.1 (**a**) has an error in labeling. (**b**) is correctly labeled. Can you spot the error in (**a**)? The original captions were: "(**a**) Average apparent quality of publications versus career age for the 4-year sample. (**b**) Average yearly publication rate versus career age for the 4-year sample (from Krumland and Gorry [25]. Used with permission)." Note to reader: The original legends are included to explain what the graphs are meant to show

After Publication

Saving Your Files

Some people save empty boxes, lengths of ribbon, odd pieces of wood, and half-empty cans of paint. They will tell you, "I might use this someday." Saving stuff is a very good idea for writers. I tend to file by project. I have a file with all the notes and quotes used for this book. If I plan to use something from this book in another project, I will make a copy for the new book or article. Items you liked, but didn't actually use, might be just what you need for your next article or book. For example, my last book was titled *The Amazing Language of Medicine* (Taylor R. New York: Springer; 2017), and I have an idea for a new book that will be along the same lines. When I come across papers or anecdotes that may be useful, I drop them in a file, unsorted for now. My files include metaphors, similes, and examples that might support my pet theories. I also keep a computer file of topic ideas that may become chapter titles or section headings. Some of these items languish for years and then turn out to be useful. That is how I happen to have this chapter's reference 6 from 1980.

Reprints

Sometime during the production process, you may be asked whether you would like to purchase reprints of your paper. Reprints are—or were—a time-honored tradition in scientific writing, and before the Internet they were an important way in which investigators disseminated their findings. Today JAMA advises authors as follows: "Published authors may acquire reprints and e-prints for their personal use such as in classroom teaching or to share with a research colleague" [27].

A century ago, C. D. Spivak, the editor of *Medical Libraries*, reported, "There is an inborn craving in the hearts of medical men for reprints of their articles." He attributed this craving to "a psychological fact, namely, that every writer wishes to give the stamp of individuality to his work." Spivak called for authors to let medical libraries be the first claimant on reprints [28].

Today, reprints are going out of fashion, and I don't buy them anymore. They have become expensive. Journals use them to generate income and seem unable to sell me a reasonably small number. Today most reprint requests arrive online and are answered by sending a PDF of the article. Each year more and more journals go to open access, and I predict that before long journal reprints, like my file of journal article clippings, will become a historical curiosity.

Criticism of Your Writing

There is an old aphorism about medical writing: He who writes stands up to be shot at. After publication of your article, chapter, or book, some readers may write letters to the editor saying, "Great job." (In fact, such letters are unlikely to be published, because they do not generate controversy.)

In Chap. 7, I told about writing book reviews. Now your book or research report is being reviewed by someone else, someone whose name you probably didn't even know. Some book reviewers may praise your work. The first edition of my book *Family Medicine: Principles and Practice* was reviewed in the *British Medical Journal* as "the Cecil & Loeb/Gray's Anatomy of family practice for the foreseeable future." Wow! Four decades later, I still feel good about this review. When you and I receive such accolades, we should savor them — because they are the exception.

Other book reviewers and letter writers have reported that I misspelled words, "missed the mark," and, in one instance, was an example of why no single physician should be the sole author of a medical book. I have endured my share of harsh criticism.

Authors of research reports are not exempted. The *New England Journal of Medicine* published a paper on physician sleep deprivation and elective surgery (Nurok M et al. NEJM. 2010;363:2577). A printed comment challenges the opinion of the authors, stating, "we believe that the solution the authors offer — mandatory disclosure — is unwarranted" (Pelligrini CA et al. NEJM. 2010;363:2673).

In response to an article titled "Candidate Performance Measures for Screening for, Assessing, and Treating Unhealthy Substance Use in Hospitals: Advocacy or Evidence-Based Practice?" (Saitz R. Ann Intern Med. 2010;153:40), a letter writer remarks: "We read Saitz's recent article with great interest. Saitz concluded that evidence is insufficient to support screening and offering counseling to hospitalized patients with substance abuse problems. He recommends that clinicians treat 70 chronic acute and chronic illnesses that are linked to unhealthy substance use and ignore the underlying cause. That would be the death of medical common sense. It would be like treating a patient with myocardial infarction without screening for hypercholesterolemia..." (Gentilello LM et al. Ann Intern Med. 2011;154:73).

In an extreme example of reader criticism and editorial response, the publishers of *Human Immunology* retracted an immunogenetics paper that some believed contained inappropriate content. Statements in the paper concerning culture, religion, and genetics were judged to be offensive. The journal editors deleted the article from the online edition of the journal and requested that medical librarians tear the article pages from their printed, often bound, issues of the journal!

The conclusion is that as a medical writer you must be able to withstand criticism. All you can do is write your article or book chapter, check everything carefully, have the manuscript reviewed by a colleague, and then submit for publication. When the paper or book appears in print, be prepared to accept the barbs, or perhaps the applause, that may come from readers and reviewers. Take pride in the fact that you have successfully navigated the review process and had your work published and that your critic has, in fact, been one of your readers.

Beyond Publication

At the beginning of the chapter, I hinted that there are more steps after publication. Some of these possibilities are presented next.

Writing Groups and Courses

The *writing group* is composed of individuals committed to improving their writing skills. There may be a formal group leader, or leadership may rotate. Generally one member presents his or her work, followed by comments by others in the group. Sometimes the group uses specific writing exercises. Fundamentally these are support groups of persons who provide one another with encouragement, while allowing members to applaud their colleagues' successes and grieve their rejections.

Grzybowski et al. describe a writing group at a hospital in Vancouver, Canada. The group met regularly over 3 years. Fifty writing projects were discussed, and 12 of those were subsequently published in indexed journals. The seven group members who attended most frequently saw an increase in their publication rate over 3 years of more than 300% [29].

In 2013, Badenhorst published *Writing Relationships: Collaboration in a Faculty Writing Group*, describing a group that began in 2009 and has, through the relationships developed within the group, evolved into "a successfully publishing community of practice" [30].

Taran describes a residents' Creative Writing Group that meets monthly at a "charming but run-down restaurant with a hipster vibe that has survived both modernization and gentrification." Here, over dinner and drinks, members of the group share pieces they have written, in a setting with live music and occasional dancing [31].

Fellowships

Fellowships offer opportunities for clinicians who want to go further with their writing and editing. Today fellowships in writing and editing are offered by the *Journal of the American Medical Association*, the *New England Journal of Medicine*, the American Medical Writers Association (see below), and other specialty organizations and publications.

American Medical Writers Association

The American Medical Writers Association (AMWA), with 5000+ members, is the leading professional organization for biomedical communicators. Membership is open to all who write, edit, or teach about writing in areas such as medical science, biotechnology, or the pharmaceutical industry.

AMWA offers continuing professional education, which includes courses and workshops. The organization publishes the *AMWA Journal*, a source of information and opportunities in the field of biomedical communication. Some recent article topics in the journal were "Of Pirates, Ghosts, and the Fool: Stumbling Toward a Unified Theory of Medical Writing" and "Creating Effective Slides." If interested in learning more about AMWA, visit the organization's web site: http://www. amwa.org.

Contests

Several journals and organizations sponsor writing contests. An example is the Lasker Foundation Essay Contest, which "engages young scientists in a discussion about the big questions in biology and medicine today, and builds skills in communicating important medical and scientific issues to broader audiences." For more information, see http://www.laskerfoundation.org/programs/lasker-foundation-essay-contest/.

In 2015, the American Medical Writers Association established the Susan Love Resident Writing Competition. The contest honors Dr. Susan Love, a well-known author on women's health topics. The submission should address some aspect of women and medicine. Details are available at https://www.amwa-doc.org/residents/awards-r/susan-love-resident-writing-competition/.

The practicing physician with writing skills and a compelling story based on personal experience—such as how to solve a troubling practice problem or deal with a difficult patient—should consider the *Medical Economics* Annual

Physician Writing Contest. The current grand prize? A $1000 Visa gift card and publication of the winning article. If interested, visit the journal web site at http://medicaleconomics. m o d e r n m e d i c i n e . c o m / m e d i c a l - e c o n o m i c s / news/2016-annual-physician-writing-contest.

There is also the Michael E. DeBakey Medical Student Poetry Award, with information available at https://www. bcm.edu/news/awards-honors-students/14th-annual-debakey-student-poetry-awards.

Contests are announced periodically and then have deadlines. Be sure to check for up-to-date information if considering a submission.

Self-Publication

Self-publication of an article, poem, or cartoon is easy. Just type the following at the bottom of the page: copyright, your name, and the current year. Then print out the document, give it to a friend, and it is published. Legally no one can copy or otherwise use this now-published document without your permission. But what I just described is not the topic of this section.

Many of us write books and then find that attaining publication is difficult. In fact, without an agent, it is almost impossible for the beginning writer to find a publisher for a trade book. Also, agents are busy and most won't read your book unless you are a previously published trade book author. Do you see the catch here? Clinical books, if timely and well written, are more likely to be published, but this process can also be challenging.

Let's assume that you are a clinician or educator who has written a book. Perhaps your book is a tightly plotted medical mystery novel, your heartfelt autobiography, or "How I Learned Neurosurgery on the Internet in Five Easy Lessons." Sadly, no publisher has recognized the literary merits and marketing potential of your book, and the information in your manuscript is getting out of date.

Then you come across the magazine advertisement that reads, "AUTHORS WANTED, Leading subsidy book publisher seeks manuscripts. Fiction, nonfiction, poetry, juvenile, religious, etc. New authors welcome." Or web surfing brings you to Amazon, which offers CreateSpace, offering to publish copies of your book on demand, sparing you an investment in inventory. You may want to visit the Barnes and Noble web site and learn about their PubIt! self-publishing portal. Other possibilities such as Tate, Lulu, Smashwords, and Trafford publishing companies can be easily found on the web.

The vanity press accepts all works without regard to quality and has the author assume all financial risk; you are hiring a company to print your book. In short, the vanity press makes money from authors, not book buyers. The subsidy press publishes the book under its own imprint and may assume some of the financial risk; the best of them, like CreateSpace, provide an ISBN (International Standard Book Number), a numeric commercial book identifier that is unique to your book. Be sure to read reviews on the web before committing to deal with any self-publishing company.

I consider self-publication seeking commercial success to be the last refuge of the desperate author. The problem is distribution. There is no publishing company with a full financial investment in your effort out there trying hard to sell your book, and you probably do not personally have the time or resources to do so. You will have copies to give your family members. You can show your book to your friends. You will almost certainly not sell many books through commercial channels or receive much in royalties. Your satisfaction with the process will depend on your feelings about seeing your name and your work in print. In 2010, my cousins Bill and Melinda and I published the illustrated history of part of our family tree, titled "Our Brown Heritage: From England Across America." We paid the full cost of publication, and anticipated (accurately) that only a few copies would be sold to family members. Yet today, in early 2018, I still find the book available online for sale from the publisher, Blurb, Inc. Our family members treasure the book and we consider the effort a success.

Here is a personal story about self-publication and another of my writing error tales: Years ago a friend and I acquired the translation rights for a medical book written in Europe for the lay public. We formed a corporation called Erbonia Books and self-published the book. We then owned a garage full of books. To our surprise at the time, no one beat a path to our garage door to buy our books. Several local bookstores stocked a few copies, largely as a favor to us, but sales were sparse. We ran magazine advertisements, but none brought enough orders to cover the cost of the advertisements. Eventually we were lucky; my partner had a friend who worked for a major publishing firm in New York City. This company bought the rights to our book and published a paperback edition that finally had national distribution. When all was said and done, we spent a lot of time and effort. Our original printing costs and advertising costs exceeded the royalties received from the real publisher. We had learned a lesson, and we disincorporated Erbonia Books. (Today, just for fun 40 years later, I looked up the title of this small paperback. A very few used copies are for sale online at prices between $79 and $144. If only I had held on to that garage load of books!)

Now and Future Medical Publishing

Medical publishing may seem staid, but it is certainly not static. In fact, it seems to be undergoing a revolutionary change at this time. With full recognition of the perils of prognosticating, let's try to envision tomorrow's medical "journal" through the eyes of today's aspiring medical writer.

I recently read the announcement of the millionth word in the English language: It is "web 2.0," denoting the second generation of the World Wide Web. The new word connotes interactivity, collaboration, and networking—all at great speed. And this is what I see as the future of medical publishing—for both journals and books. Wolpert writes of the stakeholder communities that enable the production of peer-reviewed literature: funding agencies and foundations, universities and other research centers, authors, and publishers. She continues, "In a system this interdependent, destabilization at any one point perturbs critically important relationships. The advent of the Internet and digital formats was just such a disruption" [32].

Today, my scientific journals—those I get by virtue of paid subscription or society membership—arrive in my mailbox and are stacked in a pile until I have time to read them. But I sense a change. Before my paper copy arrives, the NEJM sends me the table of contents online, and I can open and read articles. The same thing happens with my specialty publications, such as *American Family Physician*. In the case of the NEJM, some items are only available online. How long will it be before the paper copies just disappear?

The transformation we are seeing has a name. It is called open-access (OA) publishing, and it will bring some profound changes to how we report research, read these reports, and respond to what we read. First about the reporting: Over the past few months, I have received e-mails inviting me to submit papers to several journals: *Medical Education Development*, *The Open Medical Informatics Journal*, and the *International Journal of Family Medicine*. I had never previously heard of any of these publications, and I was intrigued to receive unsolicited invitations to contribute, flattering indeed after decades of working very hard to find homes for articles I had written. What these periodicals all have in common, of course, is that they are open-access journals.

Open access describes barrier-free scientific communication that is digital and available without cost to anyone online. Articles published in an open-access journal are typically subject to limited or no copyright restrictions, meaning that clinicians, educators, and students can download, copy, and share the articles without the current restrictions we face. How is this possible? The answer is that authors, their institutions, or the sponsors of research studies fund most open-access publishing.

A good example of pure OA journals is the Public Library of Science (PLoS) group of publications, with a flagship publication *PLoS ONE*, an interactive open-access journal for the communication of peer-reviewed scientific and medical research, with a very respectable Impact Factor of 3.53. (For comparison, the *Journal of General Internal Medicine* currently has an Impact Factor is 3.49.) The current fee charged to an author or author's institution to publish a paper in *PLoS One* is $1495, used to cover the cost of peer review, professional editing, and electronic distribution. There is also *PLoS Medicine* with a per paper fee of $2900. PLoS journals offer a complete or partial fee waiver if authors or sponsors cannot pay the publication fees.

On the way to exclusively open-access journals, we currently have hybrid journals, with *British Medical Journal* (BMJ) as an example. In 2010, the BMJ initiated a publication fee of £3000 (about US $3746) for each published research article. These articles are then both printed in a traditional journal format and distributed online in an OA mode. The BMJ has a waiver policy for authors who cannot pay.

In addition to speedy dissemination of information, online OA offers some other advantages, although some of what I describe next may be yet to come. Illustrations can be presented with a "Download to a PowerPoint Friendly Image" option. Instead of the fixed-image, silent illustrations found in print journals, OA has the potential to present graphics with motion and sound. And can images with depth be far behind? The citation list can provide hyperlinks to each paper cited.

We may even see a paradigm shift in how papers are reviewed, moving much of the emphasis from prepublication review by so-called experts to postpublication review. This idea is championed by Smith, who tells how the posting of findings to be judged by the research community is already used in the fields of high energy physics and astronomy [33].

Open-access publishing may also help minimize the conflict of interest, described above, that journal editors face when they consider a study they know might bring their journal a huge profit in paper reprints—if published. Might this ethical dilemma become a thing of the past when there is open-access online?

Here is another potential benefit for those of us who search the medical literature often. As an example, I came across online an interesting research report in a recent issue of the *New England Journal of Medicine* comparing thresholds for repair of abdominal aortic aneurysms in England and the United States (Karthikesalingam A et al. NEJM. 2016:375:2051). The study was funded, in part, by the National Institutes of Health. You could access the abstract online, but, if you were not a subscriber, you would have been required to pay a fee to read the full article. I am aware that NIH-funded studies must be available by OA after 1 year. Nevertheless, since you paid for the study as a taxpayer, why must you pay again to read the full results while data are timely? Open-access publishing may just solve this problem.

If online publishing is faster, cheaper, and more user-friendly than print, how could anyone speak against it? Authors have had some reservations, aside from the publication fees. Some consider OA journals to be inferior caliber, an argument that is partly countered by the respectable Impact Factors of the PLoS journals. On the other hand, supporting the concern is a study by Davis et al. involving 1619 research articles and reviews in 11 journals published by the American Physiological Society. They report: "No evidence was found of a citation advantage for open access articles in the first year after publication" [34]. The future success of OA journals will depend, in some measure, on convincing medical authors that these publications are high quality and are respected by their peers, which will include how articles in these publications are assessed in promotion and tenure decisions.

Not unexpectedly, both commercial and nonprofit publishers are very wary of OA journals. Commercial publishers, some with huge investments in hardware, high production costs, and substantial profits tied to advertising and reprints, feel threatened. They question the viability of the "author-pay" model. So-called nonprofit publishers, most linked to clinical specialty societies, often provide much of the financial support of these specialty societies, and I suspect that they fear their demise if they must compete with OA journals.

On balance, we all know what happens to an idea whose time has come. We are already seeing our traditional 10-pound medical reference books move online. Journals will surely follow, in some way. JAMA now publishes more articles online than ever before [35]. The future is electronic publication, searchable storage of readable electrons in open virtual libraries, and instant, free access to today's scientific information for all. As you read this, electronic publication is replacing paper. Two questions remain: How will journal and book publishers adapt? And how can today's medical writer prepare for the open access future?

The Dark Side of Open-Access Publishing

On December 16, 2016, I received an unsolicited invitation, from the journal editor himself, to submit a paper to the *Archives of Community Medicine and Public Health*, based in India. The journal was especially seeking case reports, and included a handy link to "Submit Paper." I became a little wary upon noting that the invitation had three subtle grammatical oddities. Intrigued, I checked out the *Archives.*

Archives of Community Medicine and Public Health exists online, published by Peertechz Publications, with a large international editorial board. I could not find an Impact Factor listed. A recent issue includes reports with titles such as "Ambulatory Monitoring of Blood Pressure in Occupational Hypertension," a very brief description of two persons whose blood pressure increased with occupational stress, a paper that would have been rejected by return e-mail by any reputable journal. I could not find this report on PubMed. Although the invitation's "Submit Manuscript" link failed to mention the fact, searching another site revealed that there is a processing fee of $1549 to see your article online [36].

As a previously published author, I receive a similar offer at least weekly. Haug, writing in the *New England Journal of Medicine*, reports, "Personally, I have been alternately amused and annoyed by these messages. A glance at the journal's name or the associated website has told me that these simply are not serious publications" [37]. But they do, actually, have a serious purpose, and that is to make money for the publisher at the expense of aspiring authors.

A librarian at the University of Colorado in Denver, Jeffrey Beall, publishes an online list of "potential, possible, or probable predatory scholarly open-access publishers." The list, available at http://beallslist.weebly.com/, is quite long. Beall describes criteria for identifying predatory open-access publishers. Just a few of these red-flag criteria are:

- The publisher's owner is identified as the editor of each and every journal published by the organization.
- No single individual is identified as any specific journal's editor.
- The journal does not identify a formal editorial / review board.
- No academic information is provided regarding the editor, editorial staff, and/or review board members (e.g., institutional affiliation) [38].

A scholarly services firm, Cabell's International in Beaumont, Texas, is reported to be creating its own blacklist of journals, which it says is launching this spring (2017). It had hired Beall as a "consultant" [39].

In case there might be bit of doubt in your mind about the existence of predatory journals, consider the work of James Bohannan reported in *Science* [40]. The author created similar reports of a bogus, but superficially credible, study, all describing how lichen (moss) can inhibit the growth of cancer cells. The names of the authors were all fictitious, and all authors were supposedly affiliated with nonexistent African institutions. Bohannan describes the scientific flaws in the papers as both obvious and "boringly bad." The papers were sent to several hundred open-access journals. By the time his paper went to press, 157 of the journals had accepted the paper, and 98 had sent rejection notices. Journals published by Sage, Elsevier, and Wolters Kluwer all accepted the submissions. A few publishers requested a submission fee; the others subscribed to the open-access "gold" model in which the author pays a fee when the paper is published.

The best of the lot was *PLoS ONE*, described earlier, whose editors raised ethical issues, investigated the fictional authors, and rejected the paper based on its lack of scientific quality.

And what did the Bohannan do when these papers were accepted for publication? He withdrew the submission without paying the fee.

Help may be on the way. According to Grant, in August 2016, the US Federal Trade Commission filed suit, "taking a journal publisher, the OMICS Group, to court, alleging the open-access operation and two of its subsidiaries misrepresent their editorial process and take advantage of academics seeking outlets for their work" [41].

The message in all of this is this: There are hundreds of the predatory journals, trolling for your paper, but only wanting the publication fee. Don't count on any meaningful peer review. Your paper, with little or no improvement in the process, will appear online, but the entry on your curriculum vitae will have the scant merit it deserves.

Hijacked Journals

What is a hijacked journal? When a cybercriminal creates a fake web site for a respectable scientific journal offering physicians and scientists a venue to publish their papers for a fee, the journal has been hijacked. A fake domain name is created, or even sometimes the legitimate journal domain name is stolen when the publisher fails to pay the required registration fee. Academicians receive e-mails inviting them to submit their papers, often to journal sites that seem to have nothing to do with the author's sphere of expertise. The temptation is great, for good reason: Bohannan estimated in November 2015 that gold open-access publishing is a $250 million market [42].

Do you think there are only a handful of hijacked journals and that you would never fall for the ruse? Just for fun, I followed the links to the fake and legitimate sites for the *International Journal of Academic Research*. I could not tell with certainty which was the authentic site. Authors beware!

Putting It All Together

Medical articles and book chapters traditionally have a "Summary" section at the end. This is it.

When you go to live theater, you get something from the performance and you give something back to the actors, musicians, and writers—applause, reviews, sometimes even esteem. I believe that sort of response happens when reading an article or, in this instance, a book. In writing this book, I have offered some facts, my best advice, and what I think are engaging personal stories. In return you have given your attention, especially since you have reached this page in your reading. In doing so, you allow me to assume that I may be some small help in your future writing successes. For me, that is the real reward of my writing effort.

Remember that writing is a continuous process. The writer does not think about the writing episodically. For a writer, the current task, and maybe the next, will always be lurking in the subconscious mind. You will be sensitive to the analogy, the anecdote, and the image that can make your work sparkle just a little. The ongoing mining of your personal experience and connectivity, cataloging ideas and images, and organizing ideas and supporting facts are all part of writing. Writing does not occur just when you turn on your computer.

In the 1987 movie *Throw Momma from the Train*, Billy Crystal plays a down-on-his-luck English literature teacher leading an adult night school course in creative writing. Danny DeVito plays a not-too-bright student aspiring to be a writer. At several key points in the movie, Crystal emphasizes to DeVito, "A writer writes!" In the end, both successfully publish their books.

I urge you to join others and me in writing. See it as an ongoing journey of education, self-discovery, and personal growth. For me, writing, and now revising, this book has been part of such a process. I hope that you have enjoyed reading it half as much as I have enjoyed creating it. I am a little sorry to see it end. But I have another project in mind to start next week.

My last offering in the book is a personal indulgence. We have all heard of Robert's Rules of Order. Here are *Doctor Taylor's Rules for Medical Writers*:

- *Be smart enough.* Yet, be well aware that being intelligent is only part of what you will need for success.
- *Be organized.* Keep files and notes, with full reference citations, whether on paper or computer. Know where things are, and take the time needed to systematize all your writing materials before putting words on the screen.
- *Be a reader.* Always read something, and seek a wide range of topics. While reading, note both what is said and how the author expresses the ideas.
- *Do not write until you have something to worthwhile to say.* Do not clutter the literature with pedantic drivel.
- *Be a good time manager.* Clinical care, teaching, or research is your day job, and it cannot be neglected. If you do so, patients, students, or your professional colleagues will suffer, and you will lose your wellspring of writing ideas. But you must also carve out regular, dependable time for writing if you are ever to finish a project.
- *Be an effective networker.* Get to know medical editors, other writers, and—if planning to edit a multi-author book—potential authors. Make the ongoing effort needed to nurture these relationships.
- *Be bold.* Don't hesitate to aim high or to propose the project that seems a little beyond your abilities. Those who take on too much, with too little time and too few resources, sometimes succeed.
- *Be persistent.* Writers endure rejection often. You must be able to bounce back and revise and resubmit, or even start over. But you must not give up on your writing. A writer writes!
- *Remember that you love to write.* If you are not finding writing enjoyable, stop for a while, but only a while. Go do

something less important but that may seem more enjoyable, such as eating, sleeping, or watching a movie. Your energy will be renewed, and you may just formulate a good writing idea in the process.

Now it's time to write it up. Have fun!

References

1. Holmes OW. Some of my early teachers. In: Holmes OW, editor. Medical essays. Boston: The Boston Society for the Diffusion of Useful Knowledge; 1842.
2. King LS. Why not say it clearly? Boston: Little, Brown; 1978. p. 5.
3. Callaham M, Wears RL, Weber E. Journal prestige, publication bias, and other characteristics associated with citation of published studies in peer-reviewed journals. JAMA. 2002;287:2847–50.
4. Norton SA. Read this but skip that. J Am Acad Dermatol. 2001;44:714–5.
5. The New England Journal of Medicine. Author Center: New Manuscripts. http://www.nejm.org/page/author-center/manuscript-submission. Accessed 15 Jun 2017.
6. Grouse LK. A rogue's gallery of medical manuscripts. JAMA. 1980;244(7):700–1.
7. von Elm D, Poglia G, Walder B, Tramer MR. Different patterns of duplicate publication: an analysis of articles used in systematic reviews. JAMA. 2004;291(8):974–80.
8. International Committee of Medical Journal Editors. Recommendations for the Conduct, Reporting, Editing, and Publication of Scholarly Work in Medical Journals. http://www.icmje.org/recommendations/. Accessed 15 Jun 2017.
9. British Medical Journal Resources for Authors. http://www.bmj.com/about-bmj/resources-authors/article-types/research. Accessed 15 Jun 2017.
10. Jha KN. How to write articles that get published. J Clin Diagn Res. 2014;8(9):XG01–3.
11. NEJM. Author Dashboard of ScholarOne Manuscripts. https://mc05.manuscriptcentral.com/nejm. Accessed 15 Jun 2017.
12. Kübler-Ross E. On death and dying. New York: Macmillan; 1969.
13. Bryson B. A short history of nearly everything. New York: Broadway Books; 2003. p. 381.

14. Smith RS. The trouble with medical journals. Medico-Legal J. 2008;76(3):79–93.

15. Charlton J, Mark L. The writer's home companion. New York: Franklin Watts; 1987. p. 28.

16. Purcell GP, Donovan SL, Davidoff F. Changes to manuscripts during the editorial process. JAMA. 1998;280(3):227–8.

17. Emerson GB, Warme WJ, Wolf FM, Heckman JD, Brand RA, Leopold SS. Testing for the presence of positive-outcome bias in peer review: a randomized controlled trial. Arch Intern Med. 2010;170(21):1934–9.

18. Okike K, Hug KT, Kocher MS, Leopold SS. Single-blind vs double-blind peer review in the setting of author prestige (Research letter). JAMA. 2016;316:1315–6.

19. Coates R, Sturgeon B, Bohannan J, Pasini E. Language and publication in "Cardiovascular Research" articles. Cardiovasc Res. 2002;53(2):279–85.

20. Cho DW. Science journal paper writing in an EFL context: the case of Korea. English for Scientific Purposes. 2009;28(4):230–9.

21. Peters DP, Ceci SJ. Peer-review practices of psychological journals: the fate of published articles, submitted again. Behav Brain Sci. 1982;5:187–255.

22. Jefferson T, Di P, Rivetti A, Baweezer GA, Al-Ansary LA, Ferroni E. Vaccines for preventing influenza in healthy adults. Cochrane Database Syst Rev. 2007;2:CD001269.

23. Wager E. Getting research published: an A to Z publication strategy. London: Radcliffe; 2010. p. 110.

24. Melander H, Ahlqvist-Rastad J, Meijer G, Beermann B. Evidence b(i)ased medicine—selective reporting from studies sponsored by pharmaceutical industry: review of studies in new drug applications. BMJ. 2003;326(7400):1171.

25. Krumland RB, Gorry GA. Scientific publications of a medical school faculty. J Med Educ. 1979;54:876–84.

26. Haug CJ. Peer-review fraud—hacking the scientific publication process. N Engl J Med. 2015;373(25):2393–9.

27. JAMA Network: reprint requests. http://jamanetwork.com/pages/reprints-and-permissions. Accessed 15 Jun 2017.

28. Spivak CD. Reprints, whence they come and whither they should go. JAMA. 1902;38:1018–9.

29. Grzybowski SC, Bates J, Calam B, et al. A physician peer support writing group. Fam Med. 2003;35(3):195–201.

30. Badenhorst CM, Penney S, Pickett S, Joy R, et al. Writing relationships: collaboration in a faculty writing group. AISHE J. 2013;5(1):1001–26.

31. Taran S. The Lisboa Café. JAMA. 2017;317:1213–4.
32. Wolpert AJ. For the sake of inquiry and knowledge—the inevitability of open access. N Engl J Med. 2013;368(9):785–93.
33. Smith RS. Reinventing the biomedical journal. J Neurosci. 2006;26(39):9837–8.
34. Davis PM, Lewenstein BV, Simon DH, Booth JG, Connolly MJL. Open access publishing, article downloads, and citations: randomized controlled trial. BMJ. 2008;337:a568.
35. Bauchner H, Fontanarosa PH, Golub RM. To JAMA authors, peer reviewers, and readers—thank you. JAMA. 2015;313(7):675–6.
36. Archives of Community Medicine and Public Health, Processing fees. https://www.peertechz.com/article-processing-fee. Accessed 15 Jun 2017.
37. Haug C. The downside of open-access publishing. N Engl J Med. 2013;368(9):791–3.
38. Beall's List of predatory journals and publishers. http://beallslist.weebly.com/. Accessed 18 Jun 2017.
39. Silver A. Controversial website that lists "predatory" publishers shuts down. Nature. https://doi.org/10.1038/nature.2017.21328. http://www.nature.com/news/controversial-website-that-lists-predatory-publishers-shuts-down-1.21328. Accessed 15 Jun 2017.
40. Bohannon J. Who's afraid of peer review. Science. 2013;342(6154):60–5.
41. Grant B. US Gov't takes on predatory publishers. The Scientist. http://www.the-scientist.com/?articles.view/articleNo/46902/title/US-Gov-t-Takes-On-Predatory-Publishers/. Accessed 15 Jun 2017.
42. Bohannon J. How to hijack a journal. Science. 2015. https://doi.org/10.1126/science.aad7463. http://www.sciencemag.org/news/2015/11/feature-how-hijack-journal. Accessed 15 Jun 2017.

Appendix A: Glossary of Medical Writing Words and Phrases

Altmetrics A measurement indicating the influence of an academic article based on the attention received on a variety of online sources.

Author Someone who has actively participated in preparation of a paper or book, and who assumes intellectual responsibility for its content. An **archival author** is an author who assumes responsibility for maintaining research and other records related to a published article, just in case questions arise in the future.

Boolean logic An approach to relationships among search terms, using AND, OR, and NOT. Boolean logic, named for British philosopher and mathematician George Boole (1815–1864), was an important building block in the development of today's digital computer.

Caption See **Legend**.

Career topic The topic that you present in writing and in lectures throughout your career, keeping up with all advances in the field. For clinicians, this is most likely to be a disease (such as hypertension), a clinical presentation (such as chest pain), or a procedure (such as retinal surgery or minimally invasive management of breast cancer).

© Springer International Publishing AG 2018
R.B. Taylor, *Medical Writing*,
https://doi.org/10.1007/978-3-319-70126-4

Copyeditor The person who makes needed improvements in grammar and syntax and then marks up a manuscript for the printer. The copyeditor is generally employed by the publisher.

Copyright The legal rights to publish, copy, sell, or otherwise use a specific intellectual property.

Cover letter Also called a **submission letter**, the cover letter is a document that should accompany every manuscript submitted to a journal, even if the manuscript is a letter to the editor.

Direct costs In grant parlance, the phrase "direct costs" refers to the price of salaries, equipment, and supplies, as well as miscellaneous expenses such as consultant fees and travel related to the project. Also see **indirect costs**.

DOI An abbreviation for **digital object identifier**, an alphanumeric label used to distinguish a publication online. For example, the identifier *doi:10.1056/NEJMoal1600931* would lead the reader to an article by Karthikesalingam et al. titled "Thresholds for Abdominal Aortic Aneurysm Repair in England and the United States" published in print in the November 24, 2016, issue of the *New England Journal of Medicine.*

Duplicate or dual publication The unethical practice of publishing the same data two or more times in different journals.

Editor The editor holds the powerful position of deciding which manuscripts are published and which "do not meet our publication needs at this time." There are also various types of editor, especially in book publishing: acquisition editors, development editors, production editors, associate editors, and copyeditors.

Electronic journal An online version of a medical publication. Some electronic medical journals are extensions of print publications. Today we see more and more freestanding electronic journals, with content that never appears on paper.

Epigraph A short quotation presented at the beginning of an article, chapter, or book, intended to set the stage for what is to come.

Funding preference, funding priority A special consideration in a request for proposal—sometimes with a social intent such as improving health care for the homeless or for pregnant women or perhaps having special capabilities such as telemedicine—that, if included in the grant proposal and approved, add points to the final grant review score, moving the application higher in the funding queue.

Galley proofs, galleys A copy of typeset matter, lacking page numbers, intended to be reviewed by the author before being converted into page proofs.

GIF Abbreviation of Graphic Interchange Format, a color image compression algorithm.

Gray (or grey) literature The locus of many trials that have not achieved primary publication in scientific journals. Here we find posters and research reports presented at scientific congresses, with descriptions found in conference abstract collections. The common thread among items in the gray literature is that they are outside the purview of conventional publishers. Thus, such items include material produced in academics, government, business, and industry disseminated in electronic formats or out-of-the-mainstream print sources.

Halftone A figure composed of shades of gray, usually a black and white photograph or a shaded drawing.

Hijacked journal A respectable print journal for which a fraudulent web site solicits manuscripts to be "published" online for profit, with the author believing the work has been published by the legitimate journal.

Impact factor The total number of citations made for a journal in a year for articles published in two previous years divided by the number of citable articles published in these years. It is used to judge the influence, and by inference the quality, of a scientific journal. See Chap. 5.

IMRAD An acronym that represents the organizational structure most often used in research reports: introduction, methods, results, and discussion. See Chap. 11.

Indirect costs Grantspeak for expenses related to administration of a project and for the price of electricity, heat, and building maintenance. At the NIH, these costs fall under the more descriptive term **facilities and administrative costs**.

International Committee of Medical Journal Editors (ICMJE) The ICMJE is a group of medical journal editors, representing a small number of diverse medical journals ranging from the *New England Journal of Medicine* to the *Journal of Korean Medical Science*. Because their first meeting was held in Vancouver, Canada, the committee was originally called the "Vancouver Group." Their chief product is the **Recommendations for the Conduct, Reporting, Editing, and Publication of Scholarly Work in Medical Journals**, described below.

JPEG or **JPG** Abbreviation of **Joint Photographic Experts Group**, representing a method that balances compression and quality of images.

Legend Also sometimes called a **caption**, the legend is the title of a figure or table and may also provide explanatory information.

Letter of intent Also sometimes called a **proposal concept paper**, the letter of intent is a synopsis of a research idea sent to test the waters with a funding agency. In a sense, the letter of intent is a "pre-application query." It asks the question: Do you think I should go to the trouble of preparing a full grant proposal for this idea?"

Line drawing, line art A figure composed of black and white lines, such as a graph, diagram, or drawing that is not shaded.

Loansome Doc A feature in PubMed that allows the user to place an electronic order through the National Network of Libraries of Medicine for the full-text copy of an article found on MEDLINE.

Markup This refers to both the process and the symbols by which copyeditors communicate specific instructions to typesetters.

MEDLINE (Medical Literature Analysis and Retrieval System Online) The US National Library of Medicine's (NLM) leading bibliographic database. It contains millions of references to journal articles in the life sciences, chiefly in biomedicine. It can be searched via PubMed or through the NLM gateway: *www.nlm.nih.gov*.

MeSH (Medical Subject Headings) The National Library of Medicine's controlled vocabulary thesaurus. It consists of sets of terms that permit searching MEDLINE at various levels of specificity.

Meta-analysis A method of combining the results of several studies into a summary conclusion, using quantitative strategies that will allow consideration of data in diverse research reports.

Monograph A specialized book, usually relatively short and generally written by one person or a small group of specialists.

National Library of Medicine (NLM) The world's largest medical library with collections in all major areas of the health sciences and the home of MEDLINE and PubMed.

Network research The process of using sequential personal contacts to find out a needed fact. The key question in network research is, "Who do you recommend that I call next?" For more details, see Chap. 3.

Offprints See **Reprints**.

Open access Publishing that is readily accessible online and free to all readers. For a discussion of open-access publishing, see Chap. 12.

Overlay A transparent sheet with graphic material to be superimposed on another page.

Page proofs A copy of typeset text presented as it will appear in print, including headings and page numbers.

Pagination The process of numbering the pages of a manuscript or book.

Parachute trial A research study that examines a question that experience and common sense have already provided us with an answer, such as: Do parachutes save lives of those who jump from airplanes?

PDF An abbreviation for **Portable Document Format**, the file format used by Adobe Acrobat.

Peer review, peer reviewer The evaluation of a submitted manuscript by individuals with appropriate credentials, usually performed without the peer reviewers knowing who wrote the manuscript or the author knowing who performed the review. A peer reviewer may also be called a **referee**.

Positive outcome bias Describing how a research study with a positive outcome—drug X was better than placebo—is more likely to be published than a study that shows no difference between items tested.

Predatory publisher A publishing firm that solicits manuscripts for presentation in online, open-access journals, accepting and "publishing" almost all submissions and charging a stiff fee for the service. The goal of the predatory publisher is to make a profit, not to advance science.

Proof A copy of a work that has been set in type, sent to authors or editors to review for errors. Proof may be galley proofs, when not yet set as pages, or may be actual page proofs of the article or book pages.

Proofreader's marks A set of symbols used to identify errors or changes on proofs. See Appendix B.

Public Library of Science (PLoS) A nonprofit organization of scientists and physicians that describes itself as committed to making the world's scientific and medical literature a freely available public resource.

Publication bias The situation in academic journals when the outcome of a research study influences the decision whether or not to publish. This has been dubbed the "file drawer effect," when research results that fail to support the original hypothesis tend to be relegated to the file drawer and the failure to publish such results introduces a bias in the literature.

Publisher The person, firm, or society who manages the business activities related to bringing books or journals to print or to a web site.

PubMed A web site that is a service of the National Library of Medicine, with more than 14 million citations for biomedical articles from MEDLINE and other sources. PubMed is discussed in Chap. 1 and can be accessed at *http://www. pubmed.com*.

RBG A color mode for images based on mixtures of red (R), blue (B), and green (G) light.

Redaction The process of word-by-word, sentence-by-sentence modification of a paper.

Referee See **Peer review, peer reviewer**.

Reprints Also sometimes called **offprints**, these are separately printed copies of individual journal articles. Journals generally offer to provide these to authors for a fee.

Request for proposal (RFP) A funding agency's invitation to submit grant proposals for a specific program.

Research report Also called a "scientific paper," the research report describes the results of a scientific study.

Review article A paper that deals with known information in a thoughtful way, but does not present new data such as the results of a clinical research study.

Running head A shorthand listing of items—usually an abbreviated title of the article or chapter that appears at the top of each page of a manuscript or book. In the case of a manuscript, the running head allows the editor to reassemble the pages if blown about by the wind. Because of the anonymity of peer review, most journals do not want author names included in a manuscript's running head.

Science Citation Index (SCI) A proprietary database of citations of published articles, the SCI is also used to calculate the journal impact factor.

Stop A unit of punctuation that breaks the flow of words. Stops include the comma, colon, semicolon, period, question mark, and exclamation mark. In Commonwealth English, the period is called a *full stop*.

Stub Heading and line captions appearing at the side of a formal table used to describe the rows of figures presented.

Target journal As you prepare an article, the target journal is number one on your publication wish list. This is where you would like your paper published, and the article's format and style should mirror those of the target journal.

Tear sheets Pages removed from a previously published book, generally used when revising—on paper—a previous edition of the book.

Trade books Books published to be sold to the general public, not to the market of professional clinicians and educators. Books for clinicians, scientists, and other scholars are called **professional books**.

Typesetting The process of composing the edited manuscript as it will appear in the final pages. This term is becoming anachronistic as publishing becomes increasingly digitized but is still commonly used.

Recommendations for the Conduct, Reporting, Editing, and Publication of Scholarly Work in Medical Journals A statement by the ICMJE, available on the Web, describing how to prepare a paper for a medical journal. The ICMJE

Recommendations were previously known as the **Uniform Requirements for Manuscripts Submitted to Biomedical Journals**. See further discussion in Chap. 1. Access the latest version at *www.icmje.org*.

URL (Uniform Resource Locator) An address for a site on the Internet. The address above, *www.icmje.org*, is a URL.

UpToDate A subscription-based web site that provided timely reviews on clinical topics: *http://www.uptodate.com*.

Appendix B: Proofreader's Marks

The following symbols are used when correcting hard copy galley and page proofs. Methods for marking digital or online proofs will vary according to the program or platform.

Mark the text	*In the margin*	*Meaning*
Now is is the time	ℯ	Delete; take out
Now is the ti me	⌢	Close up
Now is the thyme	ℯ⌢	Delete and close up
Nowis the time	#	Insert space
Now ∧ is the time	eq #	Equal space between words
Now the time	is	Insert word(s)
It is time We	⊙	Insert period
It is time but	∧	Insert comma
It is time we	;	Insert semicolon
High energy pump	=	Insert hyphen
Smith 1977 stated	⟨ / ⟩ /	Insert parentheses
Smiths statement	⌄	Insert apostrophe
Evaluation of ln e ∧	⌄	Insert as superscript
The value of E$_{max}$	$\widehat{max}$	Make subscript
the v^{a}lue	≡	Straighten line(s)
all cases. ∧ The value ⌐	¶	Make new paragraph
⌐ of most data …	(no ¶)	No paragraph – run in
Ten of value is	(tr) //	Transpose
⊏ E$_{max}$	⊏	Move left as indicated
E$_{max}$ ⊐	⊐	Move right as indicated
now is the time	(cap)	Capital
Smith (1977) said	(s.c.)	Small capitals
Now is The time	(l.c.)	Lower case
(Now) is the time	(Rom)	Roman type
Now is the time	(ital)	Italic
now is the time	(cap ital)	Capital italic
Now is the time	(b.f.)	Boldface type
S (1977) stated	(sp)	Spell out
Now is the time	(stet)	Let stand as is

Appendix C: Commonly Used Medical Abbreviations[1]

Abbreviation	Meaning
ACE	Angiotensin-converting enzyme
ACTH	Adrenocorticotropic hormone
AIDS	Acquired immunodeficiency syndrome
ALT	Alanine aminotransferase (SGPT)
ANA	Antinuclear antibody
AST	Aspartate aminotransferase (SGOT)
bid	Twice a day
BP	Blood pressure
bpm	Beats per minute
BS	Blood sugar
BUN	Blood urea nitrogen
CBC	Complete blood count
CHD	Coronary heart disease
CHF	Congestive heart failure
Cl^-	Chloride
CO_2	Carbon dioxide
COPD	Chronic obstructive pulmonary disease
CPR	Cardiopulmonary resuscitation
CSF	Cerebrospinal fluid
CT	Computed tomography
cu mm	Cubic millimeter

[1] This list may be used in your medical writing. No specific permission form is required for use, but please give full credit to this book as the source.

© Springer International Publishing AG 2018
R.B. Taylor, *Medical Writing*,
https://doi.org/10.1007/978-3-319-70126-4

CXR	Chest X-ray
d	Day, daily
dL	Deciliter
DM	Diabetes mellitus
ECG	Electrocardiogram
ESR	Erythrocyte sedimentation rate
FDA	United States Food and Drug Administration
g	Gram
GI	Gastrointestinal
Hb	Hemoglobin
HDL-C	High-density lipoprotein cholesterol
HF	Heart failure
Hg	Mercury
HIV	Human immunodeficiency virus
HMO	Health maintenance organization
hr	Hour
hs	Hour of sleep, at bedtime
HTN	Hypertension
IM	Intramuscular
INR	International normalized ratio
IU	International unit
IV	Intravenous
K^+	Potassium
kg	Kilogram
L	Liter
LD or LDH	Lactate dehydrogenase
LDL-C	Low-density lipoprotein cholesterol
mEq	Milliequivalent
mcg	Microgram
mg	Milligram
min	Minute
mL	Milliliter
mm	Millimeter
mm^3	Cubic millimeter
MRI	Magnetic resonance imaging
Na^+	Sodium
NSAID	Nonsteroidal anti-inflammatory drug
po	By mouth *(per os)*

PT	Prothrombin time
PTT	Partial thromboplastin time
q	Every
qd	Every day, daily
qid	Four times a day
qod	Every other day
RBC	Red blood cell, red blood count
SC	Subcutaneous
sec	Second
SGOT	See AST
SGPT	See ALT
STD	Sexually transmitted disease
TB	Tuberculosis
tid	Three times a day
TSH	Thyroid-stimulating hormone
U	Unit
UA	Urine analysis
WBC	White blood cell, white blood count

Appendix D: Methodological and Statistical Terms Used in Research Studies

The following is a list of terms commonly used in writing research protocols, grant applications, and reports of clinical studies.

Absolute risk This is the probability of something occurring, such as myocardial infarction or death, without reference to any special context, such as comparison to another setting.

Absolute risk reduction (ARR) Typically referring to adverse events, absolute risk describes the probability of an event in the population under study, and ARR is the arithmetic difference in the rates of events between study and control groups. It is the inverse of the **number needed to treat (NNT)**. **Relative risk reduction (RRR)** is the percentage difference in outcomes between the study and control groups. Here is an example: If a treatment, such as use of an antiplatelet agent, decreases the risk of a stroke from 2 per thousand to 1 per thousand, then the absolute risk reduction is 1/1000. And in this scenario, the **relative risk reduction** (described below) is 50%.

Bias Also called **systematic error**, bias describes something that might confound the validity of a study. One example is **exclusion bias**, which occurs when persons with specific characteristics, such as a coexisting disease, are excluded from a study sample. Another type of bias is **attrition bias**, in which there is a pattern that arises among persons who drop out of

© Springer International Publishing AG 2018
R.B. Taylor, *Medical Writing*,
https://doi.org/10.1007/978-3-319-70126-4

a study. There is also **nonresponse bias**, **recall bias**, **referral bias**, and **selection bias**.

Case–control study A comparison of a group of subjects with a disease or outcome of interest with a group without the disease or outcome of interest, seeking a probable cause for the disease or outcome in the study (case) group that is absent in the control group. In other words, this study design starts with the disease or outcome—such as stroke—and looks back to identify antecedent events, exposures, or risk factors.

Cochrane Collaboration A network of physicians and scholars who perform systematic reviews and meta-analyses of randomized clinical trials and other research studies. The results of their efforts are found in *The Cochrane Database of Systematic Reviews*, which can be accessed at: *http://www. cochrane.org/*. The name commemorates the British physician and epidemiologist Archie Cochrane (1909–1988), who advocated for systematic summaries of best evidence to improve the effectiveness and efficiency of care.

Cohort A defined group of people (subjects). A study group and a control group might each be called a cohort. A study cohort may or may not share one of many types of attributes: age, race, exposure to a disease, presence of a disease, use of a drug, or something else.

Cohort study Sometimes called incidence or longitudinal studies, cohort studies are observation research that involves examination of a study group (who received an intervention or were exposed to a risk) versus a control group. In contrast to a case–control study, a cohort study starts with the exposure and follows subjects to determine the outcome. A long-term follow-up of a group of persons accidentally exposed to radiation in an industrial accident versus a control group of unexposed persons would be a cohort study.

Confidence interval (CI) An estimate of reliability. For example, an author describing a "95% CI" is saying that if things are done the same way 100 times, we would expect similar results in at least 95% of instances.

Crossover trial A method of comparing interventions in which subjects in two cohorts each complete one course of treatment and then are switched to the other.

Cross-sectional study Observation research involving disease in relationship to other variables in a specific population at a specific time. Most such research involves a one-shot survey of subjects.

Data mining, data dredging This occurs when a large database is explored searching for some sort of reportable conclusion.

Effectiveness An expression of the extent to which an intervention yields a desired outcome.

Generalizability The extent to which research findings and conclusions can be extrapolated from the sample studied to the population at large.

Hazard ratio (HR) According to the National Cancer Institute, the hazard ratio describes how often a particular event happens in one group compared to how often it happens in another group, measured over time. In cancer research, hazard ratios are often used in clinical trials to measure survival at any point in time in a group of patients who have been given a specific treatment compared to a control group given another treatment or a placebo, generating the familiar "survival curves." In this setting, a hazard ratio of 1 means that there is no difference in survival between the two groups. A hazard ratio of greater than 1 or less than 1 means that survival was better in one of the groups.

Incidence, incidence rate A measurement of the number of previously unaffected persons who develop a condition during a particular period of time, such as a year, 5 years, or even a lifetime. Knowing the incidence of a disease helps us understand the likelihood that a disease will occur in a given person over a given time frame. For example, think of a cruise ship carrying 1000 passengers on a weeklong voyage. If, during that voyage, 95 persons develop acute gastroenteritis, then the incidence of that disease in that population of passengers for that 7-day time interval is 95/1000 or 9.5%.

Likelihood ratio (LR) The odds that a given test result would be expected in a patient with the specific disease compared to the chances that the same result would be expected in a patient without the disease in question. The LR is helpful in assessing the probability that a specific diagnostic test will be useful. It does so by providing a direct estimate of how much a test result will change the odds of finding a disease and incorporates both the sensitivity and specificity of the test. The likelihood ratio for a positive test result is sensitivity/1-specificity. The likelihood ratio for a negative test result is 1-sensitivity/specificity. A LR less than 1 indicates a lower likelihood of disease, while a LR greater than 1 indicates a higher likelihood of disease. Tests with LRs less than 0.2 or greater than 5.0 tend to be the most useful clinically.

Meta-analysis A type of **systematic review** that involves quantitative methods and rigorous pooling of data from applicable clinical trials. Perhaps the best known of the meta-analyses are the reports from the Cochrane Collaboration.

Mixed methods research Research that combines quantitative and qualitative methods in a single study. Mixed methods research has been called the third research paradigm.

Nonresponse bias Commonly seen in survey research, nonresponse bias occurs when those who complete the survey differ in some meaningful way from those who do not.

Null hypothesis (H_0) An assertion that no statistical significance exists in a set of given observations. It is presumed to be true until statistical evidence nullifies it for an alternative hypothesis.

Number needed to treat (NNT) The number of persons who must receive an intervention in order for one more person to benefit. It can be calculated as the inverse of absolute risk reduction (1/ARR). The other side of the coin would be the **number needed to harm (NNH)**.

Odds ratio The odds ratio is a descriptive statistic used to assess the risk of a particular outcome, typically a disease, if a certain risk factor or event is present. Thus it is a relative measure of risk, telling us how much more likely it is that someone who is exposed to the factor being studied will develop the disease or other outcome as compared to someone who is not exposed.

Posttest probability The proportion of patients with a particular test result who have the target disorder. In deciding whether to recommend a specific test—for example, a magnetic resonance scan in a patient with back pain—knowing the posttest probability will help the clinician decide if the test result is likely to make a difference in the treatment of the patient.

Precision An expression, often described as a **confidence interval**, of the paucity of random error.

Predictive value A ratio, stated as a percentage, of the patients with a positive test for a disease who actually have the disease (**positive predictive value**). Predictive value is strongly affected by the prevalence of a disease, even if the sensitivity and specificity of the test remain constant. There is also **negative predictive value**, the probability that a person with a negative test does not have the disease in question.

Pretest probability A measurement of the likelihood of a positive test result determined before the result of a test is known. For example, if we know, hypothetically, that in a large population of 50-year-old asymptomatic women, the vitamin D level will be low in 9% of subjects, this figure represents the pretest probability of finding a low vitamin D serum level in the next asymptomatic 50-year-old woman tested.

Pretest/posttest case series An observational study in which outcomes are measured in subjects before and again after exposure to some sort of intervention. Clinician researchers are fond of using this method to measure clinician behavior, such as prescribing a certain therapy before and after being exposed to new information.

Prevalence A measurement of the total number of cases of the disease in the population at a given time. It may be stated as a percentage: the total number of cases in the population (the numerator) divided by the number of individuals in the population (the denominator). Hypertension, for example, is often stated as having a 28–30% prevalence in the US population. Prevalence tells us how common a disease is. In contrast, incidence tells us how many new cases occur in a given time frame.

Primary outcome The finding considered most clinically relevant in assessing the effect of an intervention. As an example, in a study of the use of a new analgesic in treating low back pain, the primary outcome would logically be back pain relief, and not, for instance, reports of improvement in general well-being or a reduced incidence of tension headaches.

Prospective study A "looking-forward" study in which the outcome event has not yet occurred. An example might be a study of what happens when a group of overweight persons are treated with a new appetite suppressant versus the outcome in a similar group of persons who do not receive the drug. Randomized trials are all prospective studies, as are some cohort studies.

p-value See **Statistical significance**.

Qualitative research Research used when traditional quantitative measurements would not be helpful. Usually employed in studies of human subjects, qualitative research explores issues, phenomena, and the reasons underlying clinical decision-making.

Randomization A process, sometimes called **random allocation**, by which subjects are assigned to groups by chance, often using a table of random numbers. At the other end of the spectrum is the **convenience sample**, which might be the next 100 patients to walk through the door.

Randomized controlled trial (RCT) The gold standard of clinical scientific research, the RCT is an experimental study design that involves random allocation of subjects and interventions. With successful randomization of subjects, study and control group have comparable characteristics (even if we don't know what the relevant characteristics are!), and selection bias is absent.

Recall bias A systematic error in a research study that occurs when evidence is collected by relying on the patient's memory. Think of a study that involves administration of a new vaccine evaluated by an interview a few months later, asking about possible side effects occurring the day after the injection.

Referral bias A type of systematic error related to who is assigned to the study group versus the control group, typically seen when patients are referred from the community to a study in a tertiary care center, and decisions are made based on patient characteristics as to who should be in which cohort. The result is a non-randomized study.

Relative risk (RR) Also sometimes called the **risk ratio**. Relative risk describes the probability of an adverse outcome occurring during a specified time interval in a study group exposed to some sort of event versus the outcome without the exposure. For example, we might be concerned with the relative risk of stroke among persons with and without hypertension.

Relative risk reduction (RRR) An expression of the degree to which an intervention decreases the probability of developing a disease, complication, or other adverse outcome. For example, we might conduct a study to see what protection against major cardiovascular events is afforded by various categories of antihypertensive agents.

Reliability The consistency of an assessment method. If the speedometer on my car happens to be set incorrectly to read 50 miles per hour (mph) when the actual speed is 60 mph, it will reflect this error every time and thus be reliable even though it is not accurate. This will make scant difference to the traffic officer who writes the summons for speeding.

Retrospective cohort study An examination of what has already happened to a group of individuals who experienced an exposure or intervention compared with an otherwise similar group who did not experience the exposure or intervention. An example of such a study might be the record review to determine the uterine cancer risk that has already occurred in women previously exposed to hormone replacement therapy (HRT) compared to a similar group with no HRT exposure. A prospective cohort study, in contrast, would follow exposed and unexposed women into the future.

Selection bias In a cohort or case–control study, selection bias occurs when, for one reason or another, study groups and control groups differ from the start. Suppose, for instance, that in a cohort study to determine the outcome of treating heart failure with a specific drug, the intervention group had far more diabetic patients than the control group. Selection bias may also be termed **allocation bias**.

Sensitivity (Sn) A measurement of the portion of items correctly detected as present. This usually has to do with tests used to detect disease. A test with 100% (also stated as 1.0) sensitivity for tuberculosis, for example, would identify all persons with the disease, and a test with 0.5 sensitivity would detect half of those infected. Compare this term with **Specificity**. A test with a high sensitivity will have few false negatives.

Specificity (Sp) A measurement of the proportions of items correctly identified as not present, often represented as the percentage of healthy people who are correctly identified as not having a particular disease. A test with 100% (or alternatively, 1.0) specificity for tuberculosis, for example, would not identify (incorrectly) anyone from the healthy group as sick. A test with a high specificity will have few false positives.

Statistical significance The term refers the likelihood that a result could occur by chance, usually expressed as a **p-value**. The smaller the p-value, the less likely it is that the findings reported are the result of chance. If the level is 0.05, then there is a 5% chance that the findings occurred by chance. A *p*-value of 0.01 thus represents a higher level of statistical significance than a *p*-value of 0.05.

Stratification The process of separating research subjects into clinically relevant subgroups for analysis. For example, we might stratify the analysis of a drug for treating hypertension by separately examining patients with and without elevated creatinine levels. This is one strategy for reducing confounding; another strategy would be to simply exclude patients with high creatinine levels from a study.

Systematic review A general term describing a look back at multiple published reports on a single topic in an attempt to answer one or more focused questions relevant to the topic. Using a reproducible search strategy in bibliographic databases and selecting all articles that meet specified criteria (e.g., sample size, randomization, or other design features) are the characteristics that make a review "systematic," in contrast to "what's in my file drawer."

Umbrella review A "review of reviews," bringing together evidence from multiple previously published review reports into a single document.

Validity A description of the extent to which a study accurately measures what the researcher set out to measure. There are various types of validity. **Face validity** is the research "sniff test": Do the study design and results reported seem to make sense? **Internal validity** has to do with the integrity of the research design. **External validity** is a description of the extent to which the study conclusions are generalizable to other populations. These all differ from **reliability**—the reproducibility of the actual measuring instrument or procedure.

Acknowledgments

Any single-author book, especially a "how-to" work such as this one, is the product of the writer's life experiences, the influence of professional colleagues, and the writings of others whom I probably will never meet in person.

In addition to my professional time in private practice and later in academic medicine, my life experiences center around my family: Anita D. Taylor, MA Ed, an accomplished author and academician, honest critic, and sharp-eyed proofreader; our children Diana and Sharon; and our four grandchildren, Francesca (Frankie), Elizabeth (Masha), Jack, and Anna (Annie).

I thank just some of the many physicians who, over the years, have helped me better understand medicine, writing, and life. In no special order, these valued persons are Doctors Robin Hull, Ray Friedman, Tom Deutsch, John Saultz, Bill Toffler, Scott Fields, Eric Walsh, Tom Hoggard, Mary Burry, Subra Seetharaman, Joe Scherger, David Warren, Takashi Yamada, Ryuki Kassai, John Kendall, and the late Peter Goodwin, Ben Jones, and Charles Visokay. Faculty colleagues Rick Deyo and Matthew Thompson helped me polish drafts of some parts of the book and, I earnestly hope, avoid egregious errors. Such faults as there are—and there surely are a few—are solely my doing.

I offer a special thanks to Coelleda O'Neil, who assisted with the manuscript preparation of my books for more than two decades. In addition, I gratefully acknowledge the excellent

© Springer International Publishing AG 2018
R.B. Taylor, *Medical Writing*,
https://doi.org/10.1007/978-3-319-70126-4

work of my Springer editor, Margaret Moore, and development editor Michael Wilt.

Finally, I am grateful to the clinicians and scientists who reported the case studies, systematic reviews, randomized trials, and other publications that provided the examples used to support my advice about *Medical Writing*.

Index

© Springer International Publishing AG 2018
R.B. Taylor, *Medical Writing*,
https://doi.org/10.1007/978-3-319-70126-4

Printed in the United States
By Bookmasters